Core Knowledge in Orthopaedics

Foot and Ankle

SECOND EDITION

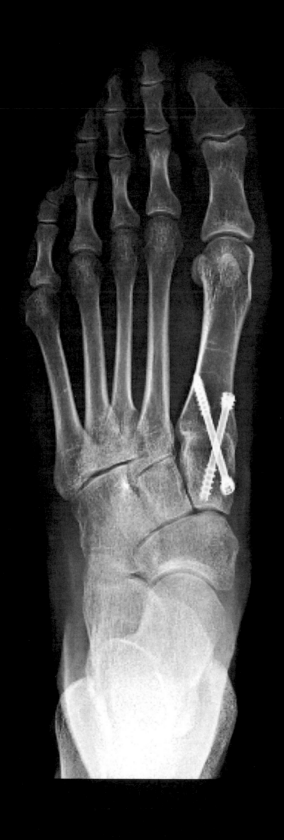

Core Knowledge in Orthopaedics
Foot and Ankle

SECOND EDITION

TEXTBOOK EDITORS

Justin K. Greisberg, MD
Professor of Orthopaedic Surgery
Columbia University Medical Center
Chief, Orthopaedic Foot & Ankle Service
New York-Presbyterian Hospital
Chief, Orthopaedic Trauma
New York-Presbyterian Lawrence Hospital
New York, New York

J. Turner Vosseller, MD
Assistant Professor, Department of Orthopaedic Surgery
Columbia University Medical Center
New York-Presbyterian Hospital
New York, New York

SERIES EDITORS

Joshua S. Dines, MD
Associate Attending, Sports Medicine and Shoulder Service
Hospital for Special Surgery, New York
Associate Professor, Orthopaedic Surgery
Weill Cornell Medicine
Assistant Team Physician: New York Mets and New York Rangers
New York, New York

Andrew J. Rosenbaum, MD
Assistant Professor
Director of Orthopaedic Research
Division of Orthopaedic Surgery
Albany Medical College
Albany, New York

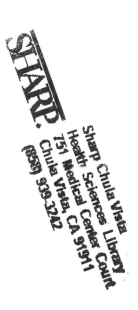

ELSEVIER

1600 John F. Kennedy Blvd.
Ste 1800
Philadelphia, PA 19103-2899

CORE KNOWLEDGE IN ORTHOPAEDICS: FOOT AND ANKLE, SECOND EDITION   ISBN: 978-0-323-56838-8

Library of Congress Control Number: 2018953136

Cover Designer: Tom M. Olson, BA
Printed in Canada by Friesens, Altona, Manitoba, Canada

Last digit is the print number: 9 8 7 6 5 4 3 2 1

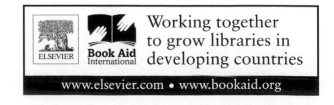

Dedications

To my parents, for making anything and everything possible.
To Dr. Peter Trafton, who always reminds us about the person connected to the cast.
To Dr. Michael Ehrlich, who taught me never to be happy with "good enough" and whose greatest satisfactions were always from the accomplishments of his residents.
To Dr. Sigvard (Ted) Hansen, who laid the foundation of modern foot and ankle orthopaedics while being a dedicated physician to each and every patient.
And most of all, to my children, who inspire me each and every day.

JKG

To my parents, Anne and Jim, whose sacrifice and love sustain me always.
To my sister, Jamie, whose steadfast friendship and strength have helped me and whose organization skills dwarf mine.
To my wife, Hariklia Bezhani, for her support, for being my sunshine every day, and to whom it is a joy to come home every day.
To Dr. Jack Delahay, who is the reason I am an orthopaedic surgeon.

JTV

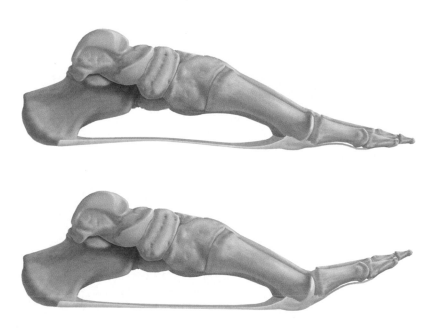

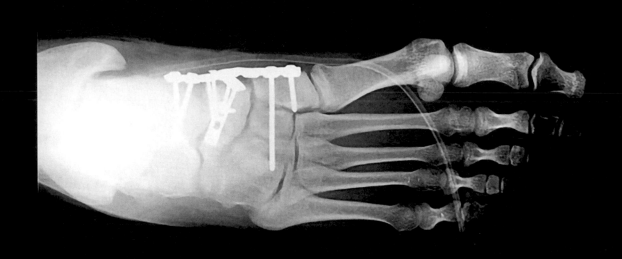

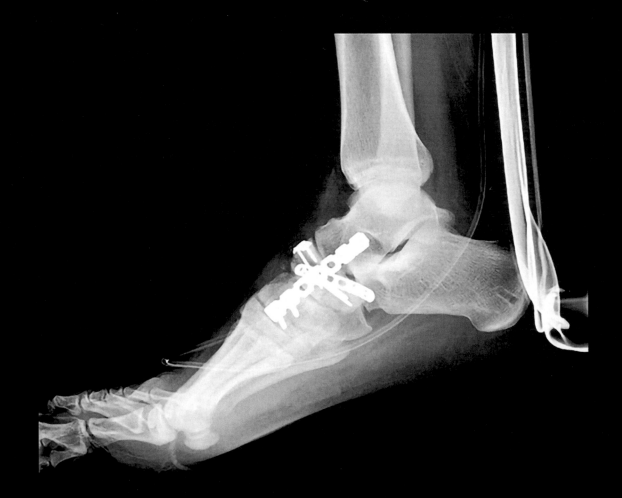

Contributing Authors

Eric S. Baranek, MD
Department of Orthopaedic Surgery
Columbia University Medical Center
New York, New York

Additional Contributors

Michael S. Aronow, MD

Mathieu Assal, MD

Eric M. Bluman, MD, PhD

Michael Brage, MD

Lloyd C. Briggs, Jr., MD, MS

Jason Cochran, DO

Peter A. Cole, MD

Gregory J. Della Rocca, MD, PhD

Craig P. Eberson, MD

Jason Heisler, DO

Dov Kolker, MD

Phillip R. Langer, MD, MS

Margaret Lobo, MD

Douglas H. Richie, Jr., DPM

Catherine M. Robertson, MD

Bruce J. Sangeorzan, MD

Jonathan Schiller, MD

Niket Shrivastava, MD

Raymond J. Sullivan, MD

Michael P. Swords, DO

Ivan S. Tarkin, MD

Richard M. Terek, MD, FACS

Steven Weinfeld, MD

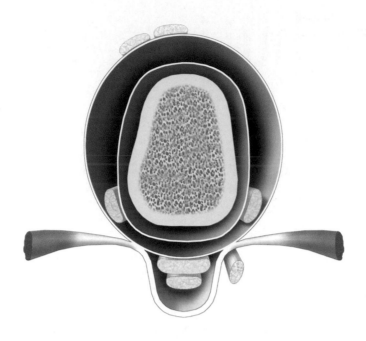

Preface

Thanks to the dedication of a few pioneering surgeons over the past 50 years, foot and ankle has risen from what was once a forgotten orthopaedic subspecialty to what is today a field at the forefront of modern medicine. Such unprecedented attention has stimulated a remarkable influx of quality research, top-notch fellowship-trained physicians, and cutting-edge innovation. This evolution has enlightened both the public and the medical community at large as to the importance of foot function. We now recognize that many of our more veteran advancements in lower extremity function, such as hip or knee replacement, depend significantly on—and are inseparable from—a well-functioning foot and ankle complex. The days of ignoring this part of the anatomy as "just a foot problem" are gone, and one need only look at the outcomes of polytrauma patients to acknowledge this. After all is said and done, these patients most often complain of their feet. Care of the foot has, partly by necessity, come a long way.

The maturation of foot and ankle into a full-fledged subspecialty of orthopaedic surgery was inevitable. This process, however, has been accelerated by certain individuals who, ahead of their time, displayed a greater appreciation of the unique attributes possessed by the foot. As any comparative anatomist will attest, the foot is what distinguishes us most as human beings. It represents the most evolved structure of our human anatomy and carries a tremendous responsibility relative to its size. These visionary surgeons were the first to incorporate these principles into clinical practice, laying the foundation for what is now the field of orthopaedic foot and ankle surgery. Nowadays, surgeons who have been inspired by the path of these leaders are fortunately commonplace, resulting in an exponential understanding of foot pathology that has revolutionized the treatment of foot problems. For example, our latest ankle arthroplasty designs are now generating cautious optimism of lasting success, improved surgical techniques have recently demonstrated more favorable and lower risk outcomes in calcaneal fracture management, and arthroscopy of the foot and ankle has now become an effective and routine tool in clinical practice.

Much of the medical research that has brought about these changes was based on retrospective case series and surgeon opinion, now referred to as level IV and V evidence. Although this has been instrumental in helping clinical science flourish, it is no longer sufficient to meet the demands of modern-day medicine. Emphasis is now, appropriately, being placed on using evidence-based medicine to drive decisions. Level I and II research (prospective, randomized trials) is emerging as the standard by which to judge all other existing information because it is less subject to bias.

With these thoughts in mind, we are pleased to compile for you this volume of *Core Knowledge in Orthopaedics*. Our goal has been to arrange an unbiased, balanced, evidence-based text broaching the most salient topics affecting foot and ankle. With the help of some of the most talented foot and ankle surgeons across the United States, we have been given an opportunity to further the visions of our founding fathers in the field of foot and ankle—for your use. We owe a great debt of gratitude to the many individuals who have devoted substantial time and effort toward this end, without whom this product could never have been completed. We hope you gain as much satisfaction in reading it as we have in putting it together.

Neither of us made this journey alone. We have each been blessed with wonderful colleagues, patients, and hospital staff, all of whom have helped create perspective for editing this text. Most importantly, though, we want to recognize our families, whose endless love and support continue to provide the inspiration, time, and motivation necessary to complete tasks like this one. This text is hence dedicated to our parents for getting us started, to our wives for keeping us going, and to our children for making it all worthwhile.

Justin K. Greisberg, MD
Professor of Orthopaedic Surgery
Columbia University Medical Center
Chief, Orthopaedic Foot & Ankle Service
New York-Presbyterian Hospital
Chief, Orthopaedic Trauma
New York-Presbyterian Lawrence Hospital
New York, New York

J. Turner Vosseller, MD
Assistant Professor, Department of Orthopaedic Surgery
Columbia University Medical Center
New York-Presbyterian Hospital
New York, New York

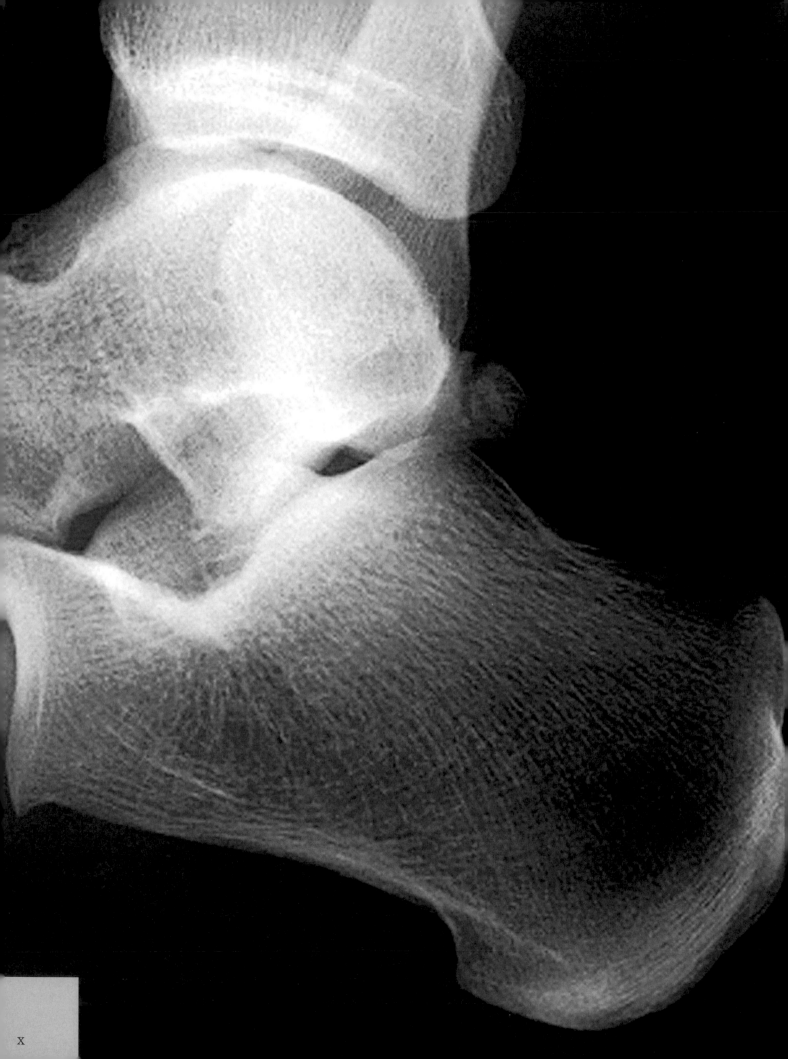

Acknowledgments

Lead Editor

Terry W. Ferrell, MS

Text Editors

Arthur G. Gelsinger, MA
Rebecca L. Bluth, BA
Nina I. Bennett, BA
Matt W. Hoecherl, BS
Megg Morin, BA
Joshua Reynolds, PhD

Image Editors

Jeffrey J. Marmorstone, BS
Lisa A. M. Steadman, BS

Illustrations

Richard Coombs, MS
Lane R. Bennion, MS
Laura C. Wissler, MA

Art Direction and Design

Tom M. Olson, BA

Production Coordinators

Emily C. Fassett, BA
Angela M. G. Terry, BA

ELSEVIER

TABLE OF CONTENTS

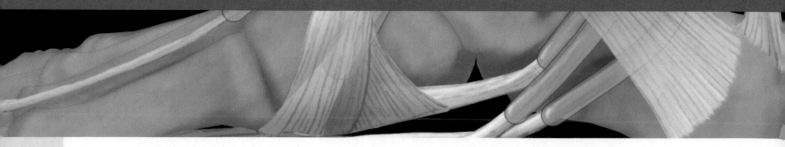

Core Knowledge in Orthopaedics

Foot and Ankle

SECOND EDITION

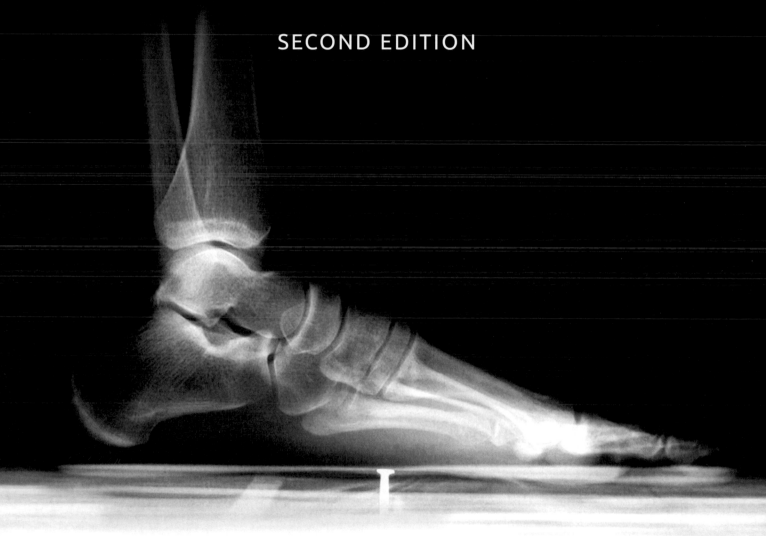

Greisberg | Vosseller

KEY FACTS

- The foot and ankle comprise a complex "machine" consisting of 26 bones and joints working together. The individual parts do not work in isolation.
- The ankle and hindfoot are 1 part of this machine, allowing the foot to adapt to uneven terrain, while the rest of the body remains upright.
- Ankle joint is the principal joint for plantar flexion/dorsiflexion. The hindfoot joints (subtalar, talonavicular, and, to a lesser extent, calcaneocuboid) provide a complex motion that can be simply thought of as inversion and eversion.
  - Ankle and hindfoot joints act as a universal joint, so the foot can be positioned on any irregular surface, while the leg remains vertical for bipedal weight bearing.
- Loss of motion from either the ankle or hindfoot will lead to overload of the other, as the joints attempt to make up for the lost motion.
  - This is why patients with ankle fusions universally develop hindfoot arthritis on x-rays at late follow-up.

- The midfoot bridges the universal joint of the hindfoot to the metatarsal heads. At the joints between the navicular, cuneiforms, and medial metatarsals, stability is much more important than flexibility.
  - Arthrodesis of these joints probably does not impair foot function at all.
- Toes, especially the 1st, provide propulsion during gait. Metatarsophalangeal motion is important in this function. Interphalangeal motion is not essential for walking.
- In the normal human foot, contraction of the Achilles pulls on the calcaneal tuberosity at a short distance from the ankle. As the ankle begins to rotate in response to the Achilles contraction, the force is transmitted across a rigid foot to the metatarsal heads, at a distance from the ankle (center of rotation). The end result is amplification of the Achilles force for propulsion.
- Overall, the human foot has changed from a flexible primate appendage used to grasp tree branches into a rigid lever for bipedal gait.

(Left) Overall schematic of the human foot is shown. The ankle and hindfoot provide flexibility. The longitudinal arch and the midfoot are important for stability. The toes remain flexible to facilitate propulsion during gait. (Right) In the normal human, the Achilles tendon acts at a short distance from the center of rotation of the ankle ➡. With a rigid arch, the short but strong Achilles contraction passes to the metatarsal heads resulting in a large displacement at the forefoot with strong propulsive forces ➡.

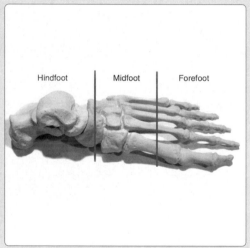

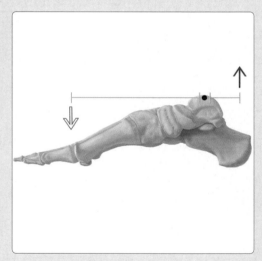

(Left) The monkey foot is well adapted for an arboreal lifestyle. The 1st ray (hallux) is mobile so that it can grasp around a tree branch. (Right) The monkey or primate foot does not have a rigid arch to act as a lever so that Achilles forces act more on the midfoot than the forefoot. The displacement of Achilles contractions ➡ are not amplified, so there is no great propulsion with bipedal gait ➡.

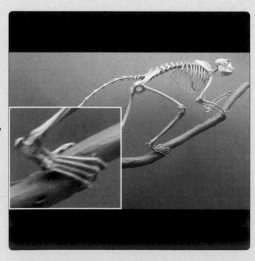

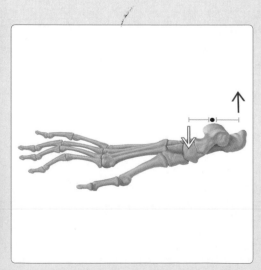

EVOLUTION OF MODERN FOOT AND COMPARATIVE ANATOMY

Evolution

- Human evolution diverged from chimpanzees ~ 5 million years ago.
- Modern apes do not have a rigid arch.
  - The lever arm for the Achilles tendon is much smaller.
  - The ape foot has less propulsive power than the human foot.
- In fact, the ape foot is better developed for grasping.
  - The 1st metatarsal is quite mobile at its articulation with the medial cuneiform, so the 1st ray (hallux) can be used to grasp tree branches.
- The foot of the modern chimpanzee or gorilla is a compromise between a weight-bearing organ and a grasping one.
  - The foot retains the mobile hallux.
- The modern human foot has a tightly packed, immobile 1st ray.
  - The hallux is no longer able to abduct because of increased rigidity at the 1st metatarsocuneiform joint.
  - Adduction of the 1st metatarsal developed along with stability of the longitudinal arch.
- Fossil footprints of a purely bipedal gait are visible from 3.7 million years ago.
  - At that time, human ancestors (*Australopithecines*) had a brain case very much like that of a chimpanzee.
- One theory proposes that development of a modern, bipedal gait was the 1st step in human evolution.
  - By freeing up the hands from any weight-bearing or tree-climbing obligations, the hands could specifically evolve for fine motor skills and tool use.
  - Such refinement in use of the hands induced rapid expansion of the cerebral cortex.
- The foot of early hominids (such as *Homo habilis* from 1-2 million years ago) probably looks very much like a modern human foot.

Longitudinal Arch

- Compared with other animals, the human foot is well adapted for prolonged walking but perhaps not as good for climbing or running.
- A key anatomical feature of the modern human foot is the longitudinal arch.
- The arch provides some shock absorption while walking and gives room for nerves and vessels to pass to the forefoot without being crushed.
- More importantly, the arch provides a long lever arm for the Achilles tendon to act on the forefoot.
  - With a stable arch, the joints between the calcaneus and metatarsals are rigid, so that Achilles tendon forces can pass from the calcaneal tuberosity to the metatarsal heads with rotation at the ankle.
- The rigid lever facilitates propulsion during gait.
- No other living primate can walk with the sustained bipedal gait of the modern human.

ANATOMY OF FOOT

- Some articulations are vital for normal function, while others are relatively unimportant for normal walking and running.

Ankle

- The tibia and fibula together make a tight socket (mortise) for the talar dome.
- The talar dome is wider anteriorly than posteriorly, so that dorsiflexion tightens up the fit of the talus in the mortise and also causes the fibula to move slightly laterally.
- The joint surfaces are highly conforming so that weight-bearing forces can be spread out over a broad surface area, minimizing joint pressures.
- Alteration in these conforming surfaces can dramatically decrease contact area and increase pressure, leading to arthritis.
  - This might occur with syndesmotic widening or intraarticular fracture.
- Widening of the mortise by 1 mm increases peak contact pressures almost 50%.
- Several studies have shown that persistent widening of the ankle mortise after injury leads to poorer outcome.
- The cartilage of the joint is relatively thick.
- About 1/6 of weight-bearing forces are borne by the fibula. The remainder passes through the tibia.
- The distal tibial articular surface (plafond) may have as much as 3° of valgus.
- The mortise is externally rotated 20-30° relative to the knee.

Ankle Ligaments

- Stability for the ankle during standing is primarily through the conforming shape of the joint surfaces.
- Collateral ligaments play a role while walking and running.
- On the medial side, the superficial deltoid ligament has fibers that pass from the medial malleolus to the talus, navicular, and calcaneus.
  - The deep deltoid is most important for stability.
    - It passes from deep inside the medial malleolus to the medial body of the talus.
  - A major source of blood supply to the talus enters the body through these medial ligaments.
- The lateral collateral ligaments include the anterior talofibular ligament (ATFL), calcaneofibular ligament (CFL), and posterior talofibular ligament.
  - The ATFL provides protection against inversion while the ankle is plantar flexed.
  - The CFL is more important when the ankle is dorsiflexed.

Distal Tibiofibular Syndesmosis

- The distal tibia has a notch posterolaterally for a snug fit with the distal fibula.
- This syndesmosis is held together by the anterior inferior tibiofibular ligament, posterior inferior tibiofibular ligament, interosseous ligament and membrane, and transverse tibiofibular ligaments.

Talus

- The talus is the center of the ankle and hindfoot "universal joint."

- A large part of the talar surface is covered by articular cartilage.
- There are no muscular attachments to the bone.
- The blood supply to the talus is somewhat tenuous.
  - The posterior tibial artery sends an artery to the tarsal canal, which enters the talus through the deltoid medially, and also through the inferior surface in the tarsal canal (between the posterior and middle facets of the subtalar joint).
  - The dorsalis pedis artery provides important blood supply through the dorsal neck.
  - The peroneal artery also sends some contributions to the sinus tarsi.
- A fracture or dislocation can easily disrupt some or all of this blood supply, leading to avascular necrosis.
- Surgical trauma can injure the blood supply to the talus as well.
  - Although avascular necrosis is rarely seen after surgery, the lack of vascularity may present as surgical nonunion.
  - With total ankle arthroplasty, surgical damage to the talus may prevent osseous ingrowth into the implant with aseptic loosening of the talar component.

Calcaneus

- In contrast to the talus, the calcaneus has abundant blood supply and soft tissue attachments.
- Fractures of the calcaneus often will have complete disruption of the blood supply to multiple fragments, yet tend to heal well.
  - Here is an old surgeons' joke: That is why it is called the "heal" (heel) bone.
- Occasionally, calcaneus fractures will show avascular necrosis but less commonly than the talus.
- The calcaneus contains a large, dense, medial projection: Sustentaculum tali.
  - The superior surface of the sustentaculum contains the middle and anterior facets of the subtalar joint.
  - The spring ligament takes its origin here.
- The posterior tibial neurovascular structures pass within a few millimeters of the medial calcaneal wall.
  - When performing a calcaneal osteotomy from the lateral side, it is important to avoid penetrating the medial wall with a saw or osteotome.

Os Trigonum

- The os trigonum is a normal bone found in many patients at the back of the ankle.
  - It may be an ununited posterior process.
- The os may articulate with the posterior facet on the calcaneus.
- It lies just deep and lateral to the flexor hallucis longus tendon.
- It may become irritated, especially in dancers who frequently go into extreme plantar flexion.
- Resection of an os trigonum can be done easily through a posteromedial approach.
  - The commonly used posterolateral approach can lead to injury of the sural nerve.

Hindfoot Joints

- The subtalar joint has 3 articular facets: Anterior, middle, and posterior.
  - The anterior and middle are often contiguous, while the posterior is larger and separate.
  - The posterior facet is saddle-shaped.
- In the past, the subtalar joint was thought to have a single axis of rotation, passing obliquely from posterolateral to anterodorsal.
  - During stance, the axis makes an angle of 41° with the ground.
- More precise biomechanical studies have shown the joint to behave more like a screw with no 1 axis of rotation.
  - As the calcaneus rotates into eversion, it also passes posteriorly.
  - Inversion is accompanied by forward translation.
- Talonavicular and subtalar motion are tightly coupled.
  - Fusion of the talonavicular joint eliminates all subtalar motion.
  - Fusion of the subtalar joint leaves ~ 25% of normal talonavicular motion.
- The calcaneocuboid joint is less critical for hindfoot motion.
  - Isolated fusion of the calcaneocuboid does not limit subtalar motion much at all and leaves 67% of talonavicular motion intact.
- The calcaneus and navicular (and the rest of the foot) rotate around the talus (peritalar motion).
  - In general, the motion between other tarsal bones is smaller and much less important than that between the talus, calcaneus, and navicular.
  - Although none of these joints have a true single axis of motion, models of hindfoot mechanics often assume they do.

Hindfoot Ligaments

- There are many interosseous ligaments in and around the subtalar joint.
- The lateral ligaments provide support against varus stresses.
  - The CFL and inferior extensor retinaculum provide some lateral support.
  - Other lateral subtalar supports include the cervical ligament and the interosseous talocalcaneal ligament.
- The spring ligament passes from the sustentaculum tali of the calcaneus to the navicular.
  - It is a key ligament in support of the longitudinal arch.
- The long plantar ligament runs from the calcaneus to the cuboid and is also an arch stabilizer.

Midfoot Joints

- The joints between the navicular and the cuneiforms have little motion.
- The metatarsocuneiform joints are very stable as well.
- There is some motion between the cuboid and 4th and 5th metatarsals.
  - This motion gives some flexibility to the lateral column of the foot, making gait more comfortable.
  - Fusion of these joints should probably be avoided.

Forefoot

- Motion at the metatarsophalangeal (MTP) joints is essential during gait, and the metatarsal heads are essential for weight bearing.
- Resection of any metatarsal head should be avoided in general.

- While standing, ~ 40% of body weight is carried through the 1st metatarsal.
  - The remainder is divided up among the lesser metatarsal heads.
- The interphalangeal joints are not important for walking.
  - They are important for grasping, although this is not an important task for the human foot.
  - Interphalangeal fusion or resection is well tolerated.
- The hallucal sesamoids reside in the tendons of the 2 flexor hallucis brevis muscles.
  - Loss of a sesamoid without repair of the flexor hallucis brevis tendon may lead to varus or valgus at the MTP joint.
  - Resection of a single sesamoid is generally well tolerated.
    - Traditional teaching is that resection of both sesamoids should not be performed.

Plantar Fascia

- The plantar fascia runs from the calcaneal tuberosity to the forefoot.
  - The main (central) band inserts both into the subcutaneous tissue in the ball of the foot and to the septa of the flexor tendons in the toes.
- The plantar fascia supports the longitudinal arch.
  - Complete division of the fascia leads to mild loss of arch height.
- With the "windlass" mechanism, extension at the MTP joints leads to tightening of the fascia and support of the arch.

Plantar Fat Pad

- The plantar subcutaneous layer consists of a specialized collection of adipose tissue within a framework of fibrous lamellae in a complex whorl pattern.
  - This fibrous frame gives the plantar fat structural support, allowing it to cushion the foot from the impact of normal walking.
  - Damage to the fat pad may occur after high-energy trauma, such as a calcaneus fracture or lawn mower injury.

Instability of 1st Ray

- The 1st ray (medial cuneiform and 1st metatarsal) is tightly packed with the rest of the foot in the normal human.
- In 1935, Dudley Morton, an anatomist at Columbia University, proposed that instability of the 1st ray was a source of trouble in the foot. He thought this trait was atavistic, implying a reversion to a more primitive state.
  - Possibly because of objections to the concept of evolution in the early 20th century, his theories were not widely accepted. Controversy continues in modern times.
- Despite continued controversy, it is undeniable that hallux valgus deformity is caused by deformity at the metatarsocuneiform and MTP joints.
  - Because the cuneiform and metatarsal do not change shape with aging, and because hallux valgus is an acquired deformity, there must be instability in the joints to create the deformity.
- Instability of the 1st ray at the metatarsocuneiform joint leads not only to hallux valgus but can also lead to elevation of the 1st metatarsal.

- Weight-bearing forces will then be transferred to the 2nd metatarsal head.
  - This is often the cause of transfer metatarsalgia.

Arch Height

- The medial longitudinal arch passes through the talonavicular, naviculocuneiform, and metatarsocuneiform joints.
- Instability or sagging at any of these joints can result in a fallen arch or flatfoot.
- Instability at the 1st metatarsocuneiform joint is seen with hallux valgus deformity.
  - Because this instability is 3D, patients with hallux valgus often have a flatfoot.
- On a weight-bearing lateral radiograph, one indicator of arch integrity is the talometatarsal angle.
  - This angle is determined by the intersection of the axis of the talus with the axis of the 1st metatarsal.
    - In the normal foot, it is ± 4°.
  - Arch height varies, but whether the arch is low or high, the talometatarsal angle should be within the normal range.
  - A talometatarsal angle outside the normal range suggests a pathologic process.

Tripod Model of Foot

- One model of foot structure depicts the foot as a tripod.
  - The 3 "legs" of the tripod are the heel, 1st metatarsal head, and 5th metatarsal head.
    - Balance between these 3 is important for foot support.
    - Elevation or depression of the 1st metatarsal will tilt the rest of the tripod.
- In some flatfeet, subluxation or sag at the 1st metatarsocuneiform joint leads to collapse of 1 leg of the tripod.
  - Without a supporting medial post to balance the foot, the hindfoot can collapse into valgus.
    - The final result is a flatfoot.
    - This has been termed forefoot-driven hindfoot valgus.
  - Collapse at the naviculocuneiform or talonavicular joints can lead to the same end result: Hindfoot valgus.
- By a similar model, plantar flexion of the 1st metatarsal will drive the hindfoot into varus.
  - This is termed forefoot-driven hindfoot varus.
    - The end result is a cavovarus foot.

Structural Diversity in Human Feet

- It is clear that there is a wide spectrum of foot shapes in modern humans.
  - Variations in arch height and 1st metatarsal alignment lead to abundant diversity.
- Interestingly, when fossil specimens from prehistoric hominids are evaluated, there is also structural diversity.
  - Rather than implying that early hominids could not walk upright, it suggests that the human foot is a work in progress.
  - It will be interesting to see whether human feet are more uniform 1 million years from now.

Importance of Joints of Foot

Joint of Foot	Importance
Ankle (tibiotalar)	Essential
Subtalar	Essential
Talonavicular	Essential
Calcaneocuboid	Not essential
Naviculocuneiform	Not essential
Metatarsocuneiform	Not essential
Cuboid-metatarsal	Essential
Metatarsophalangeal	Essential
Interphalangeal	Not essential

Hindfoot Mechanics

With hindfoot eversion (pronation), axes of talonavicular and calcaneocuboid joints are parallel; this alignment effectively unlocks those joints and allows them to flex

When hindfoot is inverted, axes of these joints are divergent; this "locks" Chopart joint, making arch rigid

During heel rise portion of gait, posterior tibial tendon inverts hindfoot, making arch rigid so that forces from Achilles tendon can be transmitted across arch to metatarsal heads; failure of posterior tibial tendon leads to arch collapse during heel rise and ineffective gait

Foot and Ankle in Gait

- As the heel strikes the ground, the ankle moves from dorsiflexion to plantar flexion (foot flat on the ground).
    - Eccentric contraction of the tibialis anterior controls the descent to foot flat.
    - Tibialis anterior rupture or peroneal nerve palsy leads to a gait pattern with uncontrolled "slapping" of the foot on the ground as the limb moves from heel strike to foot flat.
- As the leg moves to midstance, the ankle dorsiflexes ~ 10°.
- Body weight passes over the foot, and strong gastrocnemius and soleus contractions move the foot to heel rise.
    - The ankle once again plantar flexes.
- The primary functions of the Achilles muscles are to decelerate tibial advance for knee stability and to stabilize the ankle so the limb can rock on to the forefoot.
    - In routine gait, they are not as important for push off.
        - As the stride is lengthened, more work is required of the Achilles.
- Untreated rupture or overlengthening of the Achilles will prevent effective heel rise.
    - Body weight is kept close to the heel rather than moving to the forefoot.
    - Stride length is shortened, and heel rise is delayed.
- The toe flexors, especially the flexor hallucis longus, are active during late stance, heel rise, and toe-off stages.
- Once the foot leaves the ground, the ankle must dorsiflex to clear the ground.
    - The 1st toe clears the ground by < 1 cm during normal gait.
    - Absence of the ankle dorsiflexors (tibialis anterior) leads to a high steppage gait, where the limb is lifted higher off the ground for clearance.
- Normal cadence for an adult is 101-122 steps per minute.
    - It is slightly higher in women than in men and much higher in small children.
    - Cadence does not change with aging, but stride length does decrease.

Ankle Stability

- Inversion injuries are the most common ankle athletic injury.
    - This is due in part to the relative strength of the medial (deltoid) ligaments relative to the lateral complex.
    - Furthermore, many athletic maneuvers tend to promote inversion.
- Stability of the ankle comes in part from static soft tissue ligaments.
    - The lateral ankle ligaments, in particular the ATFL and CFL, provide some mechanical constraint to inversion.
- The ATFL and CFL are not stout enough to prevent uncontrolled inversion.
    - Rather, their role may be more as proprioceptive sensors than simple static restraints.
    - When the ankle begins to roll into inversion, the ATFL suddenly stretches.
    - In a reflex similar to the patellar deep tendon reflex, stretch of the ATFL leads to reflexive contraction of the peroneal tendons.
        - Peroneal activation prevents uncontrolled ankle inversion.
- The peroneal tendons also have stretch mechanoreceptors, and these may be more important than the ligaments in providing position sense.
    - Reflex contraction of the peroneals in response to sudden stretch of ankle mechanoreceptors is referred to as "closed-loop" control.
    - Stretch receptors in the ligaments and tendons send a signal to motor cell neurons in the spinal cord with reflexive contraction of the peroneal muscles.

- ○ Peroneal closed-loop reaction time may be too slow to prevent inversion injuries during athletic activity.
- There also appears to be "open-loop" controls, consisting of preactivation of stabilizing muscles in anticipation of upcoming stress.
  - ○ In other words, an athlete learns through training and experience to activate appropriate stabilizing muscles at just the right time.
- Perhaps in the real world, open-loop preactivation fires appropriate stabilizing muscles for the anticipated stress, and then closed-loop stretch reflexes fine-tune the balance as needed.

SELECTED REFERENCES

1. Hansen ST: Functional Reconstruction of the Foot and Ankle. Philadelphia: Lippincott Williams & Wilkins, 2000.
2. Astion DJ et al: Motion of the hindfoot after simulated arthrodesis. J Bone Joint Surg Am. 79(2):241-6, 1997
3. Olson TR et al: The evolutionary basis of some clinical disorders of the human foot: a comparative survey of the living primates. Foot Ankle. 3(6):322-41, 1983
4. Morton DJ.: The Human Foot: Its Evolution, Physiology, and Functional Disorders. Morningside Heights: Columbia University Press, 1935

(Left) *The foot* ➡ *of the chimpanzee is adapted for flexibility, not stability.* **(Right)** *From left to right are the chimpanzee, gorilla, and human feet. Both the chimpanzee and human have a medially angulated hallux with flexibility, not stability. The hallux is packed in tightly with the rest of the forefoot in the human, providing stability and propulsion for gait. The primates have a mobile hallux for grasping, while the human foot is tight for weight bearing.*

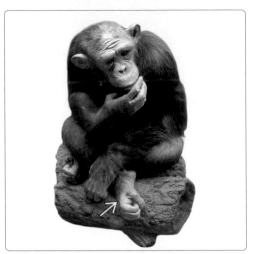
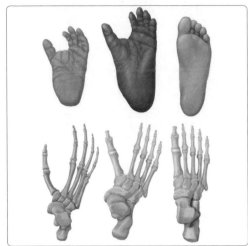

(Left) *Dorsiflexion of the toes* ➡ *tightens the plantar fascia* ➡, *strengthening the toes and supporting the longitudinal arch. This is known as the "windlass" mechanism.* **(Right)** *View shows the talus from above. Note the talar dome* ➡ *and talonavicular joint* ➡. *The articular facets are shaded. Note that the talar neck is relatively medial, and there is a lateral shoulder* ➡ *and process* ➡.

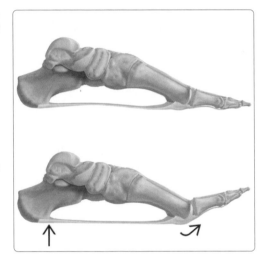
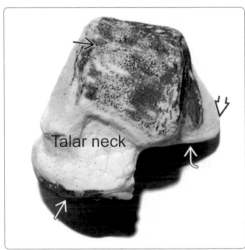

Talar neck

(Left) *A lateral view of the talus shows how the talonavicular joint* ➡ *is contiguous with the anterior facet of the subtalar joint* ➡. *The function of these joints in providing complex hindfoot motion is closely linked. Also note the lateral process* ➡ *and the posterior facet of the subtalar joint* ➡. **(Right)** *View of the calcaneus from the lateral side is shown highlighting the subtalar facets* ➡ *and calcaneocuboid joint* ➡.

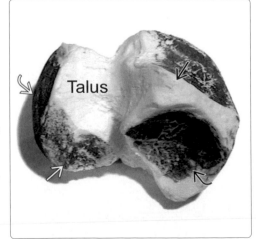
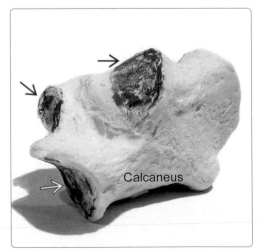

Talus

Calcaneus

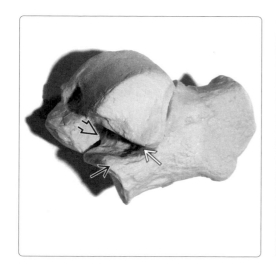

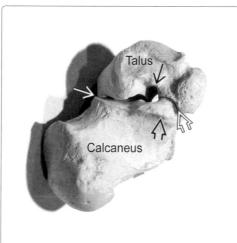

(Left) *This lateral view of the subtalar joint shows how the sinus tarsi ⇨ is formed as the space between the lateral process of the talus ⇨ and the anterior process of the calcaneus ⇨.* **(Right)** *Medial view of the subtalar joint is shown highlighting the posterior facet ⇨, anterior/middle facets ⇨, tarsal canal ⇨, and sustentaculum tali ⇨.*

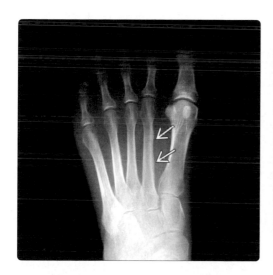

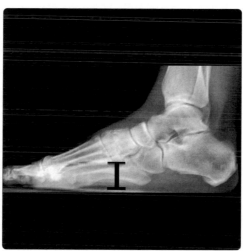

(Left) *Patient with mild hallux valgus pain under the 2nd metatarsal head and instability of the 1st metatarsal is shown. The metatarsal instability or hypermobility leads to long-term overload of the 2nd ray, evident as 2nd metatarsal cortical thickening ⇨. Also, note how the 2nd MTP joint is slightly deviated medially (compared with the smaller MTP joints). This is a subtle clue to 2nd MTP overload with synovitis.* **(Right)** *In some feet, the arch will be "high" with a large distance between the medial cuneiform and floor.*

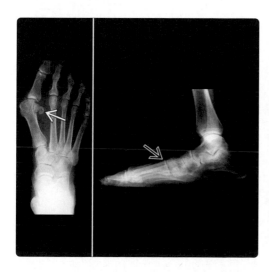

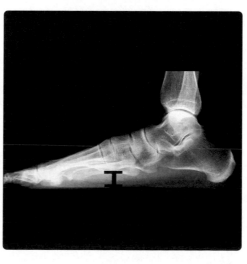

(Left) *Patient with hallux valgus, medial deviation of the 1st metatarsal ⇨, and a flatfoot deformity is shown. Dorsal angulation of the 1st MTC joint is clearly visible ⇨. This sagging of the medial column of the foot allows the hindfoot to fall into valgus, thus making a flatfoot.* **(Right)** *Other feet show a "low" arch. In these images, the talometatarsal angle is close to normal. These are variants of normal feet, not flatfeet. A pathologic flatfoot will show collapse of arch and increased talometatarsal angle.*

KEY FACTS

- A thorough physical examination includes the following components:
  - Inspection
  - Palpation
  - Assessment of motion
  - Strength testing
  - Examination of vascular status
  - Stability assessment
  - Evaluation of alignment
  - Assessment for gastrocnemius contracture
  - Assessment of 1st-ray mobility
- Inspect for swelling, scars, skin condition, pigmented lesions, calluses, and shoe condition.
- Describe all tenderness anatomically.
- Proper positioning of the foot and limb is essential for an accurate and reproducible physical exam, particularly during assessment of motion, stability testing, and when evaluating the gastrocnemius and 1st-ray mobility.

- Radiographic stress testing can allow the clinician to precisely quantify any instability.
  - Comparison to the contralateral side can be more easily performed in the office.
- Weight matters; heavy patients who lose weight can eliminate foot pain.
- Are there any other joints involved? The patient's problem could be an inflammatory arthropathy.
- Does the patient smell of smoke? Nicotine inhibits bone and wound healing, leading to higher surgical complication rates.

(Left) *Heavy callusing under the 1st metatarsal head suggests a cavus foot.* **(Right)** *Equinus measured with hindfoot in neutral and knee extended is shown. The examiner's thumb is over the medial navicular to maintain neutrality of the hindfoot.*

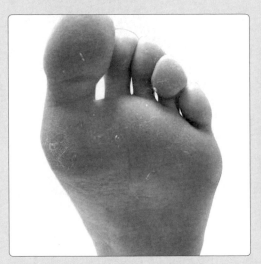
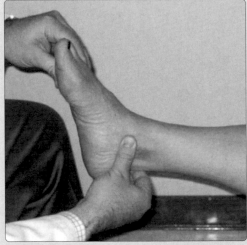

(Left) *Improved dorsiflexion with knee bent implies gastrocnemius equinus.* **(Right)** *Anterior drawer test of the ankle is shown. Stabilize the tibia and translate slightly plantar flexed foot anteriorly.*

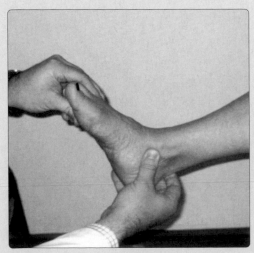
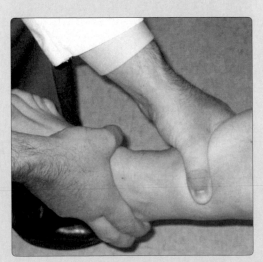

INSPECTION, PALPATION, AND MOTION

Inspection

- Examination may begin with the patient sitting on an elevated table with the leg at eye level for the physician.
- The location and amount of swelling is noted.
  - Swelling may be diffuse from peripheral edema.
  - Swelling may be focal as with inflammation of tendonitis or single-joint arthritis.
- Previous wounds are noted in order to understand the role of previous injury or surgery in current pathology.
- Pigmented lesions should be noted.
  - Subungual hematomas are common.
  - A pigmented subungual lesion that does not grow out with time raises the possibility of melanoma.
- Is the skin shiny, "wooden," &/or with loss of hair?
  - This could indicate an underlying vasculopathy.
- Is the skin tight with poor flexibility?
  - This is seen with chronic hyperglycemia.
- Does the patient have calluses?
  - Calluses are the clue to where the patient is bearing the most weight.
- It is normal to have mild callusing under the 1st metatarsal head or the heel.
- Callusing under the 2nd metatarsal head is an indirect sign of 1st-ray hypermobility/instability.
- Heavy calluses under the 1st metatarsal head may be present in the cavus foot.
- Thick calluses under the heel will be seen with calcaneus deformity from a weak Achilles.
- Calluses under the navicular may be seen with a collapsed arch (pathologic flatfoot).
- Look at the shoes.
  - Many patients with forefoot deformities will be wearing shoes that are too small for the deformity.
    - A switch to proper-fitting shoes may relieve symptoms.
  - Wear under the lateral shoe suggests cavus or varus alignment, while medial wear is visible with valgus or flatfoot deformity.
    - Some wear on the heel lateral to midline is normal for many people, though.

Palpation

- Most structures in the foot are superficial and directly palpable.
- Describe the tenderness anatomically.
  - For example, instead of saying "lateral foot or ankle tenderness," say where it is exactly.
  - Is it the base of the 5th metatarsal, the anterior process of the calcaneus, the peroneal tendons, the distal fibular tip, or the anterior talofibular ligament?

Motion

- Begin with knee motion.
  - Misalignment in the knee can overload the foot with secondary pain.
  - Stiffness in the knee may be present and may make mild foot deformities or mild ankle stiffness more symptomatic.
- Plantar flexion and dorsiflexion of the foot is mainly through the ankle, although in many cases, up to 1/3 of perceived ankle motion is actually through the subtalar and (especially) transverse tarsal (talonavicular and calcaneocuboid) joints.
- Subtalar motion is a complex motion with contributions from the 3 hindfoot joints (talocalcaneal, talonavicular, and calcaneocuboid).
  - The motion is described as inversion and eversion.
  - Hindfoot motion is not purely in the coronal plane.
    - It is a complex motion that is best measured by comparing with the contralateral side.
  - The motion is normal if it is fluid and equal to that of the unaffected side.
- Limitations of hindfoot motion are important to note.
  - A patient with a flatfoot deformity and a "fixed" hindfoot has moderate to severe restriction of subtalar motion, which implies arthrosis or perhaps peroneal spasticity.
    - This finding may determine whether a joint-sparing or fusion surgery is indicated for flatfoot reconstruction.
  - An arthritic ankle with decreased subtalar motion may not be a great candidate for an isolated ankle fusion, as this may place more stress on an arthritic joint.
- All the metatarsophalangeal (MTP) joints normally have good motion, especially in extension.

GASTROCNEMIUS CONTRACTURE

- When checking ankle dorsiflexion, gastrocnemius contracture may limit passive ankle dorsiflexion.
  - Because the gastrocnemius origin is above the knee on the femoral condyles, a contracted gastrocnemius will limit ankle dorsiflexion with the knee extended but not flexed.
- Normally, passive ankle dorsiflexion should be at least 5° or 10° past neutral.
  - When examining the patient's right foot, the examiner's right hand cups the heel with the thumb on the navicular tuberosity.
  - The left hand is wrapped around the metatarsal heads to keep them level.
- It is essential to keep the hindfoot neutral or just slightly inverted.
  - Because of the oblique axis of the subtalar joint, hindfoot eversion will also dorsiflex the forefoot, masking any gastrocnemius equinus.
- Passive ankle dorsiflexion is checked 1st with the knee extended.
  - The normal ankle dorsiflexes 5° or 10° past neutral.
  - Then the knee is flexed, and dorsiflexion is checked again.
- Limitation of ankle dorsiflexion with the knee extended that corrects with knee flexion indicates gastrocnemius contracture.
- Limitation of dorsiflexion in all knee positions means that both the soleus and the gastrocnemius are contracted.

STABILITY

- Anterior drawer and talar tilting tests check for lateral ankle ligament stability.

- The anterior drawer test is done by stabilizing the tibia with one hand and applying an anterior force to the hindfoot with the other hand.
  - The normal ankle will have little translation with a solid end point.
  - The anterior drawer tests the anterior talofibular ligament.
- The talar tilt test assesses the calcaneofibular ligament.
  - The talus is tilted into inversion, but it is important not to confuse hindfoot inversion with talar tilting relative to the tibia.
- For each of these tests, the result should be compared with that for the other side.
- Both these ankle tests are best done with radiographic imaging to precisely quantify the degree of instability.
  - It also may be helpful to perform these tests with the patient under anesthesia to prevent muscle contraction.
- For ankle injuries, external rotation stress testing is important.
  - Pain with external rotation of the foot relative to the leg suggests an injury.
  - External rotation stress x-rays are the best test for mortise integrity when evaluating malleolar or syndesmotic injuries.
- There can be instability of the MTP joints, especially the 2nd.
  - This is checked by noting the inferior-superior motion of the phalanx on the metatarsal head with stressing.

1ST-RAY MOBILITY

- The ideal human foot has evolved to have stability in the 1st ray, especially at the 1st metatarsocuneiform joint.
  - This stability gives strength to the medial column, supporting the arch of the foot.
- Instability at the 1st metatarsocuneiform joint can be 3D, giving rise to a flatfoot, transfer metatarsalgia, &/or hallux valgus.
- Assessing 1st-ray stability is difficult.
  - Several devices have been designed to measure 1st-ray stability.
  - However, these devices are not available for regular clinical use.
- Stability of the 1st ray can be checked on routine physical examination.
  - When examining a right foot, the examiner's left thumb is placed under the lesser metatarsal heads.
  - The examiner's right thumb is placed under the 1st metatarsal head.
  - Both thumbs apply an equal upward force to the forefoot.
  - Normally, the 1st metatarsal head should remain even with the 2nd.
  - With hypermobility of the 1st ray, the 1st metatarsal head will elevate well above the 2nd.
- Some physicians recommend checking the overall plantar-dorsal translation of the heads, but the important finding clinically is elevation of the 1st metatarsal above the 2nd.
- A callus beneath the 2nd metatarsal head is indirect evidence of 1st-ray instability.

STRENGTH

- Strength of all the muscle groups is assessed and rated on a 1-5 scale.
  - 1 is a flicker of muscle contraction.
  - 2 is strength unable to overcome gravity.
  - 3 is strength able to overcome gravity.
  - 4 is mildly weak.
  - 5 is normal.
- It is important to note strength when evaluating neuromuscular patients.
  - If a muscle is to be transferred, it will generally lose 1 grade of strength.
  - If a muscle that is graded as 4/5 is transferred for another function, the final strength may be too low to be useful.
- When patients are asked to plantar flex the foot, some patients will push the 1st ray down more than the others.
  - This is due to **overdrive of the peroneus longus** and is commonly seen with cavus feet.
  - The dynamic plantar flexion of the 1st ray tends to drive the hindfoot into varus.
  - This process is termed **forefoot driven hindfoot varus**.
- Some patients will show toe extension when asked to dorsiflex the ankle.
  - This phenomenon, termed **extensor recruitment**, results when the long toe extensors are recruited to assist the tibialis anterior.
  - It may appear in patients with a tight gastrocnemius.
  - In theory, the chronic overactivity of the long toe extensors may lead to clawing of the toes.

VASCULAR EXAMINATION

- Check dorsalis pedis and posterior tibial pulses.
  - The ankle-brachial index can be calculated.
- Look for indirect signs of vascular trouble:
  - Loss of hair
  - Ischemic ulcers
  - "Wooden" skin

SENSATION

- Checking for light touch sensation is obvious and can help when defining previous traumatic nerve injuries.
- However, most diabetic patients with neuropathy will have intact light touch sensation.
  - It is the loss of protective sensation that is important.
  - The Semmes-Weinstein monofilaments are used to check protective sensation.
  - The traditional test is to use the 5.07 (10 g) monofilament on 5 sites on each foot.
  - A recent study found good sensitivity with the use of a smaller force (4.5 g) under the 1st metatarsal head (Saltzman et al 2004).
- The dorsal columns can be checked in patients with neurologic disease by testing proprioception at the 1st MTP.

ALIGNMENT

- The patient should stand with both shoes off and both legs visible to a point above the knees.
  - Knee alignment is assessed.
- While looking at the patient from the front, a preliminary judgment about foot alignment can be made.
  - The foot should appear under the leg, not out to the side (as in a valgus flatfoot).
- If the heel is seen medial to the ankle, a varus heel is present.
  - This has been termed the **peek-a-boo heel**, because it "peeks" out from behind the ankle.
- The patient is then viewed from behind.
  - The heel should be in neutral to slight valgus alignment.
- With a planovalgus (flatfoot) deformity, the forefoot will be abducted.
  - The examiner will see the lesser toes lateral to the leg.
  - This has been called the "too many toes" sign.
- The heel rise test is then performed to test for posterior tibial tendon function.
  - While standing on 1 leg, the patient rises up on to the forefoot.
  - A normal posterior tibial tendon will bring the heel into varus with no pain.
  - If the heel remains in valgus alignment, or the patient feels pain along the medial hindfoot, then it is likely there is dysfunction of the posterior tibial tendon.
- For the patient with a varus hindfoot (cavus deformity), the Coleman block test is performed.
  - The foot is placed with a block (or a phone book) under the heel and the lateral forefoot.
  - The medial forefoot is allowed to hang over the side.
  - As weight is applied by the patient, the 1st metatarsal will be able to drop below the level of the block.
  - With a flexible hindfoot, the heel will fall into valgus as the 1st metatarsal falls below the level of the rest of the foot.
    - This is termed **forefoot-driven hindfoot varus**.
  - If the hindfoot is stiff, the heel will remain in varus, and no correction will be attained.
- The Coleman block test is based on the tripod model of foot structure.
  - The 1st ray supports the hindfoot.
  - Plantar flexion of the 1st ray drives the heel into varus, and dorsiflexion of the 1st ray allows the heel to fall into valgus.

SELECTED REFERENCES

1. Manoli A 2nd et al: The subtle cavus foot, "the underpronator". Foot Ankle Int. 26(3):256-63, 2005
2. Saltzman CL et al: 4.5-gram monofilament sensation beneath both first metatarsal heads indicates protective foot sensation in diabetic patients. J Bone Joint Surg Am. 86-A(4):717-23, 2004
3. DiGiovanni CW et al: Isolated gastrocnemius tightness. J Bone Joint Surg Am. 84-A(6):962-70, 2002
4. Morton DJ. et al: Dorsal hypermobility of the first metatarsal segment: Part III. In The Human Foot: Its Evolution, Physiology, and Functional Disorders. Morningside Heights: Columbia University. 187-195, 1935.

(Left) *An overactive peroneus longus plantar flexes the 1st metatarsal more than the others.* (Right) *This patient has developed claw toes from increased activity of the long toe extensors over time. The foot uses extensor recruitment to "help" ankle dorsiflexion.*

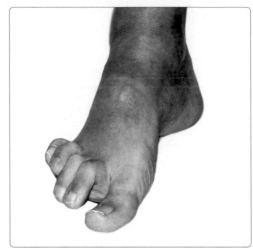
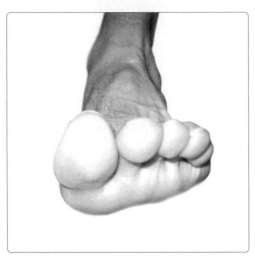

(Left) *The patient's left foot shows a peek-a-boo heel. The heel on the normal right foot is not visible from the front.* (Right) *The valgus heel is lateral to the leg* ➡. *The neutral heel appears under the leg* ➡. *The varus heel will be medial to the leg* ➡.

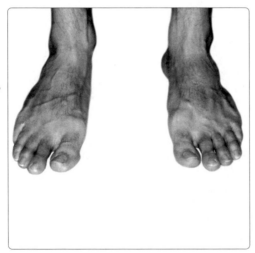
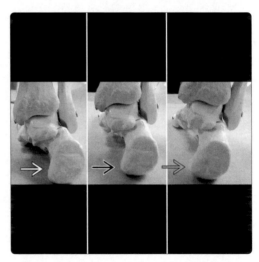

(Left) *"Too many toes" on the patient's left foot is associated with increased forefoot abduction due to posterior tibial tendon insufficiency.* (Right) *Double-limb heel rise test is shown. Both heels are inverting properly.*

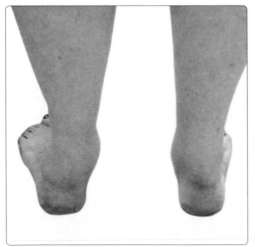
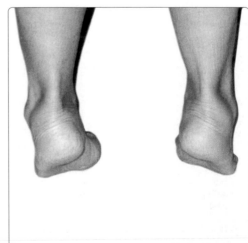

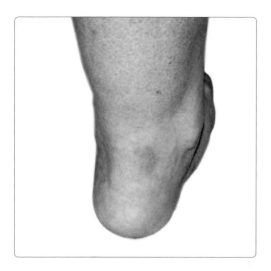

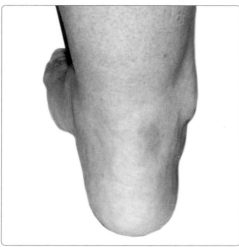

(Left) *The patient has a cavus foot with heel varus.* **(Right)** *With a block under the heel and lateral forefoot, the 1st metatarsal can "drop down," so the heel shifts to a more neutral alignment. This is consistent with forefoot-driven hindfoot varus in this patient.*

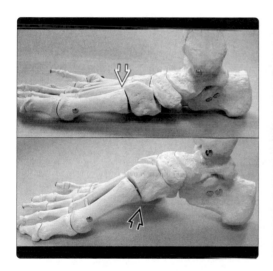

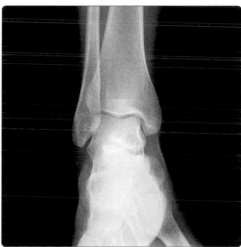

(Left) *With an unstable 1st ray, the medial column collapses, and the hindfoot can fall into valgus ⮕. The foot with a plantar flexed 1st ray drives the hindfoot into varus ⮕. This is commonly seen with many cavus feet.* **(Right)** *Routine non-weight-bearing AP view of the ankle is obtained with the patient supine, the heel on the cassette, and the toes pointed upward. The x-ray beam is directed at the center of the ankle joint. The talus overlaps the distal fibula obscuring the lateral ankle mortise. (From IA: MSK, 2e.)*

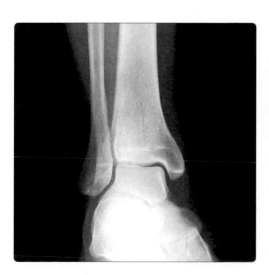

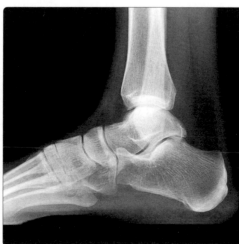

(Left) *Non-weight-bearing ankle mortise view (oblique) is obtained with the patient supine and the foot internally rotated ~ 15°. The lateral ankle mortise is now visualized. (From IA: MSK, 2e.)* **(Right)** *Non-weight-bearing lateral view of the ankle depicts both the calcaneus and talus in profile. The posterior, medial, and lateral malleoli are superimposed over one another and over the talus, potentially obscuring fractures at those locations. (From IA: MSK, 2e.)*

KEY FACTS

- The use of orthotic devices varies in a fairly significant way depending on the training and background of the prescribing practitioner.
  - Various practitioners, including orthopaedic surgeons, podiatrists, physical therapists, and more, prescribe orthotics for various pathologies, and there are widely varying opinions about best practices.
  - With that being said, there are pathologies that unquestionably benefit from orthotics, and there are many themes in terms of types on inserts that are appropriate.
- In certain pathologies, orthotic devices are an indispensable component of nonoperative treatment.
  - A stiff insert can be beneficial in hallux rigidus as well as midfoot arthritis and in recovery from metatarsal stress fractures.

- Metatarsalgia ± hammer toes can be treated with a metatarsal pad often with some success. The accompaniment of a Budin splint may impart a greater success rate.
- An arch support of some description is typically a large part of nonoperative treatment for the symptomatic flatfoot.
- A cavus foot with a supple hindfoot may be manipulated into a better position with a relief underneath the 1st metatarsal head.
- Differences of opinion with regard to orthotics largely center over the relative ubiquity of their need, i.e., many practitioners agree that their directed use is appropriate, while promoting them as a panacea for all manner of ills is likely inappropriate.

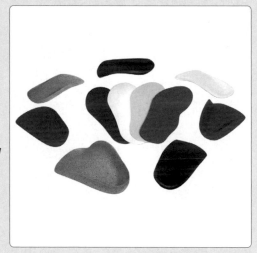

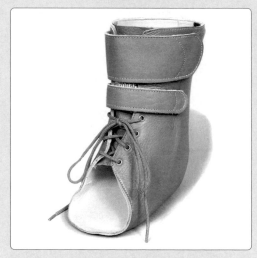

(Left) *This picture shows all manner of accomodative orthoses. These inserts are meant to support the foot in its position, as opposed to pushing it into a more desirable position.* **(Right)** *An Arizona brace is a solid ankle-foot orthosis that is rigid and accomodative. It is custom made for patients, although it can be bulky and make getting shoes on difficult.*

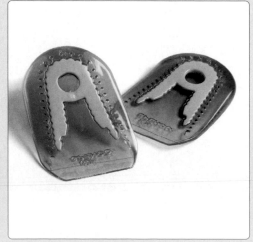

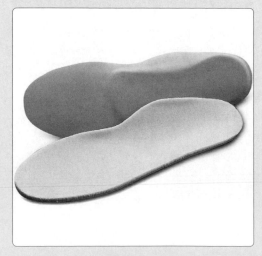

(Left) *This gel heel pad can provide some relief of pressure in pathologies, such as plantar fasciitis. It is simply a cushion to relatively offload the heel area without providing much structural integrity.* **(Right)** *These contoured cushioned insoles are used more for comfort than to directly influence any particular pathology. These inserts are "off the shelf" and can be used for general comfort or in mild pathology.*

INTRODUCTION

- Orthosis is an externally applied device used to modify the structural or functional characteristics of the musculoskeletal system, an apparatus used to support, align, prevent, or correct deformities or to improve the function of movable parts of the body.
- During static stance and ambulation, the lower extremities are subjected to external forces and moments. During normal function, these forces and moments are resisted or controlled by internal structures of the body. When internal structures fail, orthoses can modify external forces and moments to allow the body to function in a "normal" manner.
- An external device used to support or improve function of the foot and ankle can take many physical forms, from a simple felt pad to a composite brace controlling foot and ankle motions. Orthotics prescribed for lower extremity pathologies include foot orthoses (FOs), ankle-foot orthoses (AFOs), knee orthoses, and knee-ankle-foot orthoses.

TYPES OF ORTHOSES

- Various types of orthoses are commonly prescribed for foot and ankle pathologies. The basic subcategories of FOs are prefabricated and custom. There are clear differences between the manufacture and design of orthoses in each category, yet advantages or benefit of one type of device over another has yet to be proven.
  - Prefabricated devices have the distinct benefit of lower cost compared with custom-fabricated foot orthotics. In addition, prefabricated orthoses can be readily stocked for immediate dispensing to the patient. The disadvantage of prefabricated orthotic devices is their difficulty in application to limb and foot shapes that fall outside the "average" range.
  - Custom molding and contouring of an orthotic device to a body segment may be the critical feature necessary for a successful treatment outcome. Yet the mechanism by which foot orthotics actually achieve their treatment effects remains poorly understood, and, thus, claims of superiority of custom vs. prefabricated devices remain speculative.
- Prefabricated FOs are available for a wide variety of clinical application. In general, these devices are used to offload specific areas of the foot, cushion the foot from impact, support the medial longitudinal arch, and provide mild biomechanical control of hindfoot movements.
- Custom FOs can be either accommodative or functional.
  - Functional orthoses are most often used with flexible feet, working to alter how foot meets floor.
  - Accommodative orthoses generally are used with more rigid deformities; rather than attempting to alter foot alignment, accommodative orthoses work to relieve pressure under bony prominences.

PREFABRICATED FOOT ORTHOSES

- The simplest types of prefabricated FOs are in-shoe pads. Felt forefoot pads are available to relieve metatarsalgia, sesamoiditis, and intractable plantar keratoses. These adjust pressure by offloading adjacent areas and increasing pressure under the pad itself. They are often placed near, but not directly under, the area of pain.
- Contoured cushioned prefabricated insoles have a wide variety of clinical application for relief of plantar foot pressures, dissipation of impact shock, and enhancement of overall foot comfort. These contoured insoles function as a softer version of a prefabricated arch support.
- Prefabricated, "biomechanical" semirigid foot orthotics are made from materials commonly used in the fabrication of more expensive custom functional FOs. These devices are contoured to an average shape of a medial and lateral longitudinal arch and generally lack any heel cup. Sometimes, posting is provided in the hindfoot to enhance pronation control.
- The goal of treatment of these devices is to provide more rigid support and motion control than with softer arch supports.

CUSTOM FOOT ORTHOSES

- Custom foot orthotic devices require fabrication to some type of model of the patient's foot. The model on which the orthosis is contoured can be a positive plaster cast, a computer-generated model, or the actual foot of the patient.
- Equally important to the value of any custom foot orthotic is the selection of material composition, which will be unique to the patient's clinical condition or biomechanical needs.
- Accommodative FOs are designed to relieve pressure on certain areas of the foot and to provide support of the foot in its compensated position. The most common use for accommodative foot orthotics is in the management of diabetic foot complications. These devices are also known as total contact orthoses and can disperse plantar pressures to the maximal foot surface area.
- Functional FOs are designed to control forces that act on the foot during the stance phase of gait. These forces are generally inversion/eversion &/or rotatory forces acting on the subtalar and midtarsal joints.
- While not part of the definition, functional FOs are often expected to correct alignment of the foot. Yet improvements of alignment with functional FOs are relatively modest, as revealed by numerous kinematic studies of these devices. Kinetic studies of FOs have confirmed that these devices can alter forces or moments acting on the joints of the lower extremity.

- A predecessor to the functional FO was the University of California Biomechanics Laboratory orthosis (UCBL). This device is still popular today in the treatment of flatfoot conditions. The UCBL is a plastic FO with a deep heel cup and steep medial and lateral flanges. The UCBL is best suited to control transverse plane subluxation of the foot by applying force against the lateral wall of the calcaneus, sustentaculum tali, and lateral aspect of the 5th metatarsal shaft. These devices have fallen out of favor due to difficulty with shoe fit and the need for multiple adjustments for comfort.
- Functional FOs were developed in the early 1960s. Several principles apply to functional orthotic development. Semirigid to rigid materials are utilized to control significant forces that occur in most foot pathologies. A mold is made of the foot to which posting can be added to address the individual deformity present.

TREATMENT EFFECTS OF ORTHOTICS

- The majority of studies of treatment effects of FOs have significant deficiencies that must be noted before any conclusions or recommendations can be made. Many studies are simple retrospective "patient satisfaction" surveys, and higher levels of evidence are generally lacking. In most cases, the type of orthosis is not described in detail, and descriptions of the foot types of the subjects are often lacking.

Effects of Foot Orthotics on Plantar Pressures

- Numerous studies have shown that FOs can significantly reduce vertical force and pressures on various areas of the plantar surface of the foot. Peak pressures can be reduced, at the most, by ~ 20% with an FO. In terms of injury, the significance of this pressure reduction remains speculative.
- FOs have been shown to decrease plantar callus size in patients with diabetes. Patients with leprosy were noted to have improved healing of plantar ulcers with custom FOs.
- A semirigid custom foot orthotic was shown to significantly reduce the incidence of femoral and metatarsal stress fractures in military recruits. A prospective 9-week study of military recruits showed that a neoprene insole reduced overuse injuries and tibial stress syndrome from 32% to 23%.

Changes in Foot and Leg Alignment

- Kinematic studies have primarily focused on the effects of foot orthotics on hindfoot alignment. Most of these studies have been performed on running athletes. These studies have demonstrated relatively modest improvements. Rather than causing noticeable change in foot and leg alignment, FOs may have other effects on kinematics.
- Semirigid and soft orthotics have shown a significant effect in reducing the velocity of pronation in both running and walking subjects. More recent studies have shown that medially posted custom FOs can reduce the overall range of pronation, maximum angle of calcaneal eversion, and range of internal tibial rotation associated with pronation.
- The results of kinematic studies have led most researchers to conclude that these devices do not function to realign the skeleton. These devices can, however, significantly alter kinetics of lower extremity segmental function, as documented by many studies on changes in joint moments with orthotic intervention.

Effect of Foot Orthotics on Joint Moments

- A key area of understanding of orthotic effects on the lower extremity has focused on joint moments. The term **moment** describes a force couple that acts at a distance from an axis of rotation of a specific joint in the body.
- Much of the recent insight into the treatment effects of FOs has been obtained by studies of joint kinetics. Reduced strain of specific anatomical structures (internal joint moments) has been measured with certain orthotic conditions, and this information can be helpful in designing treatment strategies.
- Wedging of shoe inserts can affect knee joint moments. External varus knee joint moments were reduced by lateral wedged shoe inserts. Also, medial compartment knee joint load was estimated to be reduced with the lateral wedged inserts. Medial arch support shoe inserts were shown to reduce lateral patellofemoral joint load during running gait. However, some studies have shown that the responses of human subjects to various types of wedging of shoe inserts are subject specific and unsystematic.
- In summary, nearly any type of shoe insert modification that applies medial wedging to the hindfoot or molding of the device to the medial arch will significantly reduce hindfoot inversion moment during the early phase of running gait. This would indicate a reduced strain of the ankle "invertors," such as the tibialis posterior muscle, and passive structures of the medial ankle, such as the deltoid ligament.

Treatment Effects of Foot Orthoses for Specific Injuries: Heel Pain Syndrome

- Subcalcaneal pain syndrome has been extensively studied in terms of response to treatment with various forms of FOs. Retrospective studies of large groups of patients receiving semirigid and rigid custom FOs report significant improvement of symptoms and high patient satisfaction.
- A well-designed prospective study showed that early-onset heel pain responded best to a program of stretching combined with a prefabricated heel pad or arch support, compared with stretching combined with use of a custom semirigid functional FO.
- However, several retrospective studies of large groups of patients with plantar heel pain have shown disappointing results with the same viscoelastic heel pad used in the aforementioned prospective study.
- A prospective, randomized study compared the results of 3 types of treatment for long-term, chronic plantar heel pain: Corticosteroid injection and nonsteroidal antiinflammatory drug, viscoelastic heel cup, and functional FOs. A larger number of patients obtained good to excellent results in the custom foot orthotic group compared with the other groups.

Treatment Effects of Foot Orthoses for Specific Injuries: Patellofemoral Pain Syndrome

- Foot orthotics have been reported to be very successful in the treatment of patellofemoral pain syndrome with a success rate between 70-80%. However, most of these studies were not randomized controlled trials, and other adjunctive treatments were utilized.
- Two randomized, controlled studies have shown that an exercise program combined with "soft" orthotics can significantly decrease patellofemoral pain syndrome.

Treatment Effects of Foot Orthoses for Specific Injuries: Balance and Postural Control

- The most consistent objective measure of foot orthotic treatment effects have been found in studies of balance and postural control.
- At least 4 different studies have shown significant improvement in balance control in patients with chronic ankle instability when FOs are utilized. Custom-molded foot orthotics have been shown to reduce postural sway in patients after acute ankle sprain and have been shown to reduce pain while running in these patients.
- Custom-molded FOs appear to reduce postural sway better than flat orthoses. Posting of orthoses appears to also enhance postural control, particularly when medial posting is applied or when pronation of the subtalar joint is controlled.

MATERIAL SELECTION

- Despite the vast array of different types of FOs available, there is not a wide range of materials commonly used in the manufacture of these devices. Material selection will usually determine the general classification of the type of orthosis: Soft, semirigid, or hard. However, there is little agreement about the true definition and criteria for these categories. A discussion of the specific materials from which orthotics are crafted is beyond the scope of this chapter. An understanding that materials can generally be classified as soft, semirigid, or rigid relates to how and why a given orthotic will be used.

INDICATIONS FOR SOFT, SEMIRIGID, AND RIGID ORTHOSES

- Table 1 outlines general indications for soft, semirigid, and rigid FOs. These suggestions are based on empiric evidence in the literature. No scientific evidence exists for the superiority of one rigidity over another in the treatment of any lower extremity pathology.
- Rigid orthoses continue to be popular for the treatment of the collapsing flatfoot. Hypermobile foot types appear to tolerate and respond best to rigid orthotic intervention, while rigid cavus feet are best suited to semirigid or soft orthotic designs.
- Soft orthoses tend to be well tolerated by all foot types initially.
- Semirigid FOs may be the best devices for most foot and ankle pathologies, as they are generally well tolerated and provide good support.

SPECIFIC INDICATIONS AND PRESCRIPTION GUIDELINES FOR FOOT ORTHOSES

1st Metatarsophalangeal Pathologies

- Conditions that cause painful range of motion of the 1st metatarsophalangeal (MTP) joint include hallux rigidus, tear of the plantar capsule ("turf toe"), and sesamoiditis. The basic strategy to alleviate pain in the 1st MTP joint involves blocking motion of the joint, although offloading the joint can be used in certain pathologies.
- In both turf toe and hallux rigidus, stopping motion of the 1st MTP joint is desirable. This can be accomplished by inserting a full-length carbon fiber plate inside the shoe. Plates are available from various manufacturers in various stiffness and toe spring design. The plate makes the shoe into a "hard-soled shoe."
- Offloading the 1st MTP joint is used to treat pathologies of the sesamoid bones. A dancer's pad offloads the plantar aspect of the 1st metatarsal head and sesamoid apparatus by extending proximal to this area.

Central Metatarsalgia

- This category includes many diagnoses, including 2nd MTP synovitis and interdigital neuroma. Foot orthotic strategies for these conditions involve either blocking motion of the lesser MTP joints or offloading the affected metatarsal head.
- Blocking motion across the lesser MTP joints is most useful for conditions like Frieberg or even stress reactions/fractures. This can be accomplished with a rocker sole possibly coupled with the application of a carbon fiber plate to the shoe.
- Many cases of bursitis, capsulitis, or callusing around a central metatarsal head are due to failure of the 1st metatarsal head to accept load during late midstance and terminal stance. Modifications can be added to the functional FO to enhance stability of the 1st ray, decreasing load under the central metatarsals. A reverse Morton extension is 1 technique to elevate the lateral metatarsals while allowing the 1st metatarsal to plantar flex. A 1st-ray cutout is an effective way to improve weight bearing under the 1st metatarsal while decreasing load under the central metatarsals.
- Direct offloading of the central metatarsals can be accomplished with accommodations placed under the area of pathology. A metatarsal pad or metatarsal "dome" will offload the metatarsal head that is located immediately distal.
- A metatarsal bar applied to an orthosis will theoretically elevate all the metatarsals from the weight-bearing surface. A metatarsal bar will also direct ground reaction forces to a more proximal location of the metatarsal, theoretically away from the area of pathology.
- When treating interdigital neuroma of the forefoot with any type of shoe insert, a potential aggravation of the condition can occur if there is any compromise of shoe fit. Cushioned, properly fitted footwear is essential in the treatment of interdigital neuromas. Any orthotic designed to treat a neuroma will fail if shoe fit is made tighter.
- For standard footwear, the insertion of a metatarsal pad proximal to the neuroma is a standard practice that has been reported to give relief for patients with mild symptoms of a neuroma.
- Foot pronation causes a distal-lateral migration of the forefoot and metatarsals during midstance and terminal stance. This motion is thought to be 1 mechanism by which the intermetatarsal nerves may be traumatized. Controlling pronation may decrease shear of the 3rd and 4th metatarsals against the plantar digital nerve in the 3rd intermetatarsal space.

- Enhancement of an FO for relief of a neuroma can be accomplished with application of a metatarsal pad or a more oblong "neuroma pad" proximal to the neuroma site to create an elevation between metatarsals 3 and 4 to theoretically lift and "spread" the metatarsals off the injured nerve.

Heel Pain Syndrome

- The majority of people using FOs for heel pain are likely self-treating with devices purchased in a drug store.
- Most healthcare professionals recommend several types of treatment before prescribing FOs for this pathology. The cornerstone of this treatment typically centers on stretching the heel cord, specifically the gastrocnemius. When FOs are prescribed to treat heel pain, prefabricated devices are usually preferred as the initial treatment.
- Cushioned inserts can be of some benefit. Any heel pad that elevates the hindfoot will conceivably decrease the tightness of the heel cord, thereby decreasing the pull on the plantar fascia.
- The primary pathology is typically degeneration of the central band of the plantar aponeurosis with plantarmedial pain at the heel. Most FO strategies are thus designed to take pressure off the central band. A vast array of prefabricated "arch supports" are available in the commercial marketplace for this purpose.
- Custom FOs are commonly prescribed. The preferred design, material composition, and posting of custom orthoses vary significantly among various disciplines and among practitioners within any discipline. This reflects poor understanding and agreement of how an FO can offload strain in the plantar fascia. Support of the medial arch and resistance to flattening are essential requirements for orthoses designed to decrease strain in the plantar aponeurosis.

Cavus Foot

- The cavus foot predisposes patients to a number of conditions that may respond to FO therapy. However, the cavus foot type can present a challenge to the practitioner, as these feet are typically somewhat stiff and therefore less forgiving and less tolerant of orthotic correction than other foot types.
- Cavus feet can be described as "cavoadductovarus" in terms of alignment, i.e., high arch, forefoot adductus, and hindfoot varus. The varus alignment of the hindfoot in stance may be the result of compensation for a plantar flexed 1st ray, or the varus position of the hindfoot may indicate a true positional deformity where subtalar joint range of motion in the direction of eversion is limited. Coleman block testing can differentiate between these 2 variants.
- When hindfoot varus is secondary to a plantar flexed 1st ray, a functional FO can be of value to reduce deformity and improve stability in gait. In this case, application of a forefoot valgus post, or a depression under the 1st metatarsal head, may allow the hindfoot to fall into eversion. This movement does require a supple hindfoot, however.

- The ability of an FO to move a hindfoot out of varus is dependent on the available range of motion of the subtalar joint. With fixed hindfoot varus, such an orthosis will not correct foot alignment. However, symptoms can improve because FOs can influence joint moments and resultant strain on soft tissue structures.
- FOs can reduce high plantar pressures seen in cavus feet by distributing ground reaction forces more evenly and by providing cushion along the plantar surface of the foot. The requirements of an FO in treating the cavus foot therefore are geared toward cushioning and reduction of plantar pressures.

Flatfoot

- There is perhaps no pathology that more evokes the need for FOs than the symptomatic flatfoot.
- Generally speaking, FOs take advantage of the flexibility that is usually present in most flatfeet to push the foot into a less flat position.
- The use of FOs in this pathology is most commonly seeking to address an issue in 1 of 2 areas: Either a deficient or tendinotic posterior tibial tendon or lateral sinus tarsi impingement. At a most basic level, posterior tibial tendinopathy occurs as a result of the tendon being placed at a relative mechanical disadvantage, trying to invert the foot against the stronger Achilles tendon. By providing an orthosis with some arch support with a medial heel post, hindfoot varus is encouraged and, simply put, the mechanical work of the posterior tibial tendon is made easier.
- In patients that have sinus tarsi impingement, the declination of the talus coupled with the calcaneus shifting into valgus causes the 2 bones to physically contact one another, obliterating the space in the sinus tarsi and causing pain. A similar FO can "open up" the sinus tarsi to some degree, decreasing the impingement and alleviating symptoms somewhat.
- AFOs have been shown to be successful in the treatment of various stages of adult acquired flatfoot and are perhaps an option in those patients that wish to avoid surgery altogether.
- Some authors advocate the use of an Arizona brace for a significantly symptomatic flatfoot. While it can provide relief, the author's experience is that patients often dislike an Arizona brace to such a degree that they just do not wear it, as it cumbersome and difficult to get a shoe over.
- An Arizona brace is perhaps most appropriate in the older patient who adamantly does not want to have surgery.

SELECTED REFERENCES

1. Healy A et al: A systematic review of randomised controlled trials assessing effectiveness of prosthetic and orthotic interventions. PLoS One. 13(3):e0192094, 2018
2. Sinclair J: Mechanical effects of medial and lateral wedged orthoses during running. Phys Ther Sport. 32:48-53, 2018
3. Williamson P et al: Pressure distribution in the ankle and subtalar joint with routine and oversized foot orthoses. Foot Ankle Int. 1071100718770659, 2018
4. Hsu JR et al: Patient response to an integrated orthotic and rehabilitation initiative for traumatic injuries: the PRIORITI-MTF study. J Orthop Trauma. 31 Suppl 1:S56-S62, 2017
5. Menz HB et al: Predictors of response to prefabricated foot orthoses or rocker-sole footwear in individuals with first metatarsophalangeal joint osteoarthritis. BMC Musculoskelet Disord. 18(1):185, 2017

Indications for 3 Different Categories of Foot Orthoses

Category	Material Composition	Indications
Soft	Plastazote Aliplast Pelite Ethylene vinyl acetate Poron	Diabetic foot Rheumatoid foot Cavus foot
Semirigid	3/8" polypropylene Subortholene (3 and 4 mm) TL-2100 SF (composite)	Sport injuries Patellofemoral pain syndrome Mild to moderate pronation
Rigid	1/4" subortholene TL-2100 "rigid"	Severe pronation (i.e., flexible collapsing flatfoot) Tarsal coalition Chronic ankle instability

Comparison of Effects of Foot Orthoses vs. Ankle-Foot Orthoses

Foot Orthosis	Ankle-Foot Orthosis
Controls foot in stance phase only	Controls foot in stance and swing phases
Indirect control on ankle	Direct control on ankle
Indirect control on tibia	Direct control on tibia
Forces applied below axis of rear foot complex	Forced applied above and below axis of rear foot complex

6. Almonroeder TG et al: The influence of a prefabricated foot orthosis on lower extremity mechanics during running in individuals with varying dynamic foot motion. J Orthop Sports Phys Ther. 46(9):749-55, 2016
7. Gabriner ML et al: The effectiveness of foot orthotics in improving postural control in individuals with chronic ankle instability: a critically appraised topic. J Sport Rehabil. 24(1):68-71, 2015
8. Garbalosa JC et al: The effect of orthotics on intersegmental foot kinematics and the EMG activity of select lower leg muscles. Foot (Edinb). 25(4):206-14, 2015
9. Sinclair J et al: Effects of foot orthoses on Achilles tendon load in recreational runners. Clin Biomech (Bristol, Avon). 29(8):956-8, 2014
10. Cameron-Fiddes V et al: The use of 'off-the-shelf' foot orthoses in the reduction of foot symptoms in patients with early rheumatoid arthritis. Foot (Edinb). 23(4):123-9, 2013
11. Newman P et al: Risk factors associated with medial tibial stress syndrome in runners: a systematic review and meta-analysis. Open Access J Sports Med. 4:229-41, 2013
12. Foot orthotics. Inexpensive is often best. Mayo Clin Health Lett. 30(2):6, 2012
13. Chevalier TL et al: Effects of foot orthoses: how important is the practitioner? Gait Posture. 35(3):383-8, 2012
14. Redmond AC et al: Contoured, prefabricated foot orthoses demonstrate comparable mechanical properties to contoured, customised foot orthoses: a plantar pressure study. J Foot Ankle Res. 2:20, 2009
15. Landorf KB et al: Effectiveness of foot orthoses to treat plantar fasciitis: a randomized trial. Arch Intern Med. 166(12):1305-10, 2006
16. Mündermann A et al: Foot orthoses affect frequency components of muscle activity in the lower extremity. Gait Posture. 23(3):295-302, 2006
17. Imhauser CW et al: The effect of posterior tibialis tendon dysfunction on the plantar pressure characteristics and the kinematics of the arch and the hindfoot. Clin Biomech (Bristol, Avon). 19(2):161-9, 2004
18. Rome K et al: Randomized clinical trial into the impact of rigid foot orthoses on balance parameters in excessively pronated feet. Clin Rehabil. 18(6):624-30, 2004
19. Mündermann A et al: Orthotic comfort is related to kinematics, kinetics, and EMG in recreational runners. Med Sci Sports Exerc. 35(10):1710-9, 2003
20. Imhauser CW et al: Biomechanical evaluation of the efficacy of external stabilizers in the conservative treatment of acquired flatfoot deformity. Foot Ankle Int. 23(8):727-37, 2002
21. Hertel J et al: Effect of rearfoot orthotics on postural sway after lateral ankle sprain. Arch Phys Med Rehabil. 82(7):1000-3, 2001
22. Chao W et al: Nonoperative management of posterior tibial tendon dysfunction. Foot Ankle Int. 17(12):736-41, 1996
23. Brodsky JW et al: Objective evaluation of insert material for diabetic and athletic footwear. Foot Ankle. 9(3):111-6, 1988

(Left) *In-shoe pads, or metatarsal pads, are shown. These "off-the-shelf" inserts can be used to offload the metatarsal heads in an effort to decrease pain from metatarsalgia.* **(Right)** *Image shows the optimal positioning of the pad in the shoe. The goal is to make it so that the weight-bearing stresses are concentrated in an area proximal to the metatarsal heads.*

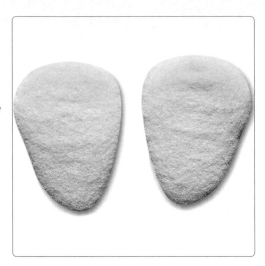

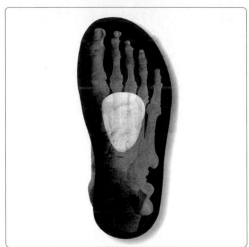

(Left) *Image shows arch pads. These pads are used to support the medial longitudinal arch. They are reasonably subtle and can be used in an effort to unload the arch.* **(Right)** *Optimal positioning of the arch pad in the shoe is shown. Given the name, the pads are meant to be placed under the arch; they can potentially alter stresses in the foot, potentially protecting the posterior tibial tendon and unloading the sinus tarsi to some degree.*

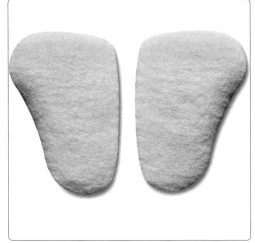

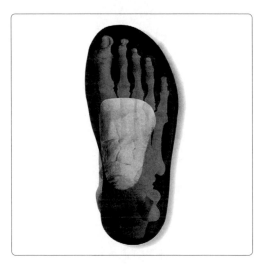

(Left) *Heel wedges are seen here; these can come in various shapes and sizes and can be helpful in a variety of pathologies.* **(Right)** *Most consistently, heel wedges can be helpful in Achilles pathology to help offload a relatively tight tendon or tight gastroc, thereby taking some pressure off the Achilles tendon, often dissipating symptoms.*

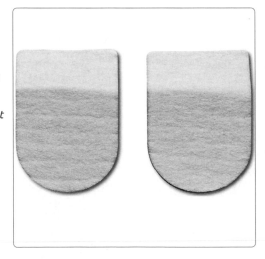

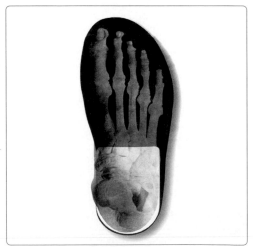

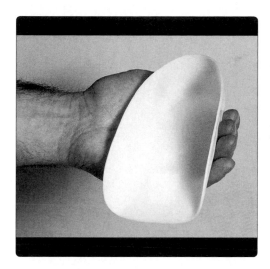

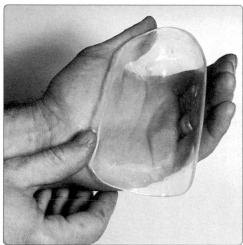

(Left) *A beginning model, which can allow for direct molding of the insert to an individual's foot, is shown.* **(Right)** *Here, another model is seen, which can once again allow for the insert to be molded.*

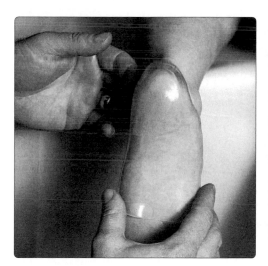

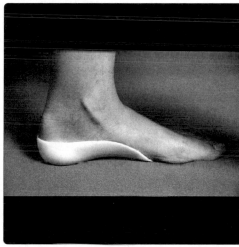

(Left) *The insert is placed on the foot to get a better sense of how the insert can be modified to better fit the patient's needs.* **(Right)** *The insert has been molded to the patient as seen in this weight-bearing view.*

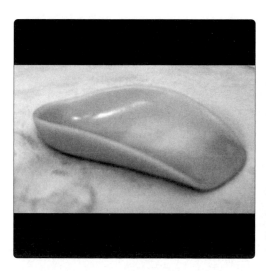

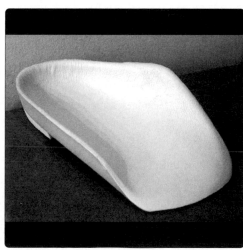

(Left) *Here, the University of California Biomechanics Laboratory orthosis, which is an off-the-shelf insert that can be used to support the medial longitudinal arch, is shown.* **(Right)** *Here, a more aggressive arch support is seen. An insert such as this one may not be tolerated well by a patient with insertional posterior tibial tendinopathy, as the rigid medial flange may impinge on the painful area.*

Flatfoot

- Arch height is widely variable in the population. A "low-arched foot" is not necessarily pathologic.
- Acquired flatfoot refers to an abnormal loss of the arch with pain.
  - Acquired flatfoot is a common end point of many etiologies.
- Posterior tibial tendon (PTT) dysfunction is the most common cause of the adult acquired flatfoot.
  - Other causes include neuropathic (Charcot) degeneration, neuromuscular disease, inflammatory disease, and trauma (fracture malunion or PTT laceration/rupture). Other factors, such as obesity, may play a role.
- Flatfoot describes the end point of a collapsed medial arch with associated deformities of the hindfoot and forefoot.
  - The hindfoot progresses into the valgus, and the forefoot supinates.
    - Peak pressures and contact forces of the associated joints, such as the subtalar joint, increase.
- In the sagittal plane, the longitudinal arch collapses with subluxation of the talonavicular (TN), naviculocuneiform (NC), or 1st tarsometatarsal (TMT) joints (or a combination of them).
- In the axial plane, the forefoot abducts, usually through the TN joint.
- In the coronal plane, heel valgus is seen.
- In 3 dimensions, the deformity is perhaps best described as dorsolateral peritalar subluxation, because the foot is subluxing dorsally and laterally around the talus.
  - Although the deformity is primarily through the peritalar joints in many flatfeet, it is important to remember that in some feet, other joints (such as NC or TMT) may be involved.
- The disease tends to be progressive. Once arch integrity is lost and collapse begins, gravity and weight-bearing forces encourage further destabilization.

(Left) The transverse tarsal joint includes the calcaneocuboid and talonavicular joints. In a simplified model, the axes of the joints are divergent in supination, locking the midfoot. When the foot is pronated, the axes are parallel, allowing motion at these joints and unlocking the midfoot. (Right) Inspection and palpation along the course of the posterior tibial tendon ➡ may demonstrate pain, swelling, and bogginess.

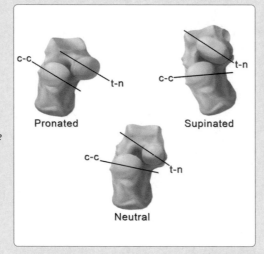
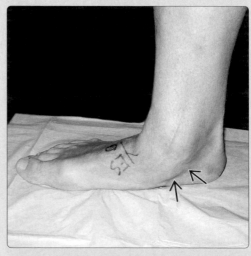

(Left) Lateral radiograph shows a large talar beak ➡. There is C-shaped sclerosis at the subtalar joint ➡. Both findings are secondary signs of a talocalcaneal coalition. (From DI: MSK Non-Trauma.) (Right) Tarsal coalition may cause a deformity that resembles the adult acquired flatfoot. CT confirms the fused medial facet of the subtalar joint ➡, while the posterior facet ➡ remains normal. This is a typical intraarticular talocalcaneal coalition, which usually only involves the medial facet. (From DI: MSK Non-Trauma.)

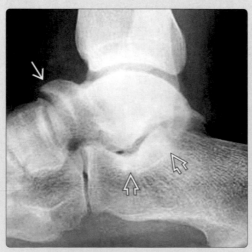
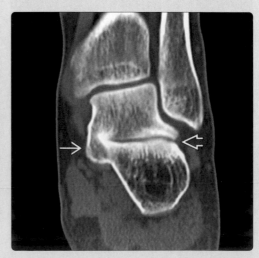

ARCHES OF FOOT

- The medial longitudinal arch comprises the 1st metatarsal, medial cuneiform, navicular, and talus.
- The lesser longitudinal arch consists of the 4th and 5th metatarsals, cuboid, and lateral calcaneus.
- A transverse arch spans the midfoot across the midtarsal joints. The 2nd and 3rd metatarsal bases are keystones and help prevent collapse.

Arch Support: Ligaments Are Key Static Supporters of Arch

- The spring ligament is an important stabilizer of the medial arch. It consists of 2 parts.
  - The superomedial calcaneonavicular (SMCN) ligament arises from the sustentaculum tali and fans out to insert on the edge of the medial navicular facet.
  - The inferior calcaneonavicular ligament runs from the anterior sustentaculum tali and inserts on the plantar aspect of the midnavicular cortex.
- The superficial deltoid originates on the medial malleolus and inserts on the dorsal edge of the SMCN ligament.
  - Its function is to serve as a check rein for the entire complex.
- The plantar fascia also contributes to arch integrity.
  - In biomechanical testing, it falls under load at 1.7-3.4 times body weight. (Hintermann 1995).
  - Division of the plantar fascia results in depression of the longitudinal arch and elongation of the medial length of the foot (Sharkey et al 1998).
    - Arch stiffness decreases by 25% (Huang et al 1993).
- The long plantar ligament runs from the anterior tuberosity of the inferior surface of the calcaneus.
  - The majority of fibers insert on the cuboid, and the more superficial fibers insert on the 2nd-5th metatarsals.
    - It is thought to be of secondary importance in arch support.

Dynamic Arch Stabilizers

- The posterior tibial tendon (PTT) is a powerful inverter and plantar flexor of the foot.
  - It locks the transverse tarsal joints [talonavicular (TN) and calcaneocuboid joints].
  - Biomechanical and electromyographic studies suggest that the tendon acts as an arch supporter during gait and loading situations.
- An imbalance between the PTT and its antagonists (tibialis anterior, peroneal longus and brevis, and triceps surae) may lead to arch collapse.
  - This occurs in muscle imbalance disorders, such as cerebral palsy.
- Extrinsic and intrinsic toe flexors also contribute to arch support but have a secondary role.
  - The flexor tendons fail under repetitive stress without a functional PTT.
- Hindfoot motion locks and unlocks the transverse tarsal joints.
  - With subtalar eversion, the transverse tarsal joints are flexible, which keep the forefoot supple to accommodate uneven surfaces.
  - When the PTT fires just prior to the heel rise portion of gait, the axes of the TN joint and calcaneocuboid joint are divergent, locking the transverse tarsal joints.
    - This creates a rigid medial column and long lever arm for forceful push-off during gait.
- In the normal gait cycle, firing of the PTT just prior to heel rise inverts the heel, bringing the Achilles vector medial to the subtalar joint.
  - Achilles contraction then supports the arch and encourages locking of the transverse tarsal joints.
    - This stabilizes the arch for push-off.

3D Deformity

- Although arch collapse is traditionally noted in the TN joint, deformity can occur with any combination of TN, naviculocuneiform (NC), &/or 1st tarsometatarsal (TMT) subluxation/collapse.
- Using the "tripod" model of foot structure, loss of the medial post of the tripod through collapse of any of these joints allows the hindfoot to collapse into valgus.
- Acquired flatfoot is a 3D deformity of hindfoot valgus, longitudinal arch collapse, and forefoot abduction.
- The talus becomes plantar flexed, the calcaneus everts, and the navicular and cuboid move to a more everted location.
- With increasing hindfoot valgus, the forefoot assumes a compensatory forefoot supination.
- The lateral column is effectively shortened as the deformity progresses.
- The talus slides anteriorly relative to the calcaneus.
- Hindfoot valgus occurs as a result of rotation through the subtalar and TN joints.
- Achilles contracture is a deforming force that can both cause and exacerbate arch failure.
  - When the heel is in valgus, the Achilles insertion lies lateral to the axis of the subtalar joint so that Achilles contraction promotes subtalar eversion and, thus, arch collapse.
- When the PTT fails to invert the hindfoot prior to heel rise, the calcaneal insertion of the Achilles remains lateral to the axis of the subtalar joint.
  - Achilles contraction then leads to hindfoot eversion.
  - The transverse tarsal joints are unlocked, and the arch can sag.
- Recurrent cycles of this dysfunctional gait can break down the static support of the arch.
- In some situations, Achilles contracture may precede any other pathology.
  - With Achilles contracture, the talus and calcaneus are plantar flexed.
  - Weight bearing places a dorsiflexion force on the forefoot.
  - Because of the oblique axis of the subtalar joint, subtalar eversion also produces some dorsiflexion.
  - In a foot with a tight Achilles tendon, subtalar eversion is necessary to produce a plantigrade foot.
  - With subtalar eversion, the PTT can become secondarily strained and eventually injured.
- Many patients with active PTT tendonitis will have a tight gastrocnemius and a low arch on the "normal" foot.
- A flatfoot deformity exacerbates Achilles contracture by maintaining the foot in hindfoot valgus and equinus.

- The Achilles may become more contracted, which further antagonizes PTT function and arch integrity with a progressive deformity.
- So, an acquired flatfoot can be caused by tightness of the Achilles (especially the gastrocnemius component) and can also result in a contracted Achilles tendon.
- In the deformity, hindfoot and midfoot joint degeneration may develop secondary to increases in joint reactive pressures.
  - With a flatfoot deformity, the subtalar joint facets sublux, so that only 1/2 of the articular surface is in contact.
  - The decrease in contact area leads to increased contact pressures (Ananthakrisnan et al 1999).

Pain From Flatfoot

- The pes planovalgus deformity alters joint mechanics as well as foot and ankle alignment.
- Pain can occur in the foot, ankle, or even more proximal locations.
  - The lower back and hip may be sore from limping or from altered gait mechanics.
  - Continued valgus stress on the knee from a valgus foot can lead to medial compartment disease.
  - Valgus foot alignment can also lead to a valgus ankle deformity with painful joint degeneration.
  - In the foot, pain may be felt medially or laterally and may arise from inflammation, tendinitis, arthritis, &/or impingement.
- In cases of PTT tendinitis, patients may feel pain only in the medial hindfoot from tenosynovitis or from a complete or longitudinal tear within the tendon.
- In an advanced flatfoot of any etiology, pain may occur over the medial malleolus and deltoid ligament, as the deltoid fibers are tensioned to oppose the worsening hindfoot valgus.

Talocalcaneal Impingement and Calcaneofibular Impingement

- With hindfoot valgus, lateral hindfoot pain can occur as a result of the calcaneus impinging on the distal tip of the fibula or lateral process of the talus.
- Cyst formation &/or sclerosis in this region, either on plain film or computed tomography (CT), should create suspicion of impingement.
- A CT imaging study compared control subjects with patients with severe deformity under 75 N of axial loading (Malicky et al 2002).
  - It determined that the prevalence of sinus tarsi impingement was 92%, and the prevalence of calcaneofibular impingement was 66% in the flatfoot group vs. 0% and 5%, respectively, in the control group.
  - The study patients who had calcaneofibular impingement also had sinus tarsi impingement.

Arthritis

- Arthritis may be the causative agent or the end result of a chronic severe deformity.
- Alteration of joint reaction forces causes abnormal loading of the subtalar, tibiotalar, transverse tarsal, and Lisfranc joints and may result in painful arthritic conditions.

Summary of Etiology of Adult Acquired Flatfoot

- If the normal balance of arch support is disturbed (such as with fracture malunion, PTT injury, or Achilles tightness), persistent abnormally directed weight-bearing forces will tax the remaining support of the arch (such as the PTT or spring ligament), leading to progressive arch collapse.
- Once the deformity is established, it may be difficult to determine which came first, the Achilles contracture, PTT dysfunction, or spring ligament rupture.
- Perhaps the most important treatment for an acquired flatfoot is prevention.
  - If the "at-risk" foot could be identified, early intervention might prevent the deformity.
  - Once the deformity is established, it is often self-perpetuating and progressive.
  - An "at-risk" foot would be one with a very tight Achilles and normal PTT function or one with severe flatfoot deformity but still normal PTT function.

POSTERIOR TIBIAL TENDON DYSFUNCTION

Tibialis Posterior Anatomy

- The muscle arises from the posterior tibia as a large muscle in the deep posterior compartment of the calf.
- The tendon travels in the medial malleolar groove and inserts broadly into the medial foot.
  - It primarily inserts onto the navicular tuberosity, but multiple slips fan out to insert into the 2nd-4th metatarsals, into the plantar surface of the cuneiforms, and on the cuboid on the lateral foot.
  - On the plantar surface, it attaches to the deep fascia, peroneal longus tendon, and long and short toe flexors.
- A zone of hypovascularity exists 40 mm proximal to the navicular tuberosity and extends proximally over 14 mm of tendon.
  - There is no mesotendon in this region, and surrounding synovial tissue is also hypovascular.
    - This area is subject to mechanical wear.
- It is possible that a transient ischemia creates tendon insufficiency and sets up the cascade of dynamic instability.
  - A diseased PTT has high relative concentrations of type 3 collagen (it is the main collagen in early tendon healing).
  - It has decreased tensile strength, which can cause tendon insufficiency and dysfunction with recurrent use.
- In an evaluation of spontaneously ruptured tendons and controls in an over-35 population, degenerative pathologic changes, such as hypoxic degeneration, mucoid degeneration, tendolipomatosis, and calcifying tendinopathy, were identified (Kannus and Jozsa 1991).
  - Of note, these changes were observed in 34% of control tendon specimens.
  - Normal tendon structure was not identified in any of the ruptured tendon specimens.
  - These findings suggest that degenerative tendinopathy is common after age 35.

Epidemiology

- It is more often seen in women between 45-65 years of age.
- It occurs with increased frequency in obese and -diabetic patients.

- About 1/2 of patients will relate a traumatic event to the initiation of symptoms.
- As previously mentioned, with PTT dysfunction, the transverse tarsal joint will not lock during heel rise. Weight-bearing forces across these unlocked joints lead to fatigue failure of the ligaments. In these cases, PTT dysfunction precedes arch collapse.
  - Weight-bearing forces across these unlocked joints lead to fatigue failure of the ligaments.
  - In these cases, PTT dysfunction precedes arch collapse.
- Arch-flattening forces, such as a tight gastrocnemius and obesity, may contribute to a flatfoot, as the repetitive forces of weight bearing cause the deformity to progress.
  - This may worsen PTT dysfunction.
- In some cases, static deformities can cause PTT dysfunction (the arch fails first).
  - The position of forefoot pronation and valgus (arch-collapse) will lead to PTT failure and worsening-deformity.
  - If the talocalcaneonavicular complex loses stiffness, the PTT insertion sites are in a valgus position.
  - Lengthening of the tendon even 1 cm reduces its efficiency as the primary dynamic stabilizer of the arch.

Posterior Tibial Tendon Disease Progression

- PTT disease progression is a continuum.
- A staging system was introduced in 1989 by Johnson and Strom that included 4 stages.
  - The system was devised to describe the clinical entity and offers guidelines for nonoperative and operative treatment.
- Unfortunately, there is no evidence that a foot progresses from one stage to the next over time.
  - It is possible that feet at stage 1 represent a different pathophysiology with a different natural history than that of a stage 3 flatfoot.
- Not all feet at any one stage are the same.
- Although treatment guidelines are often listed by stage, it is important to assess each foot individually.
  - Treatment, especially surgical, cannot be generalized.

Stage 1

- Pain and swelling occur along the course of the tendon and are defined as tenosynovitis or tendinosis.
- Tendon length is unchanged.
- The subtalar joint is flexible.
- The heel inverts on single toe rise, and there is no loss of strength.
- There is no deformity; arch height remains unchanged.
- Radiographs are normal.
- Magnetic resonance (MR) imaging will demonstrate edema around the tendon and occasional intrasubstance degeneration.
  - Exuberant tenosynovitis may be a hallmark of an inflammatory or rheumatic etiology.

Stage 2

- The tendon is elongated and enlarged and is functionally incompetent.
- On tendon inspection, there are partial tears, and there is evidence of degeneration.

- The patient may be able to perform a single limb heel rise, but the heel does not invert.
- The foot assumes a pes planovalgus appearance.
  - The arch is collapsed, the hindfoot is in valgus, the forefoot is abducted, and the subtalar joint is everted.
- The subtalar joint remains flexible, and the deformity is passively correctable.
- The Achilles tendon will be contracted.
- There will be a too many toes sign.
- Radiographs demonstrate an increased lateral talocalcaneal angle, decreased calcaneal pitch, and lateral peritalar subluxation.
- MR demonstrates tendon degeneration, possible discontinuity, and changes in the spring ligament.

Stage 3

- Tendon degeneration is pronounced, and it is attenuated or ruptured.
- Single-limb heel rise is often impossible, and the heel cannot be inverted with heel rise.
- The deformity is severe and may be fixed.
- The subtalar joint may be rigid.
- The forefoot is abducted and may be supinated.
- The navicular is in a laterally subluxed position.
- Pain may occur both medially and laterally.
- The too many toes sign is grossly positive.
- Radiographs demonstrate peritalar subluxation, plantar flexion of the talus, and, often, degenerative changes in the subtalar and transverse tarsal joints.
  - Lateral impingement may cause a fibular stress fracture.
- MR is not needed to assess the tibial tendon but may give information about the degree of degeneration of the hindfoot joints.
- CT may also be helpful in assessing degeneration of the midfoot and hindfoot joints.
  - Weight-bearing CT, if available, can give more information about the 3D deformity.

Stage 4

- Stage 4 includes all findings in stage 3 along with valgus angulation of the talus at the tibiotalar joint secondary to deltoid failure and lateral ankle erosion.
- Radiographs will demonstrate a plantarflexed valgus talus as well as tibiotalar degenerative arthritis.

Other Etiologies of Adult Acquired Flatfoot Deformity

- Rheumatoid or other inflammatory arthropathies can cause PTT dysfunction.
  - Arthrosis can occur at any of the hindfoot or midfoot joints primarily.
    - Subluxation of these arthritic joints will lead to a flatfoot, independent of PTT function.
  - Inflammatory arthritides can also affect tendons with all the symptoms of PTT dysfunction.
- **Posttraumatic deformity**
  - Soft tissue trauma as an etiology of flatfoot is often a subtle diagnosis, as the end-stage deformity, forefoot abduction, and hindfoot valgus are the same.
  - Malunion from navicular, Lisfranc, 1st metatarsal, and calcaneus fracture can cause settling of the medial longitudinal arch, creating a flatfoot deformity.

- o Flatfoot secondary to midfoot (Lisfranc) malunion is secondary to loss of medial column stability, often at the TMT joint.
  - At the level of the midfoot, the longitudinal arch will break, and the forefoot will drift into abduction.
  - Hindfoot valgus is a secondary compensatory change.
- o A PTT laceration or traumatic rupture will also lead to arch collapse as dynamic support of the arch fails, causing muscle imbalance and eventual arthrosis.
- **Neuropathic deformity**
  - o The characteristic flatfoot deformity has been described in the diabetic neuropathic population, spinal cord patients, and those with Hansen disease and other neuropathic conditions.
  - o Charcot neuroarthropathy in the midfoot causes collapse of the medial arch, often with marked deformity.
    - In these cases, it is not PTT dysfunction but rather a loss of the normal bony architecture.

Tarsal Coalition and Peroneal Spasm

- Peroneal spasm can be a sign of disease in the peritalar region.
- Protective contraction of any or all of the muscles bridging the peritalar joints may be induced in response to a peritalar insult.
- Patients with a hindfoot coalition have been traditionally thought of as having spastic peroneal tendons.
  - o However, the majority of these patients do not have spasm, and peroneal spasm has been identified in patients without tarsal coalitions.
  - o These patients should be examined for other peritalar lesions.
- A patient with a tarsal coalition classically will have a unilateral flatfoot, decreased motion, vague foot pain, and peroneal spasm.
  - o However, the foot may be normally shaped with no peroneal spasm.
  - o The typical patient presents only with hindfoot pain.
    - The astute clinician will detect a lack of hindfoot motion.
- The coalition may be osseous, cartilaginous, or fibrous, and it may be complete or incomplete.
- Plain x-rays may show dorsal talar beaking.
- CT examination of the foot can diagnose a coalition.
  - o Fibrous coalitions require a high index of suspicion when analyzing the CT.
- The most common coalition is between the calcaneus and the navicular.
- A middle facet subtalar coalition is the next most common tarsal coalition.
- Once diagnosed, involved joints should be investigated for arthritic changes.
- Coalition resection is appropriate treatment in a nondegenerated calcaneal-navicular coalition.
- Subtalar arthrodesis may be necessary for subtalar coalitions, as decreased motion, deformity, and peroneal spasm probably exist at the time of diagnosis.

Physical Examination of Flatfoot

- The physical examination comprises inspection, palpation, range of motion examination, and dynamic strength testing.

- **Inspection**
  - o Arch height in comparison with the contralateral side should be noted.
  - o The too many toes sign confirms forefoot abduction deformity.
    - When viewed from behind, the abducted forefoot will show more toes visible lateral to the leg than normal.
  - o **Heel rise testing**
    - In the normal foot, elevation of foot to a tiptoe stance requires a functional PTT to invert the subtalar joint.
      - □ If normal, this will bring the heel into varus.
    - Comparison of the affected and unaffected foot can confirm if the PTT is insufficient by an asymmetric heel position on double heel rise testing.
    - An inability to rise up on the affected foot indicates PTT insufficiency or dysfunction.
    - It can also serve as a stress test if the patient is unable to perform more than 1 or 2 single heel rises.
- **Motion examination**
  - o The flatfoot is diagnosed as either flexible or rigid based on subtalar motion.
    - A rigid deformity implies muscle spasm, advanced arthritis, or a coalition.
  - o To examine for an Achilles contracture, the subtalar joint must 1st be reduced to a neutral starting position.
    - This also allows the examiner to appreciate the degree of forefoot varus and the rigidity of the deformity.
- **Palpation**
  - o Tenderness can occur over the course of the PTT, plantar fascia, or spring and deltoid ligaments.
  - o Tenderness may also occur on the lateral hindfoot as a result of calcaneofibular or talocalcaneal impingement.
  - o Peroneal or tibialis anterior spasm may coexist in patients with a tarsal coalition.

Imaging Studies

- Weight-bearing anteroposterior and lateral views of the foot and an anteroposterior view of the ankle are essential aids in diagnosis.
- **Anteroposterior foot**
  - o The degree of abnormality in talar alignment can be assessed.
    - The talus becomes increasingly uncovered as the navicular subluxes laterally.
  - o The TN coverage angle can determine the degree of uncovering that has occurred.
- **Lateral foot**
  - o It confirms the loss of alignment between the 1st metatarsal and talus.
  - o Subluxation or sagging is identified at the TN and the NC joints.
  - o The talus assumes a plantar flexed configuration, and the calcaneal pitch decreases as the deformity progresses.
- **Anteroposterior ankle**
  - o Talar tilt is determined in this view.
  - o Stage 4 disease is characterized by tibiotalar subluxation secondary to deltoid insufficiency.
  - o Degeneration at the midfoot and hindfoot joints can be determined by observing subluxation and loss of joint space, osteophyte formation, and sclerosis.

- ○ Dorsal talar beaking or bossing, if observed, may be suggestive of a coexisting tarsal coalition.
- MR is a sensitive and specific test in the determination of PTT pathology.
  - ○ It provides insight into the morphology and internal structure of the tendon.
  - ○ Another use of MR is to evaluate the mid- and hindfoot for underlying disease when determining surgical treatment.
  - ○ Its expense must be considered, as most tendinosis can be determined by history and physical examination.
- Ultrasound is a noninvasive, less expensive modality by which the PTT can be examined.
  - ○ Ultrasound can diagnose increased tendon diameter and increased peritendinous space and compare it with the contralateral side.
  - ○ Ultrasound diagnosis of stage 1 PTT dysfunction correlates with surgical findings.
- Simulated weight-bearing CT may be useful to better understand the 3D deformity but hard to obtain in many medical centers.
- Weight-bearing CT may be most helpful when assessing deformity of the stage 2 flatfoot.
  - ○ Although there are no strict criteria, weight-bearing CT may aid in surgical planning, especially for medial column fusions and calcaneal osteotomies.
- Non-weight-bearing CT will more accurately show the presence of radiographic arthritis than plain films.

TREATMENT

General Principles

- A treatment protocol is devised based on the etiology of the disease.
  - ○ Different treatment modalities are acceptable for the various stages of disease.
- Understanding the etiology of the deformity will dictate the treatment protocol.
  - ○ The treatment plan for a rigid flatfoot secondary to tarsal coalition will differ greatly from that of a patient with disease secondary to rheumatoid arthritis.
- The goal of all treatment modalities is the elimination of pain, both long and short term, and restoration of normal foot biomechanics and orientation.
- Most clinicians argue for a trial of nonoperative treatment prior to surgical intervention.
  - ○ In some cases, such as in a young patient with early deformity and a high likelihood of progression, earlier surgery may halt the disease and avoid progressive joint degeneration.

Nonoperative Treatment

- In flexible flatfoot deformities, the goal of nonoperative treatment is to restore normal foot orientation and alleviate pain.
  - ○ Antiinflammatory medications may be helpful.
    - – The goal of this treatment is to decrease the inflammation and synovitis surrounding the PTT.
  - ○ Cortisone injections may further jeopardize the PTT and should be avoided.

- ○ With PTT tendonitis, rest with short leg casting (or a removable cast boot) often breaks the cycle leading to deformity and provides pain relief by controlling the symptoms of tendinitis or tenosynovitis.
  - – Weight bearing is allowed only if it does not cause pain.
- ○ After cast removal, a full-length medial arch support is required to maintain PTT support and foot alignment.
  - – Bracing and orthotics are designed to control progressive heel valgus.
  - – By reducing the calcaneus to neutral, the transverse tarsal joint is stiffened, and forefoot abduction is decreased.
- ○ A full-length medial arch support with a medial heel wedge and medial column post will reduce the subtalar joint.
  - – This may allow the tendonitis to recede, thus relieving early flatfoot pain.
- ○ In a more severe but flexible flatfoot deformity, a molded ankle-foot orthosis (AFO) ± an articulation may be necessary.
- ○ A University of California Biomechanics Laboratory (UCBL) orthotic is more rigid and provides lateral buttressing of the forefoot to help control severe but flexible abduction deformities of the forefoot.
- In rigid flatfoot, the goal of bracing is to support the foot in situ for pain control and correction of any remaining flexibility of the foot.
  - ○ Bracing requires use of an accommodative device custom molded to the foot deformity.
  - ○ Both articulated and nonarticulated custom-molded AFO braces are used.
    - – Often, a rocker bottom sole is required in a nonarticulated AFO.
  - ○ Skin compromise may occur in a brace that provides too much correction in a patient with a rigid -deformity.
  - ○ In severe rigid deformities that involve the tibiotalar joint, solid AFOs, such as an Arizona brace, are the only orthotic option.
  - ○ Once arch collapse has occurred, nonprotected weight bearing will exacerbate the deformity and lead to secondary degenerative arthritis in the affected joints.
  - ○ Bracing and orthotics should probably be tried for several weeks before proceeding to operative intervention.
    - – Surgical management is indicated for failure of a well-fitting orthotic to control symptoms.
  - ○ A study by Chao et al (1996) assessed the results of bracing.
    - – 67% of patients (33/49) were treated successfully with UCBL orthosis or AFOs, 24% of patients had fair to poor results but did not seek surgical intervention, and 9% went on to require surgical management.
    - – The average time of orthotic wear was between 3-6 months for the groups that were not successfully treated with orthotics.

Surgical Principles

- The sources of pain must be addressed, not just the shape of the arch.
  - ○ If there is tendon pain, then that should be addressed with tendon repair and augmentation.

○ If there is pain from osseous impingement, arch alignment must be improved to decompress the painful areas.

○ If there is pain from arthritis, the affected joints should probably be fused.

- Surgery should halt the progress of the disease so that no future surgery is needed.

○ In most cases, Achilles tendon (or gastrocnemius) lengthening is an important step to decrease arch-flattening forces and to protect the reconstructed PTT.

- Any deformity should be realigned, even if not necessary for short-term pain relief.

○ Persistent deformity will place abnormal stresses on the subtalar joint, ankle, and, to a lesser extent, knee with progressive joint degeneration.

Surgical Options for Stage 1 Posterior Tibial Tendon Dysfunction

- Active PTT disease with a preserved arch is treated by repairing and augmenting the tendon.

- Achilles tendon (especially gastrocnemius) contracture will increase stress on the tendon and may lead to deformity.

○ Surgical lengthening will aid in balancing the deforming force.

- At this early stage, bone work may be avoided.

○ However, in the patient with obesity, or with degenerative or inflammatory disease, consideration should be given to a medial sliding calcaneal osteotomy.

– This osteotomy moves the insertion of the Achilles tendon to a point medial to the subtalar joint axis, so that the Achilles can further support PTT function.

– When the Achilles pulls medial to the axis of the subtalar joint, it will promote hindfoot inversion.

- For the tendon repair, a medial approach is utilized to inspect the retinaculum, tendon sheath, and tendon.

- Tendon debridement is performed if intratendinous tears or nodularity is encountered.

○ Diseased tendon is excised, and a side-to-side repair is performed with nonabsorbable suture and buried knots.

- The flexor digitorum longus (FDL) and flexor hallucis longus (FHL) are most commonly used to augment the diseased PTT.

○ Advantages of using the FDL include in-phase -functioning of the FDL, excursion of the tendon, and proximity of the FDL to the PTT tendon sheath.

– There is probably no morbidity to transferring the FDL, even in the active patient.

○ The advantages of using the FHL include greater tendon strength and girth in comparison with the FDL.

- After tendon debridement and augmentation, the foot is protected for 6 weeks in a weight-bearing cast or cast boot.

○ The patient is gradually advanced to regular activities and kept in a medial arch support.

- There have been many studies evaluating the results of surgical debridement and augmentation of stage 1 disease (Teasdall and Johnson 1994, Mann 2001).

○ Most patients get better, but a small minority require augmentation &/or bony realignment.

Surgical Options After Arch Collapse and Prior to Degenerative Changes

- Bony realignments are used in conjunction with PTT debridement and augmentation to protect the soft tissue repair and to correct the underlying deformity.

- The goal is to realign the foot without sacrificing essential hindfoot joints (subtalar, TN).

○ This is done with osteotomies &/or fusions of nonessential joints.

○ These hindfoot-sparing procedures cannot overcome advanced collapse of the hindfoot joints, especially when degenerative changes are present.

- While most surgeons agree that bony realignment and medial soft tissue augmentation is the appropriate surgical intervention in a flexible flatfoot, there is wide variation in the method chosen to achieve correction.

○ Bony procedures include medializing calcaneal osteotomy, lateral column lengthening, &/or medial column stabilization.

○ These procedures are always combined with soft tissue balancing, including gastrocnemius or Achilles lengthening, and PTT reconstruction.

Medial Sliding Calcaneal Tuberosity Osteotomy

- The combination of medial displacement calcaneal osteotomy and a medial soft tissue reconstruction is currently a popular treatment for patients with a milder, flexible deformity and PTT dysfunction.

- Medial displacement calcaneal tuberosity osteotomy corrects hindfoot valgus directly.

○ More importantly, the osteotomy translates the insertion of the Achilles tendon so that the tendon runs medial to the axis of the subtalar joint.

○ The Achilles tendon then becomes an inverter of the hindfoot, locking the arch and assisting the posterior tibialis.

○ The shift to a more anatomical orientation also decreases the valgus vector from the peroneal brevis and enhances function of the peroneal longus as a plantar flexor of the 1st metatarsal.

– This should decrease the abduction moment on the forefoot.

- The flatfoot deformity is only partially corrected with medial calcaneal osteotomy.

○ The procedure inconsistently improves arch height and partially improves TN coverage.

- A recent clinical outcome study by Myerson et al (2004) demonstrated excellent pain relief (97%) and improvement in function (94%).

○ Subtalar motion was normal in 56 patients, decreased in 66 patients, and moderately decreased in 7 patients.

○ In most studies, radiographic correction with medial displacement osteotomy and PTT reconstruction yields inconsistent and incomplete correction of alignment. However, in this study, radiographic correction was significant in all 4 radiographic parameters.

Medial Column Stabilization

- In some flatfeet, medial column collapse occurs at the 1st metatarsocuneiform or medial NC joint.

- o In these feet, loss of medial column support (loss of the medial post of the tripod) leads to secondary hindfoot valgus.
- o In these feet, selective realignment of the metatarsocuneiform &/or NC joints may be performed.
- These feet can be identified by observing collapse of these joints on the lateral weight-bearing radiograph.
- In some cases, realignment of the medial column joints will result in excellent correction of the arch.
  - o This is relatively rare.
- In others, addition of a calcaneal osteotomy may be necessary.

Lateral Column Lengthening or Arthrodesis

- Because the subtalar joint acts like a screw, hindfoot eversion (valgus) of the flatfoot causes the calcaneus to move posteriorly, relative to the talus.
  - o Although the calcaneus is not truly "short," the anterior edge of the bone appears shorter than the talus on weight-bearing anteroposterior radiographs.
- Lengthening of the calcaneus (in the lateral column of the foot) drives the rest of the foot around the talus, through the TN joint.
  - o The end effect of such lateral column lengthening is to rotate the flexible flatfoot back around the talus, leading to impressive arch correction.
- Such lengthening can be done by inserting a structural graft of bone into an osteotomy of the anterior process of the calcaneus or into the calcaneocuboid joint (distraction arthrodesis).
  - o When the lateral column is lengthened through the anterior process of the calcaneus, the osteotomy may pass through the middle facet of the subtalar joint. Such an intraarticular osteotomy is undesirable, at least in theory.
  - o When the lengthening is done through the calcaneocuboid joint (lengthening arthrodesis), the nonunion rate is higher.
  - o In either case, nonunions can occur, so rigid internal fixation is necessary.
- Malunion/malpositioning of the lengthening (or just overlengthening) can lead to fixed forefoot varus with the 1st ray not touching the ground.
- Lateral column lengthening dramatically increases calcaneal pitch.
  - o It should probably not be used for feet in which the pitch is normal prior to surgery.
- The procedure was first described by Evans in 1975 for treatment of deformity secondary to multiple causes (poliomyelitis, idiopathic calcaneal valgus, rigid flatfoot, talipes equinovalgus, and traumatic division of the PTT in childhood).
  - o He reported that the operation was a success in all cases.
- Mosca in 1995 reported his results of the Evans osteotomy.
  - o Twenty-nine of 31 patients had a satisfactory clinical result with creation of a medial arch, decreased talar head prominence, decreased medial pain, and decreased hindfoot valgus.

- Radiographic studies have demonstrated that lateral column lengthening improves talar head coverage by the navicular, reduces forefoot abduction, diminishes hindfoot valgus, and improves sagittal alignment of the arch (Sangeorzan et al 1993).
- Realignment of the lateral column effects foot alignment in several ways.
  - o The peroneal longus lever arm is lengthened.
    - This makes the muscle a more powerful 1st metatarsal plantar flexor and restores forefoot alignment.
  - o The plantar fascia is lengthened.
    - This increases the static support of the arch.
  - o The Achilles tendon insertion shifts medially.
    - This decreases its antagonizing effect on the PTT.
- An outcome study by Toolan et al (1999) reviews the results of lateral column lengthening and PTT augmentation in 36 patients (41 feet).
  - o Five out of 6 radiographic parameters were improved significantly.
  - o Complications included nonunion of the calcaneocuboid joint (20%); sural nerve paresthesias (32%); and additional surgical procedures (71%), such as removal of hardware, revision of fixation, and revision procedures, including triple arthrodesis and medial osteotomies.
  - o 88% were less painful or pain free, and 85% of patients rated their result as satisfactory; 93% stated that they would have the procedure again if the circumstances were similar.
- In recent years, a variation of the calcaneal Evans osteotomy has been described with a "step-cut" instead of a straight cut.
  - o The osteotomy is a Z shape with more overlap of cancellous bone after lengthening.
  - o Most still use bone graft to fill it in, but in theory, a structural graft may not be needed. There are no proven benefits in outcome thus far, probably because the nonunion rate for a traditional lateral column lengthening with structural allograft has a very low nonunion rate.
  - o There are no proven benefits in outcome thus far, probably because there is a very low nonunion rate for the traditional lateral column lengthening with structural allograft.
  - o Although nonunion of calcaneal osteotomies is rare, there may be some graft collapse and loss of correction with traditional lateral column lengthening, and the step-cut procedure may reduce the risk of malunion.

Combining Medial and Lateral Procedures

- In many feet, a combination of procedures may be needed.
  - o The presumption is that the best long-term results will come from more accurate restoration of normal foot structure.
  - o Lateral column lengthening or medial displacement osteotomy may be combined with metatarsocuneiform &/or NC realignment and fusion.
- A combination of both medial and lateral column procedures is indicated for a patient with hindfoot valgus, low calcaneal pitch angle, and transverse tarsal joint sag.
  - o It is able to correct all aspects of the forefoot and hindfoot deformities in a flexible flatfoot (Chi et al 1999).

- Some surgeons advocate a procedure to include medial calcaneal slide plus lateral column lengthening along with a medial column procedure.
  - Whether this provides better outcomes is not clear.

Compensatory Forefoot Supination

- In many flatfeet, collapse of the hindfoot will lead to supination of the forefoot (relative elevation of the 1st ray).
  - As the hindfoot everts, the 1st ray must supinate or elevate to stay even with the floor.
  - If this did not occur, the 1st ray would be driven into the floor.
- After successful hindfoot realignment, many flatfeet will have an elevated 1st ray (compensatory forefoot supination).
  - In these cases, 1st metatarsocuneiform plantar flexion arthrodesis or opening wedge cuneiform osteotomy (Cotton procedure) can be added to the reconstruction.

Selective Fusions

- Over the years, some surgeons have used isolated TN or subtalar fusions to correct the less severe, flexible flatfoot.
- Double fusion (TN and calcaneocuboid) has also been advocated.
  - Short-term clinical series have shown favorable results.
- Because any of these procedures eliminate the majority of hindfoot motion, there may not be any benefit over triple arthrodesis.
- More importantly, for the less severe flatfoot with more flexible deformity (stage 2 posterior tibial tendonitis), the hindfoot-sparing procedures may lead to better function.
- Of course, for the rare foot with isolated arthritis of 1 hindfoot joint, isolated fusion of that joint should result in a good outcome.
  - A good example is a patient with posttraumatic arthritis of the TN joint after a navicular fracture.

Spring Ligament Reconstruction

- All of the osteotomies are working around the underlying problem with the acquired flatfoot: The loss of ligament stabilization of the arch.
- The spring ligament (calcaneonavicular) is the main supporting ligament.
- Limited results have been reported of spring ligament reconstruction techniques.
  - Simple imbrication of the attenuated spring ligament will not be successful.
  - The original Miller procedure combined routing of the anterior tibial tendon along the medial column (but distal to the spring ligament) along with fusion of the NC joint.
  - Sections of the PTT can be fixed into the plantar talar head or sustentaculum of the calcaneus as a spring ligament reconstruction.
  - Alternately, allograft can be placed through bone along the spring ligament.
  - Osteotomies to support the arch and decrease tension along the graft are performed at the same time, and it is not clear what the role of spring ligament reconstruction will be.

Surgery for Advanced Flatfoot

- Triple arthrodesis is historically the "gold standard" procedure for a rigid flatfoot.

- Arthrodesis of the subtalar, calcaneocuboid, and TN joints is performed with realignment of those joints.
  - In the absence of degenerative changes, the calcaneocuboid joint is sometimes spared.
    - Most of the correction comes though subtalar and TN joints.
- "In situ" fusion, without realignment, is never appropriate.
  - Persistent residual deformity can adversely affect adjacent joints (ankle).
- Long-term outcome studies have shown a high incidence of degenerative disease in neighboring joints, such as the ankle and midfoot.
- Because of the stiffness that results from triple arthrodesis, it is generally reserved for patients with hindfoot stiffness or arthritis that could not be managed with hindfoot-sparing procedures.
- Hindfoot fusion is also appropriate for patients with severe deformity, which might be beyond the ability of joint-sparing procedures to correct.
- In one large outcome study, 67 procedures were done on 57 feet with an average follow-up of 44 years (Saltzman et al 1999).
  - Many of the study subjects had neuromuscular disease, not flatfoot.
  - Fifty-four patients (95%) were satisfied with the result of the operation, although 78% had some residual deformity, 13 patients had a pseudoarthrosis, and 37 patients had ankle pain.
  - All ankles had degenerative changes on radiographs, and arthritic findings were noted at the NC and TMT joints in the majority of patients.
- Because the most important joints are directly realigned, triple arthrodesis usually leads to good realignment of the hindfoot.
- It is important to remember that many cases of advanced, rigid flatfoot will have secondary forefoot supination.
  - Realignment of the hindfoot without attention to the forefoot will result in an elevated 1st metatarsal.
  - Residual forefoot supination can be corrected by plantar flexing and fusing the 1st metatarsocuneiform joint.

Ankle Valgus

- Realignment and pantalar fusion can be performed for the most severe valgus deformities.
  - It results in a stiff, straight foot, which is an improvement from a stiff, deformed foot but certainly not ideal.
- Papa and Myerson (1992) presented the results of 21 patients who underwent a pantalar fusion.
  - 81% reported improvement, but 95% of patients had lasting pain following the procedure.
  - Those patients who underwent a tibiotalocalcaneal fusion (TN joint left free) instead of a traditional pantalar fusion were more mobile following the procedure.
- An alternative solution is a 2-stage reconstruction.
  - Hindfoot realignment and fusion (generally triple arthrodesis) is performed initially.
  - At the 2nd stage, 3-6 months later, total ankle arthroplasty is performed.
- Total ankle arthroplasty offers the potential for some motion but has a relatively high complication rate, especially in the foot with severe preexisting deformity.

Some Causes of Acquired Flatfoot

Posterior tibial tendon (PTT) dysfunction: Most common cause

Achilles tendon or gastrocnemius contracture: May cause secondary PTT dysfunction

Inflammatory arthritis: Can cause subluxation of hindfoot joints &/or PTT tendonitis

Calcaneus or cuboid fracture malunion

Peroneal muscle spasm: In neuromuscular disease

Neuropathic deformity: Can cause severe deformity

Coronal plane angulation in knee, tibia, or ankle: Drives foot into valgus, but foot deformity is secondary

Posterior Tibial Tendon in Gait Cycle

After heel contact, posterior tibial tendon (PTT) serves as shock

In midstance, PTT initiates inversion of hindfoot; this hindfoot inversion forces axes of calcaneocuboid and talonavicular joints to become nonparallel, thus locking these joints and rendering foot rigid for push-off

In propulsive phase, PTT initiates hindfoot inversion; Achilles tendon vector shifts medial to subtalar axis of rotation, which secures hindfoot inversion and transverse tarsal joint position; this optimizes lift and forward propulsion, and PTT accelerates and assists heel lift

Stages of Flatfoot and Clinical Findings

	Stage 1	Stage 2	Stage 3	Stage 4
PTT disease	Tendinosis	Elongated, functionally incompetent	Elongated, functionally incompetent	Elongated, functionally incompetent
Deformity	Normal	Flexible pes planovalgus deformity	Severe and rigid	Similar to stage 3 but includes valgus
Pain location	Along PTT	Medial ± lateral	Medial + lateral	Medial ± lateral
Too many toes sign	Absent	Positive	Positive	Positive
Heel rise testing	Normal	Heel will not invert	Unable to perform	Unable to perform
Radiographs	Normal; MR is positive for PTT tenosynovitis	Increased lateral talocalcaneal angle, decreased calcaneal pitch, and lateral peritalar subluxation	Peritalar subluxation, plantar flexed talus, and degenerative changes in subtalar and transverse tarsal joints; lateral impingement may cause fibular stress fracture	Stage 3 findings and plantar flexed valgus talus as well as tibiotalar degenerative arthritis

Physical Examination

(1) Visualize both legs from knee down

It is important to assess overall limb alignment, not just alignment of foot

(2) Observe heel alignment with patient standing with feet parallel, shoulder width apart

Look for heel valgus and forefoot abduction compared with contralateral foot

(3) Inspect and palpate course of posterior tibial tendon (PTT) for tenosynovitis

Also palpate plantar fascia, deltoid ligament, spring ligament, peroneal tendons, and lateral hindfoot

(4) Look for inability to perform single heel rise or lack of heel inversion in symptomatic foot

Inability to perform < 10 heel rises is type of stress test and may indicate PTT weakness

(5) Test inversion and eversion muscle power of both feet

Accurate assessment requires stabilizing leg with 1 hand in order to eliminate any hip abduction or adduction

(6) Examine gastroc-soleus complex for contracture with subtalar joint in reduced position

Reducing subtalar joint allows examiner to appreciate degree of forefoot varus and rigidity of deformity

(7) Evaluate subtalar motion

In early stages, hindfoot will be supple and easily reduce

In stages 3 and 4, this maneuver may be painful if secondary subtalar arthrosis exists or impossible in rigid deformity

Treatment of Adult Acquired Flatfoot by Stage of Disease

Stage	Findings	Treatment
1	No deformity; pain and swelling	Casting, arch support, PTT debridement
2	Flexible deformity; "too many toes" sign	Bracing: Arch support, AFO, UCBL; PPT augmentation; medial/lateral column fusions and osteotomies
3	Rigid deformity	Bracing: AFO, UCBL; fusions (selective or triple)
4	Rigid deformity; ankle arthritis	Bracing: Solid AFO; salvage fusion (pantalar or tibiotalocalcaneal)

PPT = posterior tibial tendon; AFO = ankle/foot orthosis; UCBL = University of California Biomechanics Laboratory orthosis.

- The foot deformity must be completely restored to minimize the valgus force across the ankle.
  - Even so, complete incompetence of the deltoid may be a problem to total ankle arthroplasty, which normally relies on a tensioned deltoid ligament to prevent tilting of the talar component.
- Hindfoot realignment and fusion, combined with total ankle arthroplasty, offers a chance for better function.

Other Procedures for Other Flatfeet

- The patient with deformity from a Lisfranc joint malunion is best treated with multiple joint midfoot realignment.
  - The 1st, 2nd, and 3rd TMT joints are fused, while the 4th and 5th are generally left mobile, even in the presence of arthritis.
  - Achilles (or gastrocnemius) lengthening is usually required.
- A calcaneal malunion is addressed by tuberosity osteotomy with subtalar fusion and lateral wall decompression.
  - The exact procedure depends on the individual anatomy and will vary.
- For the patient with advanced Charcot deformity, open reduction and internal fixation with arthrodesis is necessary.
  - Bone resection to reduce dislocations may be necessary.
- A surgeon will occasionally meet a patient with a congenitally severe flatfoot, symmetric on both feet.
  - These feet do not have a coalition and could be considered a form of dysplasia.
  - Although lateral column lengthening is often employed in treating these patients, results are mostly anecdotal.
- Long-term outcome studies for most of the modern flatfoot surgeries are not available.

SELECTED REFERENCES

1. Myerson MS et al: Treatment of stage II posterior tibial tendon deficiency with flexor digitorum longus tendon transfer and calcaneal osteotomy. Foot Ankle Int. 25(7):445-50, 2004
2. Malicky ES et al: Talocalcaneal and subfibular impingement in symptomatic flatfoot in adults. J Bone Joint Surg Am. 84-A(11):2005-9, 2002
3. Mann RA: Posterior tibial tendon dysfunction. Treatment by flexor digitorum longus transfer. Foot Ankle Clin. 6(1):77-87, vi, 2001
4. Ananthakrisnan D et al: Subluxation of the talocalcaneal joint in adults who have symptomatic flatfoot. J Bone Joint Surg Am. 81(8):1147-54, 1999
5. Chi TD et al: The lateral column lengthening and medial column stabilization procedures. Clin Orthop Relat Res. 81-90, 1999
6. Saltzman CL et al: Triple arthrodesis: twenty-five and forty-four-year average follow-up of the same patients. J Bone Joint Surg Am. 81(10):1391-402, 1999
7. Toolan BC et al: Complex reconstruction for the treatment of dorsolateral peritalar subluxation of the foot. Early results after distraction arthrodesis of the calcaneocuboid joint in conjunction with stabilization of, and transfer of the flexor digitorum longus tendon to, the midfoot to treat acquired pes planovalgus in adults. J Bone Joint Surg Am. 81(11):1545-60, 1999
8. Sharkey NA et al: Biomechanical consequences of plantar fascial release or rupture during gait: part I–disruptions in longitudinal arch conformation. Foot Ankle Int. 19(12):812-20, 1998
9. Chao W et al: Nonoperative management of posterior tibial tendon dysfunction. Foot Ankle Int. 17(12):736-41, 1996
10. Hintermann B: [Dysfunction of the posterior tibial muscle due to tendon insufficiency.] Orthopade. 24(3):193-9, 1995
11. Teasdall RD et al: Surgical treatment of stage I posterior tibial tendon dysfunction. Foot Ankle Int. 15(12):646-8, 1994
12. Huang CK et al: Biomechanical evaluation of longitudinal arch stability. Foot Ankle. 14(6):353-7, 1993
13. Sangeorzan BJ et al: Effect of calcaneal lengthening on relationships among the hindfoot, midfoot, and forefoot. Foot Ankle. 14(3):136-41, 1993
14. Papa JA et al: Pantalar and tibiotalocalcaneal arthrodesis for post-traumatic osteoarthrosis of the ankle and hindfoot. J Bone Joint Surg Am. 74(7):1042-9, 1992
15. Kannus P et al: Histopathological changes preceding spontaneous rupture of a tendon. A controlled study of 891 patients. J Bone Joint Surg Am. 73(10):1507-25, 1991
16. Johnson KA et al: Tibialis posterior tendon dysfunction. Clin Orthop Relat Res. 196-206, 1989

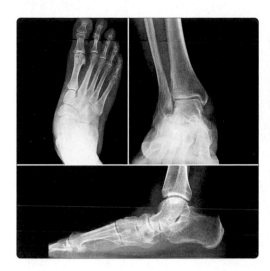

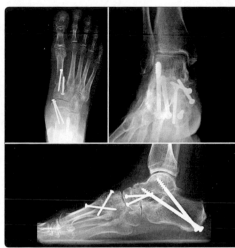

(Left) *A 57-year-old man with a severe deformity and medial and lateral pain, who has failed orthotic management, is shown.* (Right) *The patient underwent fusion of the talonavicular and subtalar joints to restore hindfoot alignment. Although a triple arthrodesis usually includes the calcaneocuboid joint, that joint was not included in this fusion because it was not necessary. Residual forefoot supination required realignment and fusion of the 1st tarsometatarsal joint. He achieved excellent alignment with this "triple" arthrodesis.*

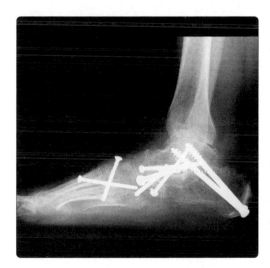

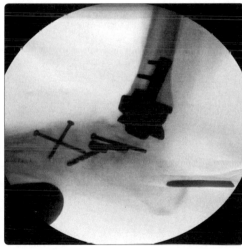

(Left) *Patient with rheumatoid arthritis and pantalar arthritis from advanced valgus deformity of the hindfoot and ankle is shown [treated with hindfoot realignment and arthrodesis of the subtalar, talonavicular, calcaneocuboid, and metatarsocuneiform joints (quadruple arthrodesis)]. Although hindfoot alignment was restored, there is now tibiotalar arthritis.* (Right) *Subsequent total ankle arthroplasty is shown. In the OR, good alignment was achieved, and a wide-based talar component was used to minimize late subsidence.*

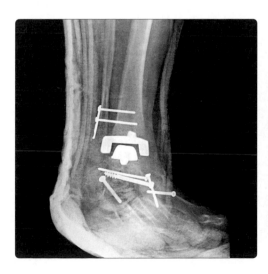

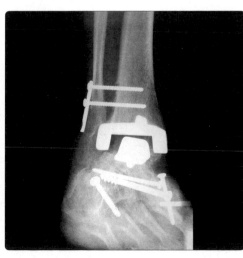

(Left) *The mortise view shows good early alignment.* (Right) *At 5 months postoperatively, the talar component is tilting into the valgus and has subsided into the talus. The patient developed severe lateral ankle impingement pain and requested revision surgery.*

(Left) *At surgery, the posterior tibial tendon is seen to be covered with inflammatory tissue (synovitis).* (Right) *With resection of the synovium, a longitudinal tear is seen* ➡.

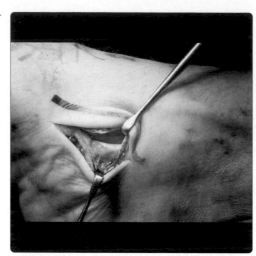
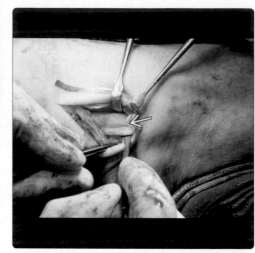

(Left) *A 62-year-old woman with a symptomatic flatfoot deformity failed nonoperative management.* (Right) *Patient was treated with Achilles lengthening, flexor digitorum longus to posterior tibial tendon transfer, medial column realignment and fusions (naviculocuneiform and tarsometatarsal), and medial sliding calcaneal osteotomy. On the anteroposterior view, note the improvement in talonavicular coverage. On the lateral, arch height and talometatarsal angle are improved.*

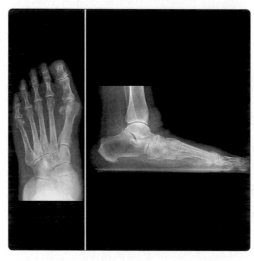
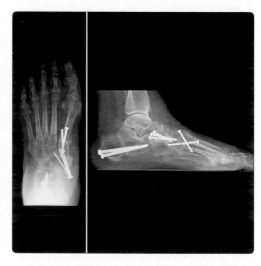

(Left) *A 55-year-old woman with a painful deformity over her lateral foot and posterior tibial tendon, severe hindfoot valgus, forefoot abduction, and arch collapse is shown.* (Right) *Patient was treated with gastrocnemius lengthening, posterior tibial tendon augmentation with flexor digitorum longus, 1st tarsometatarsal realignment and arthrodesis, and lateral column lengthening (through the anterior process of the calcaneus). She has substantial correction at 1 year post reconstruction.*

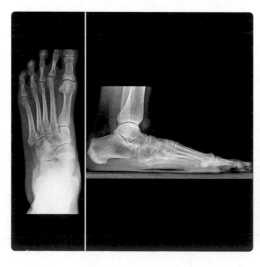
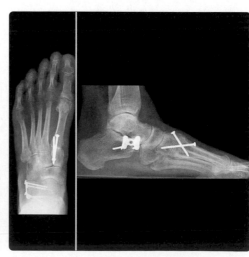

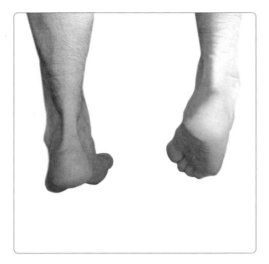

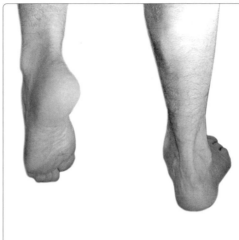

(Left) *Single heel rise testing is shown. The elevation of the foot to the toes requires a functional posterior tibial tendon. When competent, the heel will invert and assume a varus orientation.* **(Right)** *Posterior tibial tendon dysfunction is confirmed by the inability to complete a single heel rise test or the inability for the heel to shift into a varus position. In this patient, attempted heel rise gets the heel only slightly off the ground, but the heel remains in valgus.*

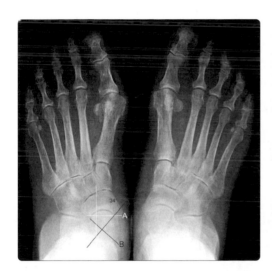

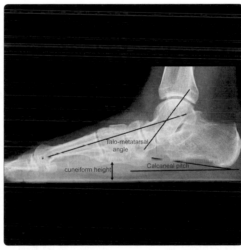

(Left) *The talonavicular coverage angle is a measure of forefoot abduction. Line A connects the articular surfaces of the navicular; line B connects the articular surfaces of the talus. Perpendicular lines are drawn to A and B through the center of the articular surface. It measures 34° in this example.* **(Right)** *A talo 1st metatarsal angle > 4° signifies pes planus (32° in this patient). The calcaneal pitch is normally 17-32° (12° in this patient). Loss of medial cuneiform-floor height is indicative of loss of arch height.*

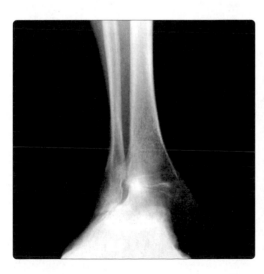

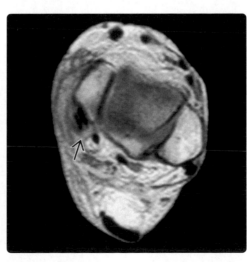

(Left) *Anteroposterior ankle is shown. An anteroposterior view of the ankle is needed to assess overall talar alignment and to evaluate for talar tilt and tibiotalar degeneration in advanced cases.* **(Right)** *MR may demonstrate intrasubstance tears within the tendon and fluid within the sheath ➡. Increased diameter may also be suggestive of tendinosis.*

KEY FACTS

- The foot is a complex "machine" consisting of many bones and joints kept in a fine balance by many extrinsic (leg) and intrinsic (foot) muscles.
- Any disruption of the precise muscle balance leads to progressive deformity of the involved joints.
- If the imbalance arises prior to skeletal maturity, bone growth will be abnormal, and bones and joints will become dysplastic.
  - The shape of the bones begins with a fixed plan but is modified during childhood based on the forces (muscular and weight bearing) on them over time.
- If the imbalance arises after skeletal maturity, bones will have an essentially normal shape, and deformity will be through the joints.
- With time, the joints can erode in response to deformity, leading to secondary "dysplasia" of the bones.
- At the level of the ankle and hindfoot, there are several muscles pairs that balance each other.

- The tibialis anterior dorsiflexes the 1st ray, while the peroneus longus plantar flexes it.
- The posterior tibial muscle inverts the hindfoot, while the peroneus brevis everts.
- The tibialis anterior and the extensor digitorum and hallucis longus all work in opposition to the triceps surae.
  - The triceps surae is by far the strongest of the leg and foot muscles.
- In the forefoot, balance between intrinsic and extrinsic flexors and extensors keeps the toes straight at the metatarsophalangeal and interphalangeal joints.
- Even when a muscle is weak, if there is no muscle to oppose it, then the weak muscle will eventually cause a deformity.
- Although muscle imbalance theoretically could lead to any imaginable foot deformity, neuromuscular deformities are generally some form of cavus.
- The neuromuscular cavus foot appears with a high arch, variable amounts of hindfoot varus, plantar flexion of the 1st ray or entire midfoot, and clawing of the toes.

(Left) *Photographs of the left foot of a patient with severe cavovarus deformity is shown. The ankle and hindfoot are in varus.* **(Right)** *Severe clawing (extension at metatarsophalangeal joint and flexion at interphalangeal joints) of the toes is evident. The toe deformity has led to injury to the 5th toenail from improper shoe fit.*

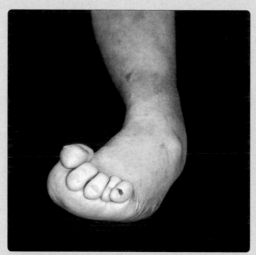 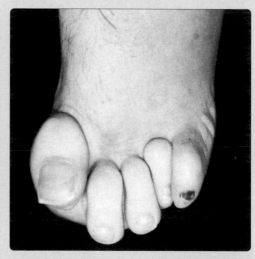

(Left) *Patient with a compartment syndrome developed intrinsic muscle atrophy and fixed clawing of the hallux and lesser toes.* **(Right)** *Lateral view of a patient's foot following a missed compartment syndrome is shown. Again note the intrinsic muscle atrophy and clawing of the hallux and lesser toes.*

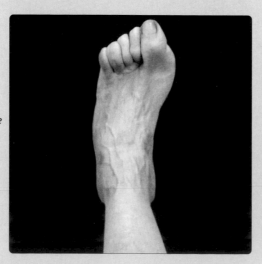 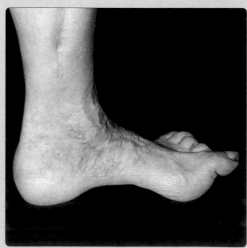

NEUROMUSCULAR DEFORMITY

- Upper motor neuron lesions, such as a stroke or cerebral palsy, lead to weakness with hyperreflexia and spasticity.
- Lower motor neuron lesions, such as poliomyelitis or traumatic nerve injury, lead to hyporeflexia.
- Muscle lesions (myopathy or untreated compartment syndrome) lead to weakness and hyporeflexia.

Symptoms From Neuromuscular Cavus Foot

- Neuromuscular imbalance leads to variably progressive deformity in the foot.
- The neuromuscular cavus foot appears with a high arch, variable amounts of hindfoot varus, plantar flexion of the 1st ray or entire midfoot, and clawing of the toes.
- Cavus or cavovarus deformity alters the distribution of pressure under the foot.
  - Focusing weight-bearing forces on smaller areas leads to higher pressures.
  - The cavus foot will have higher pressures under the heel and metatarsal heads.
- Patients may complain of pain &/or callusing in these high-pressure spots.
- If the hindfoot is in varus, then pressure may be focused on the 5th metatarsal.
  - This can cause pain and callusing and, in extreme cases, 5th metatarsal stress fractures.
- The high arch may make shoe fitting problematic.
- Shoe-fitting problems may also arise if clawing of the toes occurs with irritation over the dorsum of the interphalangeal joints.
- Clawing of the toes pulls the metatarsal fat pad distally.
  - It also uncovers the metatarsal heads and can lead to metatarsalgia.
- A varus hindfoot predisposes to ankle sprains, which is even more of a problem when the peroneus brevis is weak.
- Weakness may cause the patient to feel clumsy and fall.
- Severe deformity prevents the foot from being plantigrade.
  - In severe cases, the patient will become nonambulatory.
- If sensory neuropathy occurs, pressure sores may develop over high-pressure areas.
- Although many neuromuscular feet will have the same general cavus shape, the specific components of the cavus will vary with the cause of the imbalance.

EVALUATION OF NEUROMUSCULAR PATIENT

History and Physical Exam

- A full history and physical is appropriate, but there are several areas that should be explored more thoroughly.
- Family history should look for history of similar disease, because many neuromuscular diseases are inherited.
- Environmental exposures should be discussed; ask about residency in an area where polio might be present.
- On examination, the overall shape and symmetry of both feet are assessed.
  - Asymmetry is more common with acquired disorders (and some spinal cord abnormalities).
  - Systemic diseases tend to create symmetric deformity.
- The position of the hindfoot is assessed.
  - While the patient is standing, the observer notes the position of the heel from behind.

- In the normal foot, the heel rests in slight valgus (just lateral to the long axis of the tibia).
  - Most neuromuscular deformities pull the heel into varus.
- If the heel is seen medial to the foot while looking at the patient from the front (the "peek-a-boo" heel), then it is in varus.
- The position of the forefoot can be assessed while the patient is seated with the legs hanging over the edge of the table.
  - With the heel straight, the metatarsal heads should be even.
  - A plantar flexed 1st ray is commonly seen with neuromuscular cavus.
- The Coleman block test is an important assessment of hindfoot flexibility when the hindfoot is in varus.
  - With the patient standing with the heel and lateral metatarsal heads on a block, the 1st metatarsal is allowed to drop medial to the block.
  - If the hindfoot is flexible, the 1st metatarsal will drop lower than the foot, and the heel will fall into slight valgus (forefoot-driven hindfoot varus).
  - If the hindfoot is rigid, the 1st metatarsal will not drop, and the heel will remain in varus.
- The alignment of the toes should be assessed, looking for the characteristic clawing [extension at metatarsophalangeal (MTP) and flexion at interphalangeal joints].
- The flexibility of the hindfoot, ankle, and toes must be assessed initially and with time.
  - Many diseases begin with a flexible deformity but become more rigid over time.
- The "quality" of the soft tissues should be assessed.
  - With longstanding deformity, the tissues may become contracted on the "concave" side of the deformity.
    - Example: Medial hindfoot in varus deformity
  - In such cases, realignment may put an unacceptable amount of stretch on these tissues.
- A full motor examination is performed, documenting the strength of each muscle group in both legs.
- A full sensory examination is listed either by dermatome or peripheral nerve, depending on the underlying pathology.
- The gait pattern must be observed.
  - A foot drop may be visible during the swing phase.
- Finally, the vascular supply to the foot should be assessed.

Imaging and Other Diagnostic Studies

- Weight-bearing radiographs are an important part of the deformity assessment.
- On the lateral view, calcaneal pitch > 30° is typical of cavus.
- The lateral talometatarsal angle will show the 1st metatarsal to be plantar flexed.
  - The 1st metatarsal may be plantar flexed much more than the other metatarsals in the cavus foot.
- Magnetic resonance (MR) imaging of the foot is rarely needed, but MR of the spine may be appropriate when the cause of deformity is not certain.
  - It might be especially useful in the asymmetric cavus foot when there is a suspicion for spinal cord lesions.
  - Unilateral progressive cavus deformity should prompt an MR to search for intraspinal pathology.

○ Cavus deformity, either unilateral or bilateral, in association with scoliosis should probably also be evaluated with an MR of the spine.

- Electromyographic tests with nerve conduction velocities (EMG/NCV) are helpful in the initial evaluation of the patient to better define the neuromuscular lesion.
  ○ EMG in cases of neuropathy show an increased amplitude and duration of response.
  ○ EMG in patients with myopathy show a decreased amplitude and duration of response with short polyphasic potentials.
  ○ Denervation or anterior horn cell loss demonstrates prolonged polyphasics, positive sharp waves, and fibrillations on EMG.
  ○ Abnormal NCV with prolonged latencies and minimal decrease in velocity suggest axonal degeneration.
- In rare cases, muscle or nerve biopsy may be needed to confirm a diagnosis.

PRINCIPLES OF TREATMENT OF NEUROMUSCULAR CAVUS FOOT

- The underlying disease must be controlled as best as possible, usually in conjunction with a neurologist.
- In cases of spasticity, medication may be helpful.
  ○ Medications include baclofen, diazepam, and dantrolene.
- Specific muscle blocks with botulinum toxin may be helpful.
  ○ This is especially so if only 1 or 2 muscles are involved.
- Once a muscle imbalance in the foot has been identified, the goal is to prevent further deformity.
- Frequent stretching by the patient must be done; otherwise, contracture will inevitably set in.
- Extra-depth shoes and orthotics will help accommodate a high-arched foot; a tall toe box will better fit claw toes.
- Custom accommodative orthotics can reduce peak pressures in the sole of the foot.
- Bracing of the weak or unstable ankle with a custom ankle-foot orthosis (AFO) can permit better ambulation and perhaps prevent further deformity.
- In patients with sensory deficits, Plastazote (or other cushioned) linings are required in the brace with frequent inspection of the skin for ulceration.

Surgery for Neuromuscular Cavus Foot

- Surgical intervention is indicated in certain situations.
- Surgery is appropriate when nonoperative treatment has failed, which most commonly means that the deformity is no longer braceable.
- Surgery is indicated in cases where an obvious muscle imbalance is expected to lead to progressive deformity.
  ○ If the muscle imbalance is corrected early, surgery may require only tendon transfers.
  ○ If surgery is delayed, a later deformity will require fusions &/or osteotomies, making the recovery longer and the final function poorer.
- The basic principle of surgical treatment is to restore muscle balance and osseous alignment.
- Muscle balance is corrected through muscle transfers, lengthenings, &/or releases.
  ○ Lengthenings weaken a muscle.
  ○ Releases (tenotomies) remove the muscle entirely.

○ Muscle transfers remove the deforming force of the muscle and redirect it to another location.
- Muscle transfers can be in phase or out of phase.
  ○ In-phase transfers take a muscle and transfer it into another muscle that normally fires during the same part of the gait cycle.
    – Example: Transfer of extensor digitorum longus to tibialis anterior
  ○ Out-of-phase transfers redirect a muscle to an insertion that is normally antagonistic.
    – Example: Posterior tibial tendon through interosseous membrane to tibialis anterior
  ○ Out-of-phase transfers are less likely to result in strong active motion in an adult.
- Osseous alignment can occasionally be corrected with capsulotomies in cases of mild deformity.
- Plantar fascia release (minimal incision or wide) can be used to "relax" the arch in some cavus feet.
- More severe deformity requires osteotomies or fusions.
- In adult patients with deformity secondary to brain injury, it may be appropriate to wait 18-24 months between injury and surgery to give enough time for any recovery.

Procedures for Clawed Hallux

- Many neuromuscular diseases result in severe clawing of the hallux, which interferes with shoewear.
- When nonoperative procedures have failed, surgical realignment can be helpful.
- A common procedure is to fuse the hallux interphalangeal joint and transfer the extensor hallucis longus to the 1st metatarsal or midfoot.

FOOT DROP

- Many different etiologies may have some degree of foot drop or weakness of the anterior compartment muscles.
  ○ Given how strong the Achilles complex is relative to the other muscles, any weakness of the anterior muscles will quickly lead to foot drop symptoms.
- Initial treatment includes regular stretching of the Achilles to minimize contracture, along with bracing.
  ○ A solid AFO can be lightweight and can have some elasticity to provide propulsion.
- If the patient declines a brace, or if the Achilles develops a fixed contracture, surgery is considered.
- Lengthening of the Achilles tendon will weaken it but will result in better balance between the Achilles tendon and the anterior muscles.
- Tendon transfers can augment dorsiflexion force when the anterior compartment is weak or absent.
  ○ This can be an in-phase or out-of-phase transfer.
- The "bridle" procedure is a complex tendon transfer designed to improve dorsiflexion.
  ○ The posterior tibial tendon is transferred through the interosseous membrane.
  ○ It is connected to the anterior tibial tendon in the anterior compartment.
  ○ The peroneus longus is rerouted into the anterior compartment as well (with its original insertion unchanged) and also connected to the posterior tibial tendon.

o These 2 insertions of the transferred posterior tibial tendon act as a bridle for the forefoot.

PERONEAL NERVE PALSY

- The common peroneal nerve (consisting of contributions from L4 to S1) courses over the posterior head of the fibula and around the lateral neck of the bone.
- This nerve branches into the superficial and deep peroneal nerves in the anterolateral compartment of the leg.
  o The course of the superficial peroneal nerve is variable.
- Injury to the peroneal nerves may occur as an entrapment neuropathy.
- More common, though, is direct or indirect trauma to the nerve with neuropraxia or axonotmesis.
  o The nerve is somewhat tethered at the level of the fibular neck, so any traction on the sciatic nerve can injure the nerve.
  o The tibial nerve is not tethered about the knee and is less vulnerable to injury.
- Peroneal nerve injury can occur during surgery, either from pressure on the nerve from poor positioning while anesthetized or from traction during the procedure.
- Peroneal nerve injury is common in thin, nonambulatory patients and is related to a poorly fitting wheelchair or poor positioning while in bed.
- Inadequate short leg cast padding can injure the nerve.
- Diabetic neuropathy or entrapment neuropathy can lead to peroneal nerve dysfunction.
- Blunt or penetrating trauma can injure the nerve.
  o A common example is a posterior hip dislocation.
- In contrast to other types of nerve palsies, peroneal nerve palsy may demonstrate a greater motor deficit than sensory deficit.

Symptoms of Peroneal Nerve Palsy

- The sensory loss is variable and rarely a problem.
- Motor loss of the anterior compartment results in a foot drop.
  o At the minimum, patients may have a high-stepping gait to avoid tripping over their foot.
  o The foot may slap the floor immediately after heel strike.

Treatment of Peroneal Palsy

- When the ankle remains flexible, these symptoms can be well controlled with an AFO.
  o Patients must stretch the Achilles frequently to prevent contracture.
- If stretching is not performed, an equinus contracture will develop.
  o Patients may partly compensate for this by obtaining an AFO with a heel lift, but this is usually not well tolerated.
- Surgery is indicated if an equinus contracture has developed or if the patient cannot achieve good function with a brace.
  o In some cases, surgery may be helpful for the patient who is not willing to wear a brace.
- The 1st step in surgery is to create an ankle dorsiflexor.
  o In the typical case, no in-phase muscles are available, so the posterior tibial tendon can be transferred through the interosseous membrane to the dorsal midfoot.

o It is probably important to replace the posterior tibial tendon function by transferring the flexor digitorum longus to the remainder of the tibial tendon on the navicular.
  – Many surgeons feel that this step is not necessary.
- Second, weaken the Achilles tendon by lengthening.
- In some patients, the transferred posterior tibial tendon will adapt with time and become an ankle dorsiflexor.
- In most patients, the muscle acts as a tenodesis, meaning it balances the Achilles and keeps the ankle neutral but does not provide much active dorsiflexion strength.

DEFORMITY FROM UNTREATED COMPARTMENT SYNDROME

- Although the standard treatment for acute compartment syndrome of the leg or foot is emergent fasciotomy, there are still many cases when that cannot be done.
- Untreated compartment syndrome leads to muscle necrosis and contracture.

Anterior Compartment

- If only the anterior compartment of the leg is involved, the patient will develop a clinical picture similar to peroneal nerve palsy with foot drop.
- In these cases, stretching and bracing can be successful.
- If surgery is indicated, transfer of the posterior tibial tendon through the interosseous membrane will provide some dorsiflexion.
- Alternately, transfer of the peroneus longus or extensor digitorum longus to the midfoot may provide better function if those muscles are viable.
- In any case, Achilles lengthening is also required.

4 Compartments

- Often, the compartment syndrome involves all 4 compartments of the leg.
  o This leads to contracture of the posterior compartments with severe equinovarus deformity over time.
  o If recognized early, bracing and stretching may prevent late contracture.
- When deformity is minimal, Achilles lengthening and bracing may be effective.
  o There are no transferable viable muscles to regain active motion.
- Once severe deformity has set in, more aggressive surgery is needed.
  o The scarred remnants of the deep posterior muscles must be resected to prevent recurrent contracture.
  o The Achilles must be lengthened or released as well.
- With fixed deformity, hindfoot &/or forefoot realignment and arthrodesis are necessary.
- In many cases, the posterior tibial nerve, vessels, and overlying skin have contracted so that dorsiflexion of the ankle is not possible, even after complete release of muscles and capsules.
  o Talectomy with tibiocalcaneal fusion is a viable option.
  o Alternatively, capsulotomies and gradual stretching with an external fixator (Ilizarov device) may be successful.

Foot Compartments

- Untreated compartment syndrome of the foot may result in claw toe deformities.

- When shoe modifications (tall toe box) cannot manage the deformity, surgical correction can be undertaken.
- Correction should include flexor tenotomy or transfer to the extensor (intrinsicplasty).
- Proximal interphalangeal arthroplasty or arthrodesis is usually necessary as well.
- Extensor lengthenings may be needed for correction of MTP dorsiflexion.

CHARCOT-MARIE-TOOTH DISEASE (HEREDITARY SENSORY MOTOR NEUROPATHY)

- Charcot-Marie-Tooth (CMT) is the most common inherited neurologic disorder, affecting ~ 15 per 100,000 people.
  - The disease was described in the 19th century by Charcot and Marie in France and independently by Tooth in England.
- CMT is a group of disorders better referred to as hereditary motor and sensory neuropathy; it affects both sensory and motor peripheral nerves.
- The disorder is inherited with autosomal dominant, autosomal recessive, and X-linked inheritance patterns.
  - It is currently subdivided into types 1A, 1B, 2, and X based on the particular genetic defect involved.
  - There are at least 17 genetic variants of the disease and probably many more.
  - In some families, all the children develop the condition, and in others, none inherit it.
  - To determine the pattern of inheritance, each CMT patient should consult a genetic counsellor.
- CMT is slowly but variably progressive and usually does not result in death.
  - Most patients have normal life expectancy with full and productive lives.
- The upper extremities can be involved with distal motor weakness.
- As expected with a peripheral neuropathy, deep tendon reflexes are decreased.
- CMT often affects the foot in very consistent ways.
  - 94% of patients have foot involvement.
  - There is characteristic weakness of the tibialis anterior and peroneus brevis.
- With tibialis anterior weakness, the peroneus longus is unopposed, resulting in plantar flexion of the 1st ray.
  - This leads to a high arch (cavus).
- A weak peroneus brevis cannot oppose the posterior tibialis.
  - This leads to hindfoot varus.
- Thus, a cavovarus foot will result.
- In some cases, an equinus deformity sets in, perhaps even prior to other deformities, because of imbalance between the tibialis anterior and the Achilles.
- Clawing of the toes may appear due to muscle imbalance in the toes as well as "overactivity" of the long toe extensors (as they are substitutes for the tibialis anterior).
- Sensory loss is less severe, but patients can demonstrate loss of 2-point discrimination and vibratory sense.

Foot Symptoms in Charcot-Marie-Tooth Disease

- Weakness of the tibialis anterior can lead to a foot drop.
  - Patients may feel clumsy or trip while running.

- Patients may walk with a steppage gait or a foot slap.
- Claw toes can interfere with normal shoewear.
- Lack of hindfoot eversion from the peroneus brevis can lead to ankle sprains and fractures.

Diagnosis of Charcot-Marie-Tooth Disease

- Family history is important.
- Nerve conduction tests show characteristics of peripheral neuropathy.
- Nerve biopsy may be helpful, especially in CMT type 1, where characteristic swelling is seen.
- Some subtypes of CMT are detectable with blood tests.

Treatment of Charcot-Marie-Tooth Disease Foot Deformity

- Physical therapy is focused on strengthening and stretching.
- Bracing with an AFO can be effective.
  - A brace can reduce ankle sprains and reduce the energy requirement for gait.
- Extra-depth shoes with a custom insert can be used as well as shoes with a tall toe box for toe deformities.
- Surgery should be considered when the deformity is not braceable (the foot is not plantigrade).
- Surgery should also be considered early on if the disease is progressing despite bracing and stretching.
  - Early surgery (tendon transfers) can be easier to recover from and leads to a better functional outcome than late surgery (fusions).
- In the earliest stages, prior to any fixed deformity, Achilles lengthening is performed.
- A tendon transfer is performed to augment the weak anterior tibial muscle.
  - If the long toe extensors are strong, they are transferred to the dorsolateral midfoot.
  - If the extensor digitorum longus is weak, the tibialis posterior is transferred through the interosseous membrane to the dorsal midfoot.
- Peroneus longus is transferred to the peroneus brevis.
- These transfers remove the deforming forces and restore some dorsiflexion and eversion.
- Perhaps the earliest osseous deformity in CMT is plantar flexion of the 1st ray.
  - If this has developed, the tendon transfers can be combined with dorsiflexion osteotomy of the 1st metatarsal or dorsiflexion arthrodesis of the 1st metatarsocuneiform joint.
- Lateral sliding calcaneal tuberosity osteotomy can be added if there is some heel varus.
- Once fixed hindfoot varus has set in, these motion-sparing procedures cannot be used.
  - In these cases of advanced osseous deformity, triple joint realignment and arthrodesis are necessary.
  - If the ankle has begun to tilt into varus, ankle arthrodesis may be necessary as well.
  - Major hindfoot fusions heal more slowly than tendon transfers and result in less optimal functional outcomes.

POLIOMYELITIS

- Although polio is almost eradicated, it still appears in some less developed areas.

Some Etiologies of Cavus Foot

Neuromuscular	Congenital	Traumatic	Idiopathic
Myopathy: Muscular dystrophy	Clubfoot residual deformity	Sequela of compartment syndrome	Variant of normal
Peripheral neuropathy: Charcot-Marie-Tooth disease, polyneuritis	Arthrogryposis	Crush injury	
Spinal cord/anterior horn cell disease: Poliomyelitis, spinal dysraphism, diastematomyelia, syringomyelia, spinal cord tumor, spinal muscular atrophy		Severe burn	
Central nervous disease: Friedrich ataxia, Roussy-Levy syndrome, cerebral palsy		Malunion of fracture	

Charcot-Marie-Tooth Disease Variants

Variant	Description
Type 1	Autosomal dominant with nerve biopsy revealing "onion" hypertrophy
Types 1A and 1B	Phenotypically similar but with different genetic defects
Type 2	Autosomal recessive, presents during adolescence
X-linked	Presents during childhood

- The end result of polio virus infection is muscle weakness.
- The particular pattern of involved muscles varies between extremities and between patients, but certain characteristic patterns are seen.
- In the foot, it is common to see longstanding weakness of the Achilles.
  - Absence of Achilles function leads to a calcaneus deformity.
    - The foot is relatively dorsiflexed with weight-bearing pressure focused on the heel pad.
  - Patients may complain of pain under the heel, sometimes with thick callusing.
- Custom insoles or AFO braces can be used to better distribute forces.
- When bracing fails to provide relief, surgery to restore strength in the Achilles can be undertaken.
- Depending on the strength of surrounding muscles, transfer of the flexor hallucis longus to the calcaneal tuberosity may be helpful.
- Because polio is often contracted during childhood, the foot may have developed in the absence of Achilles strength.
  - By maturity, the calcaneal pitch will be very high with marked plantar flexion of the forefoot (very high arch).
  - In such cases, consideration can be given to performing a dorsiflexion osteotomy of the midfoot or calcaneal tuberosity osteotomy.

SURGICAL PROCEDURES FOR SEVERE DYSPLASTIC CAVUS FOOT

- When the neuromuscular imbalance is severe and longstanding (especially when acquired during growth), the shape of the bones may not be normal.
  - Joint realignment and arthrodesis may not restore a normal shape to the foot.
  - In these more unusual cases, osteotomy(ies) ± fusion are needed.

- For severe heel varus, a lateral closing-wedge (Dwyer) osteotomy will help.
  - A lateral sliding calcaneal osteotomy may preserve Achilles strength better and is technically easier to perform.
- With a very high calcaneal pitch, a dorsal sliding calcaneal tuberosity osteotomy will decrease pitch.
- For severe equinovarus, Lambrinudi triple arthrodesis is indicated.
  - In this procedure, wedges of bone are removed from the joints to allow better positioning during fusion.
- For severe cavus deformity, dorsal closing-wedge osteotomies across all metatarsals, or across the cuboid and cuneiforms, will decrease forefoot plantar flexion.
- In many of these cases, extensive plantar fascia release will be necessary because the fascia is contracted in the severe cavus foot.

SUMMARY OF CAVUS FOOT SURGERY

- Begin with muscle balancing: Transfers, releases, lengthenings.
- Capsulotomies and plantar fascia release may be necessary in some feet.
- Moderate cavus deformity will benefit from 1st metatarsal dorsiflexion osteotomy &/or lateral sliding calcaneal osteotomy.
- Ankle &/or hindfoot realignment and arthrodesis may be necessary in the most severe cases.

SELECTED REFERENCES

1. Ledoux WR et al: Biomechanical differences among pes cavus, neutrally aligned, and pes planus feet in subjects with diabetes. Foot Ankle Int. 24(11):845-50, 2003
2. Giannini S et al: Surgical treatment of adult idiopathic cavus foot with plantar fasciotomy, naviculocuneiform arthrodesis, and cuboid osteotomy. A review of thirty-nine cases. J Bone Joint Surg Am. 84-A Suppl 2:62-9, 2002
3. Sammarco GJ et al: Cavovarus foot treated with combined calcaneus and metatarsal osteotomies. Foot Ankle Int. 22(1):19-30, 2001

(Left) *The hindfoot deformities of the patient with a missed compartment syndrome were corrected with triple arthrodesis combined with an extensor digitorum longus transfer.* **(Right)** *The forefoot deformities were corrected with a Jones procedure (fusion of the hallux interphalangeal joint with extensor hallucis longus transfer).*

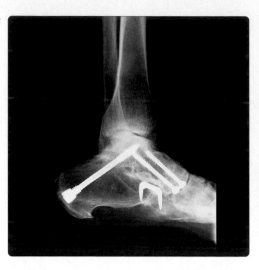
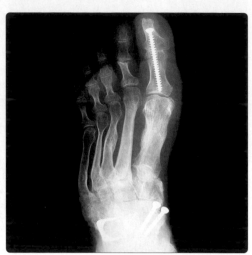

(Left) *Illustration of the 1st metatarsal closing-wedge osteotomy is shown. A dorsally based wedge of bone is removed, ~ 1 cm distal to metatarsocuneiform joint ⊡.* **(Right)** *Postoperative illustration demonstrates dorsiflexed 1st metatarsal after proximal osteotomy. Plantar fascia release may be necessary.*

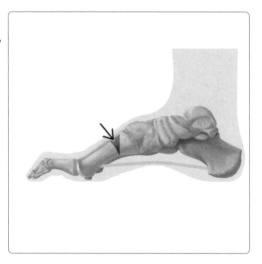
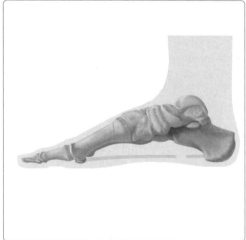

(Left) *Photograph of a patient with Charcot-Marie-Tooth disease with an equinus contracture, plantar flexion of the 1st ray, and claw toe deformities is shown.* **(Right)** *Lateral radiograph shows the cavus deformity.*

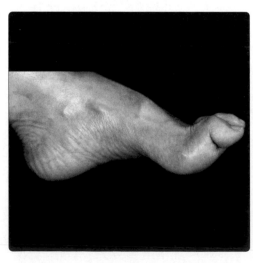
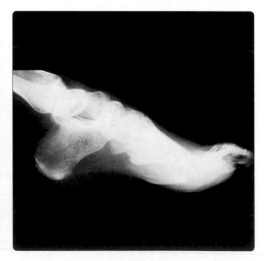

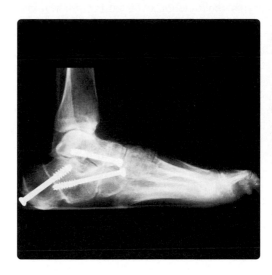
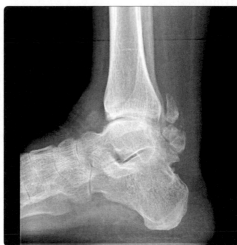

(Left) *Postoperative radiograph demonstrates the optimal correction after plantar fascia release, dorsal displacement of the calcaneus, and arthrodesis.* **(Right)** *This woman had polio as a child. Note the increased calcaneal pitch, characteristic of patients with longstanding Achilles weakness. Because of the relative weakness of the Achilles, she bears most of her weight on the heel. She has suffered from plantar heel pain for years with thick callusing of the skin. A custom orthosis has been only mildly helpful.*

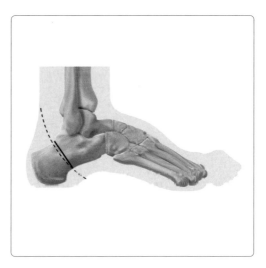
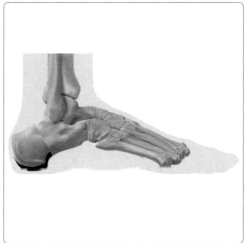

(Left) *Calcaneal slide osteotomy is shown. Neuromuscular disease can lead to abnormally high calcaneal pitch.* **(Right)** *Dorsal calcaneus displacement is shown. Calcaneal tuberosity is moved dorsally to lower the longitudinal arch.*

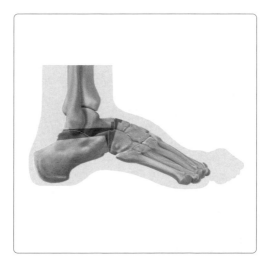
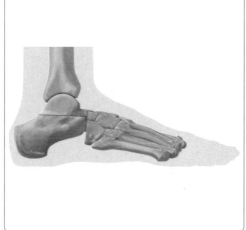

(Left) *Triple arthrodesis to correct severe cavovarus deformity may require resection of wedges of bone. Lateral closing in the subtalar joint is combined with mortising the navicular into the head of the talus. A lateral wedge is removed from the calcaneocuboid joint to correct forefoot adduction.* **(Right)** *Position of foot postoperatively is shown. Height reduction of longitudinal arch and forefoot abduction are the goals of this procedure.*

KEY FACTS

- Diabetes mellitus is a multisystem disease resulting from defects in insulin secretion &/or resistance to insulin action, which culminates in systemic hyperglycemia, which can have negative effects, especially when chronically elevated.
  - The total prevalence of diabetes in the USA was 30.3 million people (9.4% of the population) in 2015, an increase of 50% since 2002. It is estimated that ~ 30% of all diabetics are undiagnosed.
- The socioeconomic costs (direct and indirect) of diabetes were ~ $245 billion in 2012, a number that has almost doubled since 2002. An estimated 50% of the total costs for a diabetic hospital admission are due to diabetic foot complications.

- Diabetic foot complications are the most common cause of atraumatic lower extremity amputations and are the leading cause of hospitalization among diabetics in the USA. Foot complications have a negative impact on the health-related quality of life of a diabetic patient, with fear of ulceration, recurrent infection, and potential lifelong disability.
- There is currently no cure for diabetes, and treatment is based on preventing and managing the complications, requiring a multidisciplinary team approach and patient compliance.

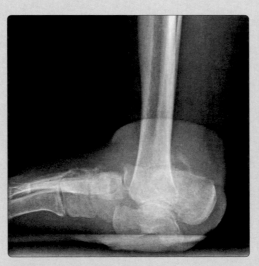
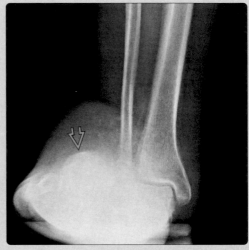

(Left) *A 64-year-old male patient with severe hindfoot Charcot and complete disassociation of the talus from the rest of the foot is shown. He was literally walking on the underside of his talus with skin breakdown in that area.* **(Right)** *The patient is essentially weight bearing on the talus directly and had a medial wound in that area. The superior surface of the calcaneus ⊟ is seen superior to the level of the ankle mortise.*

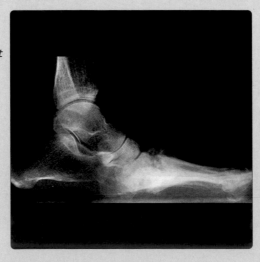
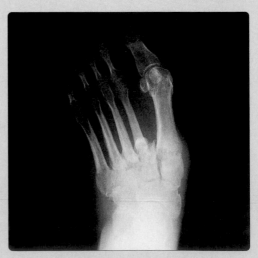

(Left) *Severe Charcot midfoot with complete collapse of the arch is shown. The plantar prominence is readily apparent here; the risk for a plantar wound is significant. An equinus contracture often plays a large role in this midfoot "break."* **(Right)** *The same patient shows essentially a dorsolateral subluxation midfoot injury in which the midfoot was the inflection point with the foot dorsiflexing and everting through the midfoot.*

DIABETIC VASCULAR DISEASE

Background

- Peripheral arterial occlusive disease is 4x more prevalent in diabetics than in nondiabetics. It tends to occur at an earlier age in diabetics, and the risk of disease increases with the duration of diabetes.
- The calcification of atherosclerotic plaques in arteries of diabetic patients is more diffuse and occurs within the tunica media of the arteries, producing a lead pipe appearance on plain radiographs (as opposed to plaques in nondiabetic patients, which are patchy and occur in the tunica intima).
- The arterial occlusion of the proximal large vessels is similar to that in nondiabetics; however, the macrovascular disease is more diffuse in diabetics distal to the popliteal trifurcation. Distal vascular procedures have proven to be helpful in diabetic patients.
- Microvascular complications of diabetes (neuropathy, retinopathy, and nephropathy) and macrovascular complications (peripheral vascular disease, coronary artery disease, hypertension, hyperlipidemia, and cerebrovascular disease) together contribute to diabetic foot problems.

Evaluation

- A detailed history should be obtained, including a history of smoking, hypertension, and hyperlipidemia. Patients with advanced disease will complain of claudication.
- Pain due to vascular claudication is usually relieved with rest. However, ischemic foot pain can also occur at rest.
- On physical examination, absent popliteal or posterior tibial pulses, thin or shiny skin, absence of hair on the foot or leg, thickened nails, and dependent rubor are all signs of vascular insufficiency.
- Any patient with signs of advanced vascular disease (such as a history of claudication, nonhealing ulcers, or nonpalpable pulses) should be evaluated by a vascular specialist.

Diagnostic Tests

- Noninvasive vascular tests include the ankle-brachial index (ABI) using Doppler ultrasound pressures, transcutaneous oxygen (TcpO2) measurement (oximetry), the absolute toe systolic pressure (plethysmography), Doppler waveform analysis, and segmental Doppler limb pressures and pulse volume recordings.
- Arterial pressure readings can be falsely elevated due to rigid arterial calcification in diabetics, which may artificially raise the ABI to > 1.00. Despite that, an ABI of < 0.80 is generally considered abnormal and < 0.45 in a diabetic patient is suggestive of limb-threatening ischemia.
- Absolute toe pressures may be more predictive of distal wound healing with toe systolic pressure < 45 mm Hg indicating poor wound-healing potential and < 30 mm Hg indicating critical limb ischemia.
- Transcutaneous oxygen measurement < 20-30 mm Hg represents poor wound-healing potential.
- When assessing Doppler waveform recordings, a triphasic waveform is normal. Biphasic (loss of reverse flow in early diastole) and monophasic waveforms suggest advanced occlusive disease. If lower extremity ischemia is strongly suspected, arteriography, magnetic resonance angiography, or computed tomography angiography should be performed to assess the vascular flow.

DIABETIC NEUROPATHY

Background

- Peripheral neuropathy is the most common cause of diabetic foot complications. The presence of neuropathy (diabetic or otherwise) greatly increases the risk of complications from any surgery.
- Diabetic neuropathy can involve the sensory, motor, and autonomic pathways.
- Diabetic neuropathy has been estimated to occur in 58% of patients with longstanding disease, although 1 study noted that close to 80% of diabetic patients having surgery had some degree of neuropathy.

Sensory Neuropathy

- The earliest finding in diabetic neuropathy is vibratory and proprioceptive loss. Signs and symptoms are variable but include paresthesias, burning sensations, hyperpathia, and dysesthesias and usually reveal a symmetric sensory loss in a "stocking-glove" distribution.
- Due to the loss of protective (pain) sensation, foot ulceration generally occurs by repetitive trauma in areas of high mechanical pressure.
- The 5.07 (10-g monofilament) Semmes-Weinstein monofilament (SWM) test of 7-10 plantar foot sites is the recommended screening test for a patient at risk for ulcer formation due to loss of protective sensation. However, up to 10% of patients who pass the SWM test may still develop skin breakdown.
- A simplified screening test has been described. If a patient cannot sense the touch of a 4.5-g/4.65 SWM when it is pressed under the 1st metatarsal head with just enough pressure to bend the filament, the patient should be considered at risk for ulceration.

Autonomic Neuropathy

- Denervation of the eccrine and apocrine glands and arteries leads to abnormal thermoregulation and interference with the normal hyperemic response to infection.
- There is decreased sweating and loss of skin temperature regulation, causing dry, cracked skin and fissure formation, which predispose to infection by allowing a portal for bacterial entry.
- Autonomic neuropathy can also cause orthostatic hypotension; cardiovascular, urinary, and gastrointestinal problems; and erectile dysfunction. It may produce chronic venous swelling, usually requiring management with compression stockings.

Motor Neuropathy

- Motor neuropathy can cause muscle weakness and intrinsic muscle atrophy in the feet. The resulting muscle imbalance leads to claw toe and other forefoot deformities.
- Metatarsophalangeal hyperextension and a distally displaced fat pad accentuate pressure under the metatarsal heads with risk for ulceration.
- Proximal interphalangeal flexion can cause pressure on the dorsum of the toe against the toe box of a shoe, and distal interphalangeal flexion can lead to increased pressure at the end of the toe, both common areas for ulceration.

Neuropathic Pain

- Although the etiology remains unclear, diabetic patients with decreased sensation may experience neuropathic pain resulting from small nerve fiber injury or from injury to the central or peripheral nervous system.
- Patients generally complain of burning or shooting pain that may be worse at night, and they may experience allodynia or anesthesia dolorosa.
- Neuropathic pain can be treated with low-dose antidepressants (amitriptyline, duloxetine), anticonvulsants (gabapentin, pregabalin), analgesics (tramadol), or local topical agents (capsaicin cream, lidocaine).
- Surgical decompression of lower extremity peripheral nerves has been reported to relieve pain and restore sensation, but this approach is controversial and should be considered experimental.

HEALING IN DIABETES

- Delayed osseous and soft tissue healing is common in diabetics. Wound-healing potential is multifactorial and is largely dependent on an individual's vascular and cardiopulmonary status, while nutritional, endocrine, metabolic, and immune status all play a significant role. Smoking and certain medications (immunosuppressant medications) can impede healing; their use should be sought.
  - Nutritional parameters suggested for successful wound healing include the following.
    - Total lymphocyte count > 1,500/microL
    - Serum albumin > 3.5 g/dL
    - Total protein > 6.2 g/dL
- Wound healing also requires adequate wound oxygenation. This can be accomplished by optimizing the patient's cardiac, renal, and vascular status; edema reduction; and occasionally using hyperbaric oxygen therapy.
- Impaired fracture healing in diabetes has been linked to defects in type X collagen expression, abnormal chondrocyte maturation, and altered expression of genes that regulate osteoblast differentiation.
- Poor glucose control and insulin deficiency will affect wound and fracture healing.
- Measurement of glycosylated hemoglobin (HbA1c) levels is the best method for medium- to long-term diabetic control monitoring (follows glycemic control over an 8- to 10-week period) with HbA1c levels of 7% or less yielding the best outcomes. HbA1c levels > 7.5% have been correlated with a higher risk of postoperative surgical site infection.

EQUINUS CONTRACTURE IN DIABETES

- Many diabetic patients develop an equinus contracture for uncertain reasons.
- Gastrocnemius contracture is assessed by measuring passive ankle dorsiflexion with the knee flexed and then extended. Limited dorsiflexion (< 5°) with the knee extended implies gastrocnemius tightness, whereas limited dorsiflexion ± knee extension implies Achilles tightness.

- An equinus contracture increases pressures across the arch and in the forefoot. This increased pressure may lead to ulceration, especially in the forefoot, and may be a contributing factor in the development of neuropathic degeneration (rocker-bottom deformity).
- Gastrocnemius or Achilles tendon lengthening decreases forefoot pressures and has been shown to decrease the incidence of forefoot reulceration in patients with previous ulcers. Gastrocnemius lengthening should be considered for any "at-risk" patient, which includes any patient with neuropathy. Achilles lengthening can be considered if the entire Achilles tendon is tight.

DIABETIC FOOT CARE AND ULCER PREVENTION

- Foot ulcers are all too common in diabetics. Prevention of ulceration through foot-specific patient education, routine foot screening examinations, routine (daily) nail and skin care (oils or creams with lanolin can be used for dry, cracked skin to help prevent skin breakdown), and use of appropriate footwear and orthoses are recommended.
- Inappropriate shoewear can cause abnormal pressure to the skin, potentially causing more dorsal ulcers. Hypertrophic nails can damage the soft tissues surrounding the nails. To help avoid an ingrown toenail, nails should be cut transversely.

Prescription Footwear

- An insensate foot in poorly fitting shoes is one of the most common causes for a diabetic ulcer.
- The optimal shoe is an extra depth shoe that will allow for a custom insole.
- Footwear options include a shoe with a padded heel counter and a wide and deep toe box, Plastizote shoe, Carville sandal (most accommodating for forefoot and hindfoot deformity), deep walking shoe, wide sneaker, or custom-made shoe.
- Insoles are the mainstay of long-term nonoperative management of the diabetic foot to decrease plantar pressure and must be made out of accommodative material. Insoles are generally custom molded with dual layers; the upper layer should consist of a soft polyethylene foam (Plastizote or Pelite), which is most effective in "force distribution" to protect the plantar skin.
- As of April 1, 2004, the Medicare Therapeutic Shoe Bill covers 1 of the following for each diabetic individual (who qualifies under Medicare part B) in 1 calendar year: 1 pair of custom-molded shoes and 2 pairs of inserts or 1 pair of extra depth shoes and 3 pairs of inserts.

FOOT AND ANKLE ULCERS

Background

- Diabetic foot ulcers are the most common diabetic foot complication, and foot infection is the most common reason for a diabetic hospitalization in the USA.
- 15% of diabetic patients will develop a foot ulcer during their lifetime. Diabetic foot ulcers precede 85% of nontraumatic lower extremity amputations and are generally preceded by the triad of neuropathy, deformity, and repetitive trauma.

Pathophysiology

- The most common risk factor for developing a diabetic foot ulcer is peripheral neuropathy. Diabetic foot ulcers commonly occur in areas of structural deformity, forming over areas of bony prominences and high pressure.
- The area of maximum soft tissue damage secondary to vertical stress and shear occurs at the edge of pressure application ("edge effect").
- Ulcers can be neuropathic or ischemic.
  - Neuropathic ulcers are caused by pressure or by shear forces and generally have a healthy bed of granulation tissue beneath a necrotic cap.
  - Ischemic ulcers with underlying vascular insufficiency are usually painful and generally have a necrotic base. Ischemic ulcers should be evaluated by a vascular surgeon for limb salvage.
- Diabetic individuals with sensory neuropathy generally lack sensation to deep pressure or pain. Loss of protective sensation due to peripheral sensory neuropathy, combined with unaccommodated structural foot deformities, commonly results in unrecognized acute or repetitive foot trauma (most commonly due to inappropriate footwear), leading to the development of ulcers with a risk of infection and possible amputation (pressure + neuropathy – ulceration).

Classification of Diabetic Foot Ulcers

- Widely used classification systems are based on wound depth and appearance.
- Neuropathic ulcers are generally not painful, whereas ischemic ulcers are often painful.
- Consider biopsy for a chronic nonhealing ulcer to rule out the possibility of a Marjolin ulcer (squamous cell carcinoma arising from a chronic wound) or malignant melanoma.

Treatment

- Assuming appropriate medical management to optimize the systemic diabetes, treatment strategy includes ulcer bed preparation, local wound care with wound dressings, and protection and offloading.
  - Ulcer bed preparation includes debridement of necrotic or infected tissue to viable margins and callus removal.
  - **Local wound care**
    - The most commonly used dressing is a normal saline moist to dry dressing, which acts to debride the superficial layer when removed.
    - Absorbents (alginate or Hydrofiber) can be used for exudative wounds.
    - Occlusive hydrocolloids, hydrogels, and debriding agents (including hypertonic saline gel) are appropriate for necrotic wounds. Foams can be used for exudative or necrotic wounds.
    - Collagen dressings can be used for granulating or necrotic wounds. Transparent films (Opsite, Tegaderm) are helpful for dry granulating wounds without exudate. Antimicrobial dressings, including iodine- and silver-impregnated dressings, have also been used.
    - Dressings with biologically active wound-healing agents may promote healing in wounds with reasonable healing potential, including those with a cellulose and collagen framework (Promogran), hyaluronic acid ester (Hyalofill), those that deliver platelet-derived growth factors [becaplermin gel (Regranex)], and those that apply living fetal foreskin cells (Apligraf, Dermagraft).
    - A negative-pressure wound dressing (vacuum-assisted closure technique) has also been used to successfully treat nonhealing diabetic wounds.
  - Protection and offloading include casts, removable CAM walkers (which can be wrapped to ensure compliance), splints, or orthoses.
    - Total contact casting (gold standard) is an effective method to heal plantar ulcers with a reported mean healing time of ~ 39 days. Total contact casts may decrease plantar pressure at the ulcer site by distributing force over an increased weight-bearing area, may reduce shear forces and vertical plantar pressures, can protect from trauma, can immobilize the ulcer edges, and can reduce edema.
    - Initially, the total contact cast should be changed every 5-14 days due to the potential for extreme changes in soft tissue swelling, and a poorly fitted cast may lead to skin abrasion. Initial non-weight-bearing status is preferred, although moderate early weight bearing only minimally reduces the time to healing of plantar ulcers and may improve patient compliance.
    - The most common complication of total contact casting is recurrent ulceration. Contraindications to total contact casting include active infection, arterial insufficiency, poor skin quality, and poor patient compliance.
    - Treatment for the "at-risk" foot (grade 0) involves patient education, regular clinical examination, accommodative footwear, and pressure-dissipating orthotics. When a structural deformity or prominence is present that cannot be accommodated by external modalities, deformity correction or removal of the bony prominence is recommended to prevent ulceration.
    - Grades 1 and 2 ulcers require debridement of the necrotic or infected tissue, local wound care, and offloading/pressure relief techniques (external or surgical). Dressings and topical treatment abet the healing process. Once the ulcer has healed, patients should use offloading devices to help prevent reulceration.
    - Surgery is indicated when external accommodative modalities are not successful. Achilles tendon lengthening may help reduce the recurrence of neuropathic plantar forefoot ulcers in patients with limited ankle dorsiflexion by reducing peak plantar forefoot pressures. A heel ulcer is the most difficult to manage and most commonly requires surgery.
    - Operative treatment is generally necessary for grade 3 ulcers and those with associated gangrene, which commonly require debridement of infected or gangrenous tissue with partial- or whole-foot amputation and culture-specific parenteral antibiotic therapy.

Infection

- Wound infections may occur as a result of abnormal white blood cell function, poor nutrition and glycemic control, and the presence of peripheral vascular disease.
- Antibiotics generally should not be used to treat a foot ulcer unless there are clinical signs of infection or underlying osteomyelitis. Infections related to superficial ulceration and cellulitis are most commonly caused by aerobic gram-positive cocci or occasionally by enteric gram-negative bacilli, which can be safely treated by a 1st-generation cephalosporin or clindamycin.
- Diabetic deep wound infections with associated necrosis or gangrene are most commonly polymicrobial with both aerobic and anaerobic ("fetid foot") organisms and can be initially treated with broad-spectrum antibiotics. Swab cultures of the ulcer or sinus tract are generally not reliable.
- Whenever bone is exposed in an ulcer, it should be considered infected. Osteomyelitis in an ulcer should be treated by surgical resection of the infected bone, in whole or in part, with antibiotic therapy.
- Soft tissue gas in a diabetic is most commonly caused by aerobic organisms or by mixed gram-negative rods, but *Clostridium perfringens* and necrotizing fasciitis, which is a surgical emergency, must be ruled out.

CHARCOT FOOT (NEUROARTHROPATHY)

Background

- Charcot arthropathy is a hypertrophic osteoarthropathy seen in patients with peripheral neuropathy.
- The 1st Charcot joint reported was due to tertiary syphilis; however, diabetes is far and away the leading cause of neuropathic arthropathy in the USA, primarily affecting the foot and ankle.
- Other causes of Charcot arthropathy include leprosy (most common vector in North America is the armadillo), myelomeningocele, spinal cord injury/cord compression, and syringomyelia (the most common cause of a Charcot joint in the upper extremity) among others.
- Diabetic Charcot arthropathy does not have a gender predilection, is more likely to occur with an increased duration of diabetes (usually > 10 years), and is bilateral in 30% of cases. The incidence is not different between patients with type 1 and type 2 diabetes. The prevalence of Charcot in diabetics is generally low with numbers quoted from below 1% up to 13%.

Pathophysiology

- Both neurotraumatic and neurovascular etiologies have been proposed. With repetitive trauma, the patient sustains a small fracture, perhaps microfracture, which worsens with persistent weight bearing in the absence of protective sensation. The neurovascular theory suggests that loss of vasomotor control leads to hyperemia, bony resorption, and weakening. Patients with Charcot arthropathy usually have good circulation.

Evaluation

- Swelling, erythema, and warmth (skin temperature usually 3-6°C higher in the acute setting) of the foot and ankle are usually present. The patient may or may not have pain.

- An acute Charcot foot is commonly confused with cellulitis. In the Charcot foot, a decrease in erythema may be seen with foot elevation, as opposed to cellulitis, where the erythema will be unchanged with foot elevation. A subacute or chronic Charcot foot commonly presents with a structurally deformed foot with collapse of the medial longitudinal arch, a rocker-bottom deformity, and bony prominences.
- Plain radiographs may not show any bony changes during the initial few weeks of acute Charcot arthropathy. Early radiographic changes include osteopenia and periarticular fragmentation.
- Later changes include bone resorption, bony proliferation with joint destruction, joint dislocation, and new bone formation. Osteolytic changes of Charcot arthropathy are commonly confused with infection. Surrounding osteopenia is generally not seen in a neuropathic fracture as opposed to infection.
- Advanced imaging studies are generally not needed, because the clinical appearance is usually what distinguishes infection from an acute Charcot foot. When needed, bone scintigraphy combined with indium-111 white blood cell scintigraphy is more specific but less sensitive than magnetic resonance imaging (without gadolinium) in distinguishing between osteomyelitis and Charcot arthropathy.

Classification

- The natural history of Charcot arthropathy can be described based on Eichenholtz stages, which incorporate clinical and radiographic evaluation
- There is also an anatomic classification of Charcot arthropathy of the foot and ankle. The most common anatomic site for the diabetic Charcot foot is the midfoot (tarsometatarsal region 60%) followed by the hindfoot (20-30%). Charcot arthropathy of the forefoot is uncommon.
- Greater deformity is associated with an increased likelihood of requiring surgery. The Charcot ankle is the most unstable and is at high risk for ulceration. It typically falls into varus with ulceration of the fibula through the skin.

Nonoperative Treatment

- Nonoperative management is the mainstay for initial treatment of the Charcot foot or ankle. Treatment goals are to achieve clinical and osseous stability (consolidation) and to prevent &/or treat associated soft tissue problems (ulcer).
- Non-weight bearing is generally recommended for the acute Charcot foot; however, protected weight bearing in a cast may be done for patients who are unable to maintain non-weight-bearing status. Rest and limb elevation are recommended to decrease acute-phase swelling.
- Offloading/immobilization methods include a total contact cast (gold standard), prefabricated removable walking braces, an ankle-foot orthosis, or a Charcot restraint orthotic walker after edema resolution. When the process has consolidated, treatment is accommodative with therapeutic footwear and orthoses geared toward protecting the foot from ulceration over bony prominences.

- The main problem that may develop during nonoperative treatment of a Charcot foot is ulceration. Increased contact pressure over a bony prominence or deformity can lead to ulceration and then possibly infection or even amputation.

Operative Treatment

- Reconstructive surgery is recommended for nonhealing or recurrent ulcers or marked instability/deformity that cannot be accommodated by nonoperative modalities. The goals of surgery are to produce a functionally stable, "braceable" plantigrade foot without soft tissue breakdown.
- For a foot that is already "braceable" or "shoeable," ostectomy and ulcer debridement may be all that is necessary. This is particularly true when the foot is well aligned and stable but with an osseous prominence causing local pressure. Realignment and fusion is needed for the unbraceable foot ± infection. Displaced ankle fractures in the neuropathic patient should also generally be treated with open reduction and internal fixation. Amputation is necessary when extensive infection makes reconstruction not feasible.
- The key to reconstructing neuropathic deformity (or an acute fracture) is more fixation and longer non-weight-bearing time, as patients with neuropathy cannot tell when they are putting too much pressure on the foot. Reconstructive surgery includes realignment and fusion. The goal is not to restore normal anatomy but rather have the foot straight with no focal pressure points (i.e., "shoeable").
- In the absence of infection, most surgeons prefer internal fixation to maintain alignment. External fixators, especially when using thin wire frames, may be helpful in cases with active infection or as an adjunct when there is significant bone loss compromising the strength of internal fixation.
- In a foot with midfoot deformity, realignment often requires resecting 1 or more dislocated midfoot bones. In the hindfoot, realignment may require resection of all or part of the navicular or cuboid. In general, fixation is obtained in those places where it will be best; joints are not necessarily respected and may be spanned if needed.
- The neuropathic ankle is difficult to manage, as much of the talus may be missing. Internal fixation can be accomplished with a retrograde intramedullary nail, a plate, or hybrid fixation.
- The complication rates for Charcot reconstruction are higher than with other foot arthrodeses. Because the alternative in most cases is amputation, the extra risk is usually worth taking.
- Following reconstruction, prolonged limb immobilization is generally recommended for at least 3 months followed by bracing for at least 12 months or perhaps indefinitely for the Charcot ankle or hindfoot. As a general rule, treatment of a fracture in the neuropathic patient should include immobilization for double the normal period of time.
- Amputations in the diabetic patient do not carry a good prognosis. After a lower limb amputation, there is a 60% 5-year mortality rate and a 50% incidence of contralateral lower limb amputation within 5 years. One study has noted that diabetic patients fear major lower extremity amputation more than death.
- It appears that diabetic patients with end-stage renal disease (ESRD) have a much poorer prognosis than those without ESRD when it comes to survival after amputation.

SELECTED REFERENCES

1. Huang YY et al: Survival and associated risk factors in patients with diabetes and amputations caused by infectious foot gangrene. J Foot Ankle Res. 11:1, 2018
2. Wukich DK et al: Patients with diabetic foot disease fear major lower-extremity amputation more than death. Foot Ankle Spec. 11(1):17-21, 2018
3. Cancienne JM et al: Hemoglobin A1c as a predictor of postoperative infection following elective forefoot surgery. Foot Ankle Int. 38(8):832-837, 2017
4. Wukich DK et al: Comparison of transtibial amputations in diabetic patients with and without end-stage renal disease. Foot Ankle Int. 38(4):388-396, 2017
5. Wukich DK et al: Neuropathy and poorly controlled diabetes increase the rate of surgical site infection after foot and ankle surgery. J Bone Joint Surg Am. 96(10):832-9, 2014
6. Larson SA et al: The pathogenesis of Charcot neuroarthropathy: current concepts. Diabet Foot Ankle. 3, 2012
7. Suder NC et al: Prevalence of diabetic neuropathy in patients undergoing foot and ankle surgery. Foot Ankle Spec. 5(2):97-101, 2012
8. Wukich DK et al: Surgical site infections after foot and ankle surgery: a comparison of patients with and without diabetes. Diabetes Care. 34(10):2211-3, 2011
9. Jeffcoate WJ: Charcot neuro-osteoarthropathy. Diabetes Metab Res Rev. 24 Suppl 1:S62-5, 2008
10. Frykberg RG et al: Diabetic foot disorders. A clinical practice guideline. For the American College of Foot and Ankle Surgeons and the American College of Foot and Ankle Orthopedics and Medicine. J Foot Ankle Surg. Suppl:1-60, 2000

Clinical Examination of Diabetic Patients

Examine both lower extremities
Observe gait
Inspect footwear and foreign objects
Record ulcer size (if present)
Palpate pulses (patients without palpable pulses or who have nonhealing ulcer require vascular evaluation)
Examine skin (feel for warmth, hair growth, examine between toes for blisters or ulceration, note skin and nail abnormalities)
Note structural deformities and bony prominences (collapsed arch of Charcot foot or tall arch with claw toes of intrinsic muscle atrophy)
Look for joint stiffness (patients with diabetes have more stiffness, less 1st-ray mobility, and less ankle dorsiflexion compared with nondiabetics, which may contribute to neuropathic ulcer development)

Risk Factors for Ulceration in Diabetic Patients

Peripheral neuropathy
Past history of ulceration or amputation
Charcot neuroarthropathy
Diabetic complications, such as retinopathy and nephropathy
Peripheral vascular disease
Poor glycemic control
Increased duration of diabetes
Trauma
Impaired visual acuity
Edema
Callus
Limited joint mobility
Structural foot deformity

Depth-Ischemia Classification of Diabetic Foot Wounds

Grade	Definition	Treatment
Depth Classification		
0	"At-risk" foot: Prior ulceration or underlying neuropathy with deformity that may lead to ulceration	Patient education; regular clinical examination; accommodative footwear
1 (Wagner grade 1)	Superficial ulceration, not infected	Offloading with total contact cast, walking brace, or accommodative footwear
2 (Wagner grade 2)	Deep ulceration with exposed tendons or joints (± infection)	Debridement; wound care; offloading; antibiotics (if infection)
3 (Wagner grade 3)	Extensive ulceration with exposed bone, deep infection, or abscess	Debridement ± partial foot amputation; offloading; culture-specific antibiotics
Ischemia Classification		
A	No ischemia	
B	Ischemia without gangrene	Vascular consultation; possible revascularization
C (Wagner grade 4)	Partial (forefoot) gangrene	Vascular consultation; possible revascularization; partial foot amputation
D (Wagner grade 5)	Complete foot gangrene	Vascular consultation; possible revascularization; major extremity amputation (below or above knee)

Modification by Brodsky of Wagner-Meggitt classification.

Coughlin MJ et al: The diabetic foot. In Surgery of the Foot and Ankle. 8th ed. St. Louis: Mosby. 911, 2007.

Ulcer Treatment Algorithm

(1) Classify the wound

(2) Is there adequate vascularity to promote healing (is there ischemic pain, vascular claudication, nonpalpable pulses, nonhealing or ischemic ulcer, or gangrene; if vascularity is in question, proceed with vascular consultation/noninvasive vascular examination)

(3) Is it infected (cellulitis, osteomyelitis, or abscess; if sterile probe through ulcer reaches bone, this is highly suggestive for presence of osteomyelitis; imaging studies include plain radiographs, bone scan/labeled white blood cell scan, or magnetic resonance imaging; if infected, admit patient to hospital; provide intravenous antibiotics and wound debridement; obtain vascular medicine &/or endocrine consult)

(4) Wound debridement and local wound care

(5) Relief of pressure: External (postoperative shoe, Plastizote shoe, walking brace, bed rest, bivalved ankle-foot orthosis, total contact cast) vs. internal (surgical reconstruction) with external postoperative support

Natural History of Charcot Arthropathy: Eichenholtz Stage

Stage	Clinical	Plain Radiographs	Management
0 ("at risk")	Neuropathic individual with acute traumatic event	No destructive changes	Initial: Foot elevation, protected offloading in cast or brace Long term: Accommodative devices (therapeutic footwear, insoles, orthoses)
1 (fragmentation)	Erythema, swelling, warmth	Subchondral fragmentation, dissolution, subluxation, dislocation	Foot elevation; protected offloading (non-weight bearing vs. partial weight bearing) in a total contact cast or brace; rule out infection, gout, rheumatoid arthritis
2 (coalescence)	Decreased erythema, swelling, warmth	New bone formation, coalescence of larger bone fragments, sclerosis	Protected offloading in cast or brace/Charcot restraint orthotic walker
3 (consolidation)	Resolution of edema, residual deformity	Bone healing/remodeling; decreased sclerosis	Accommodative devices (therapeutic footwear, insoles, orthoses)

Surgical indications include acute dislocation, osteomyelitis, nonhealing or recurrent ulcer, or deformity that cannot be accommodated by nonoperative management.

Schon LC et al: The management of neuroarthropathic fracture-dislocations in the diabetic patient. Orthop Clin North Am. 26(2):375-92, 1995.

Charcot Arthropathy: Anatomic Classification

Type	Anatomic Location	Clinical Relevance
1	Midfoot (tarsometatarsal)	Most common; relatively stable with development of rocker-bottom deformity and plantar prominence
2	Hindfoot (subtalar/Chopart)	Unstable
3A	Ankle	Most unstable; at risk for malleolar ulceration; longest time to heal
3B	Calcaneus	Fracture of posterior tuberosity of calcaneus may lead to pes planus
4	Multiple regions	More extensive pathology
5	Forefoot	Metatarsophalangeal joints usually involved, with infection

Coughlin MJ et al: The diabetic foot. In Surgery of the Foot and Ankle. 8th ed. St. Louis: Mosby. 948, 2007.

(Left) *A 65-year-old female patient with ankle Charcot and severe loss of bone from both the talus and the plafond is shown. She had almost lost the ability to walk due to fear of falling down.* (Right) *The talar neck and head are maintained, although most of the body is gone.*

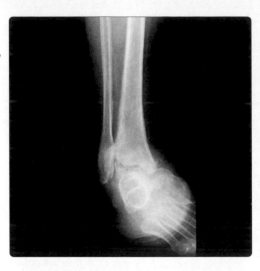
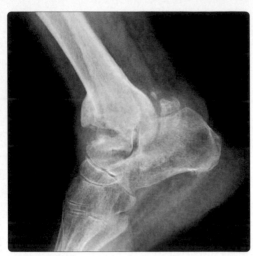

(Left) *Coronal CT shows the varus deformity as well as loss of the talar body.* (Right) *Once again, the loss of the talar body is seen with anterior impaction of the plafond.*

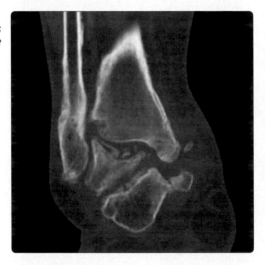
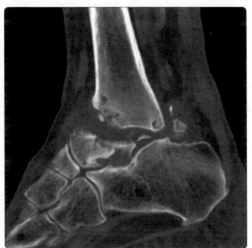

(Left) *Tibiotalocalcaneal fusion was performed with maximal fixation utilizing 2 plates and 2 fully threaded screws.* (Right) *Lateral image after arthrodesis is shown. The patient healed well and was able to ambulate without difficulty after fusion.*

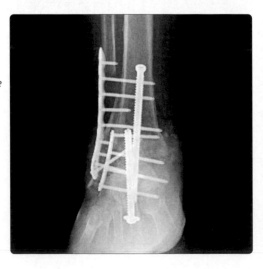
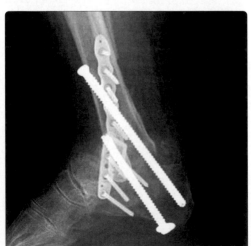

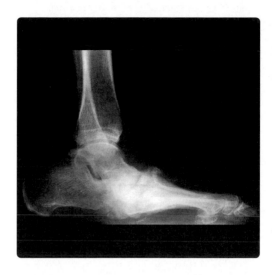

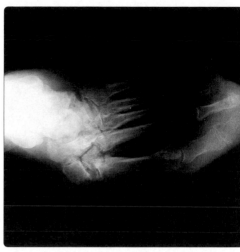

(Left) *A 58-year-old female patient who had a long history of diabetes is shown. She was no longer able to fit into any shoe. Her foot shows Charcot degeneration of the hindfoot and forefoot with marked deformity.* (Right) *AP view of the foot shows severe midfoot degeneration and severe deformity with significant loss of normal bony architecture. The patient essentially had a nonfunctional foot with a high risk for wound breakdown, given the bony prominence.*

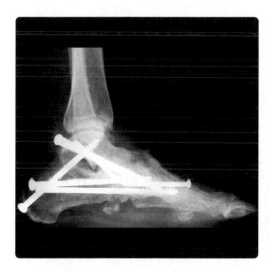

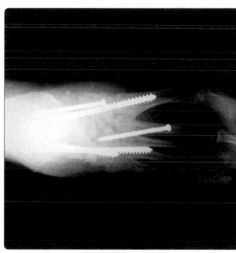

(Left) *Realignment and fusion were performed through 2 incisions. Use of long, noncannulated screws in multiple planes helps to maximize the strength of fixation. Surgeons should be very conservative postoperatively with up to 3 months of non-weight bearing after surgery.* (Right) *Given the slow healing in diabetics coupled with a lack of protective sensation, the risk of nonunion is very high in these types of surgeries. Patients need to be counseled accordingly early and often.*

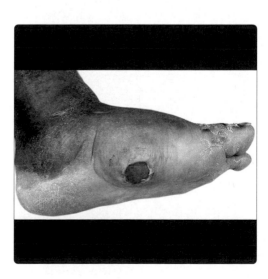

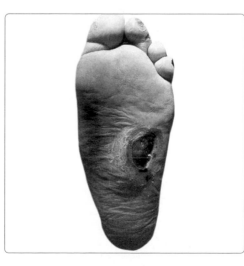

(Left) *This wound is one that you would expect from a foot with a rocker-bottom deformity. The plantar prominence in the midfoot coupled with a patient's impaired sensation ultimately causes the wound.* (Right) *A grade 2 deep, nonhealing ulcer in a Charcot foot with a plantar lateral prominence is shown. The combination of bony prominence, impaired sensation, and possible arterial insufficiency all contribute to and perpetuate the wound.*

KEY FACTS

HALLUX VALGUS

- Hallux valgus is defined principally by the intermetatarsal angle; the distal metatarsal articular angle can also weigh on treatment decisions; the hallux valgus angle is the least relevant to treatment.
- Etiology is likely multifactorial with genetics playing a large role.
- Associated symptoms (metatarsalgia, hammer toes, etc.) are very relevant and can sway treatment decisions.
- Surgery is ultimately done in order to relieve pain; the goals of surgery should always be made explicitly clear to patients.
- Various operative treatment options exist, all with relative merits and downsides.
- Generally speaking, metatarsal osteotomies have the advantage of relatively rapid healing allowing early weight bearing, although they can be limited in terms of their deformity correction capacity.

- Tarsometatarsal fusion, or the Lapidus procedure, allows for maximal deformity correction and potentially protecting the 2nd ray, although it is a bigger operation with a longer recovery and a greater risk of nonunion.

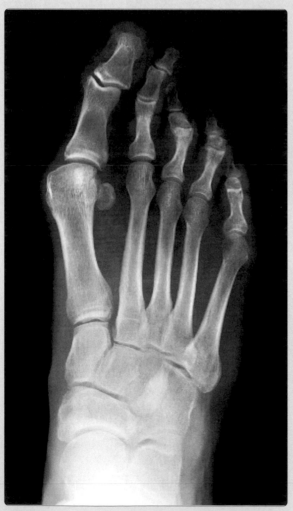

A 53-year-old male patient with longstanding symptoms of hallux valgus is shown. There are no 2nd ray symptoms.

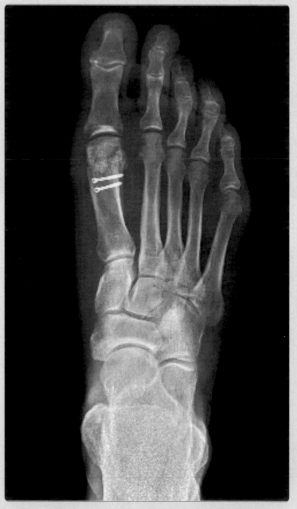

Patient underwent an extended plantar limb chevron osteotomy with a small medial closing wedge to address the distal metatarsal articular angle.

TERMINOLOGY

- The term bunion is a colloquial one for the medial prominence of the big toe. Bunion comes from the old French word buigne, which literally meant swelling.
- While the term bunion is often used in lay parlance, surgeons more appropriately refer to the deformity as hallux valgus with hallux referring to the 1st ray and valgus referring to the deformity seen at the 1st metatarsophalangeal (MTP) joint.
- Hallux valgus can be broken down into its component parts and is typically described by a set of radiographic angles, all from a standing anteroposterior radiograph.
  - The principle defining angle that defines hallux valgus is the intermetatarsal angle. This angle essentially describes the metatarsus primus varus or the inclination of the 1st metatarsal away from the 2nd. The intermetatarsal angle is typically < 9°. Surgery for hallux valgus most often seeks to address an elevated intermetatarsal angle.
  - The hallux valgus angle is used less frequently in clinical decision-making. It is measured as the angle subtended by the long axes of the 1st metatarsal and the 1st proximal phalanx and is normally < 15°.
  - The final, and perhaps most subtle, angle that defines the deformity is the distal metatarsal articular angle (DMAA). This angle essentially measures the degree to which the articular surface is offset from the longitudinal axis of the 1st metatarsal.

EPIDEMIOLOGY

- The age of onset of a bunion can be difficult to fully define from a population standpoint, as it is quite variable. Patients can present for evaluation ranging in age from early teens to the 9th decade of life. Moreover, given a pathology where the symptoms may not always match the degree of deformity, the age at which the patient develops deformity may be less relevant. The development of symptoms could very well have more to do with external factors, such as shoes.
  - One study did note that the average age of onset of deformity was 31, and the average duration of symptoms in a group of surgical patients was 5.3 years.

- While patients certainly can present with bilateral deformity, the rate of bilaterality is not well defined.
  - Some authors have noted close to 90% bilaterality, however, although the course, both from a deformity development and pain development standpoint may not be synchronous.

- There is a female preponderance with many studies quoting over 90% female patients, although there is significant variability in the literature with regard to the male:female ratio. Shoewear may account for this difference to some degree, although the overt causes are not entirely clear.

  - In 1 study of 600 elderly patients, the rate of hallux valgus was found to be 58% in women and 25% in men. The development of hallux valgus was correlated with low BMI and high heel use between ages 20-64 in women; it was correlated with a high BMI and pes planus in men.
  - Another study noted a 15:1 female:male ratio with males generally having more severe deformity and more commonly having an increased DMAA, while a 3rd study noted little sex difference between groups of elderly patients with 58.0% of males having hallux valgus and 66.5% of females.
  - It is possible that these studies, despite their widely disparate numbers, are simply assessing different patient populations in which the incidence is quite different.
- There is not a direct correlation between the degree of deformity and pain; some patients can have severe deformity with little pain, while others have mild deformity and significant pain. For most surgeons, pain is a strict indication for any surgery.

ETIOLOGY

Intrinsic Factors

- Genetics
  - Clearly, genetics play a role and likely a primary role. One study of Korean monozygotic twins, dizygotic twins, and siblings found the genetic influence on hallux valgus to be substantial.
- Ligamentous laxity
  - This may affect the 1st tarsometatarsal joint, leading to medial deviation of the 1st metatarsal.
- Osseous anatomy
  - Some have suggested, although the evidence remains in question, that a relatively rounded 1st metatarsal head may make for relatively less stable MTP articulation, potentially being more apt to end in hallux valgus.
- Pes planus
  - Superiorly directed pressure from the ground may lead to some degree of metatarsal-cuneiform instability. Abduction of the forefoot can lead to a valgus moment on the toe, altering the pull of the abductors and adductors and pushing the toe into greater valgus.
- Equinus contracture
  - This is somewhat similar to pes planus in that the contracture necessitates rolling to the outside of the foot with toe off, placing a valgus moment on the toe.

Extrinsic Factors

- Influence of shoes
  - Sim-Fook and Hodgson looked at shoewearing and nonshoewearing groups of Chinese patients in the 1950s, noting a 33% rate of hallux valgus in the shod group vs. < 2% in the unshod.
  - Other studies in various indigenous peoples have noted that hallux valgus certainly occurs, although it is much less apt to be symptomatic.
  - To what degree shoes play a role in the development of hallux valgus is a subject of some debate. However, that shoes in general, and certain shoes especially, can make hallux valgus more symptomatic is generally accepted.
- Prolonged weight bearing over time

○ No overt correlation has been found between the development of hallux valgus and excessive walking or occupation.

- It is very possible that hallux valgus represents a grouping of conditions that all have a similar endpoint. There may be several disparate mechanisms that all end at more or less the same point, although this theory remains to be tested.

ASSOCIATED SYMPTOMS

Metatarsalgia

- At a basic level, metatarsalgia simply implies pain associated with the metatarsals. Practically speaking, this term is meant to represent pain in the forefoot underneath the metatarsal heads. This pathology can exist ± symptomatic pathology in the 1st ray, although they will often be concomitant and related. If the 1st ray bears insufficient weight for any number of reasons, then that weight can be transferred typically to the 2nd or 3rd metatarsal heads, a phenomenon termed transfer metatarsalgia.

Hammer Toes

- Hammer toes are defined by a combination of flexion at the proximal interphalangeal joint (PIP) and extension at the distal interphalangeal joint. Pain can come from either the prominence of the PIP on the top of the shoe or from the end of the toe contacting the ground or the shoe.

HISTORY AND PHYSICAL EXAMINATION

History

- Most frequently, patients come in complaining of deformity and pain about the median eminence on the medial aspect of the big toe, although the pain can be plantar or dorsal as well. The timecourse can be gradual or relatively acute. The principle areas of pain and any associated symptoms should be sought and defined.

Physical Examination

- The foot should be inspected to look for deformity as well as the presence and distribution of any callosities that may be present.
- As above, direct palpation should be used to define and confirm painful areas.
- Motion at the 1st MTP joint should be assessed and compared to the contralateral side. Laxity of the 1st tarsometatarsal joint should also be sought, although this can be difficult to measure objectively. Also, generalized ligamentous laxity should be assessed using the Beighton score.
- Neurovascular exam should specifically define any sensory deficit and confirm adequate blood flow.

RADIOGRAPHIC EXAMINATION

Radiographs

- As above, weight-bearing anteroposterior, oblique, and lateral radiographs should be obtained.
- The angles as laid out above should be measured, as these angles will help define the most appropriate surgical options.

TREATMENT

Nonoperative

- Nonoperative treatment is fairly limited for hallux valgus. Typically, the most effective treatments will consist of shoewear modifications in an effort to decrease the pressure on the deformed big toe or to accept the relative width of the foot. Wide toe box shoes are most appropriate.
- Toe splints or toe spacers, etc. do not alter the deformity, although they can sometimes decrease the prominence when the splint is on the foot. They do not alter the natural history of the disease.

Operative

- The presence of pain is necessary in order for surgery to be considered. Surgery for cosmesis alone is inappropriate and not warranted. Further, patients should understand that being able to return to narrow, high-heeled shoes postoperatively is not a goal of surgery. The surgeon needs to have a frank conversation with the patient laying out what are and what are not appropriate goals of surgery. This discussion ensures that all parties are on the same page; a patient with unrealistic goals is likely to be an unhappy patient.
- There are literally over a hundred different types of operations that have been described in an effort to correct a bunion, although they will all generally incorporate a soft tissue reconstruction at the MTP joint, termed a modified McBride procedure. There may be no other 1 procedure in orthopaedics in which there are so many different types of options all with the same ultimate goal. With that being said, there are a couple of different general categories of surgeries that are performed, and so we will discuss the options in that way. We will cover 4 basic types: Distal metatarsal osteotomy, proximal metatarsal osteotomy, Lapidus procedure (tarsometatarsal arthrodesis), and MTP arthrodesis.
- Modified McBride procedure
  ○ This procedure at a basic level consists of releasing the tight lateral structures and tightening down the lax medial structures. The procedure consists of sectioning the transverse metatarsal ligament that runs from the 2nd metatarsal to the lateral sesamoid as well as the adductor tendon from the lateral sesamoid and the phalanx. The median eminence is resected, and the medial capsule is plicated with the toe held in a reduced position.
  ○ This procedure can rarely be used in isolation, although concern about early recurrence limits its effectiveness in this capacity. This procedure is almost always combined with some sort of bony correction in an effort to get a more lasting correction.
- Distal metatarsal osteotomy
  ○ In general, a principle advantage of distal osteotomies is that they heal readily, and so patients do not need to be non-weight bearing for protracted periods of time. Nonunion is rare. An increased DMAA can be addressed readily with a simple modification of the osteotomy to take a medial wedge. These osteotomies are most appropriate for mild to moderate deformity.

- The disadvantages of these osteotomies principally lies in their limited power to correct deformity. More severe deformity is likely best treated with another option.
- Proximal (or shaft) osteotomy
  - The discussion of advantages and disadvantages for these osteotomies is similar to that for distal osteotomies with a few differences.
    - Proximal osteotomies have more power to correct deformity. They may have a slightly increased risk of nonunion relative to distal osteotomies.
    - Proximal and shaft osteotomies can be prone to their individual complications depending on the individual osteotomy.
      - Osteotomies, such as the Ludloff, can get dorsiflexion malunions if allowed to weight bear without sufficient healing present, leading to issues with transfer metatarsalgia.
      - Scarf osteotomies can get "troughing," whereby the cortical bone does not maintain apposition leading to decreased superoinferior dimension of the 1st metatarsal, or height, which also may cause issues with transfer.
- Lapidus procedure
  - The Lapidus procedure consists of an arthrodesis of the proximal 1st metatarsal to the medial cuneiform. The advantages and disadvantages of this procedure are in many ways the opposite of the distal metatarsal osteotomy.
  - The Lapidus procedure has the most power to correct deformity of any operation for hallux valgus. Moreover, a Lapidus keeps the 1st metatarsal bone straight, whereas most metatarsal osteotomies make the 1st metatarsal crooked to make it look straight.
  - However, the Lapidus procedure is a more significant operation with a greater potential for nonunion.
  - Theoretically, a Lapidus could herald a lower rate of recurrence with fusion of the 1st tarsometatarsal joint.
- 1st MTP arthrodesis
  - This procedure is likely most appropriate in those patients that have hallux valgus with some degree of arthrosis in the 1st MTP joint.
- Akin procedure (phalangeal osteotomy)
  - An Akin is a medial-based closing wedge osteotomy that is used primarily to addresses any hallux valgus interphalangeus; it can often supplement a hallux valgus procedure.
  - These osteotomies heal readily and therefore do not slow down recovery when added to any other bunion procedure. The need for an Akin osteotomy is typically assessed once a more definitive operation has been performed.
- Complications
  - Hallux varus
    - Hallux varus is commonly associated with overaggressive medial reefing or overresection of the median eminence.
    - If recognized early, an aggressive taping protocol can be initiated in an effort to push the toe back into a more normal position.
    - Surgical options include extensor hallucis longus transfer for a passively correctable deformity or a 1st MTP arthrodesis if it is not correctable.

SELECTED REFERENCES

1. Maniglio M et al: Surgical treatment of mild to severe hallux valgus deformities with a percutaneous subcapital osteotomy combined with a lateral soft tissue procedure. Foot Ankle Spec. epub ahead of print, 2018
2. Golightly YM et al: Factors associated with hallux valgus in a community-based cross-sectional study of adults with and without osteoarthritis. Arthritis Care Res (Hoboken). 67(6):791-8, 2015
3. Gutteck N et al: Immediate fullweightbearing after tarsometatarsal arthrodesis for hallux valgus correction–Does it increase the complication rate? Foot Ankle Surg. 21(3):198-201, 2015
4. Lee CH et al: Genetic influences on hallux valgus in Koreans: the healthy twin study. Twin Res Hum Genet. 17(2):121-6, 2014
5. Nguyen US et al: Factors associated with hallux valgus in a population-based study of older women and men: the MOBILIZE Boston Study. Osteoarthritis Cartilage. 18(1):41-6, 2010
6. Coughlin MJ et al: Hallux valgus: demographics, etiology, and radiographic assessment. Foot Ankle Int. 28(7):759-77, 2007
7. SIM-FOOK L et al: A comparison of foot forms among the non-shoe and shoe-wearing Chinese population. J Bone Joint Surg Am. 40-A(5):1058-62, 1958

(Left) *This patient has hallux valgus with a mild to moderately increased intermetatarsal angle. The patient also has an increased distal metatarsal articular angle; note how the articular surface of the metatarsal head is offset laterally relative to the long axis of the 1st metatarsal. Any correction should take this offset into account.* **(Right)** *Preoperative lateral image is shown. The lateral x-ray is often less relevant in surgical decision making, although one can look for any elevation of the 1st ray.*

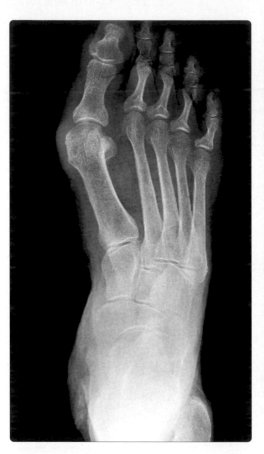
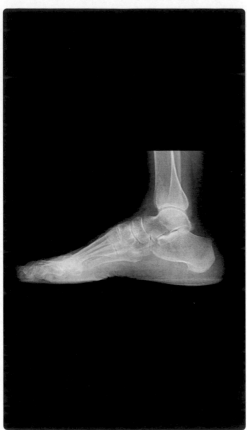

(Left) *Postoperative AP image shows correction of both the intermetatarsal angle and the distal metatarsal articular angle. Although there is still some soft tissue swelling medially in this early postoperative patient, the bony prominence has been removed.* **(Right)** *Postoperative lateral image shows the single screw fixing the metatarsal osteotomy in this non-weight-bearing image.*

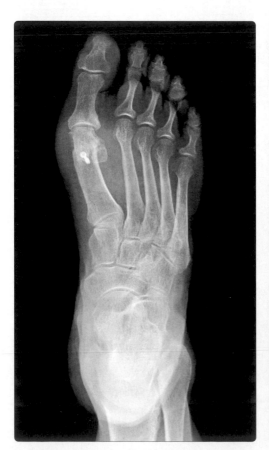
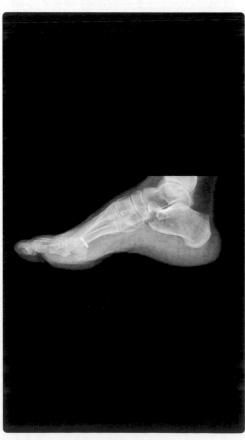

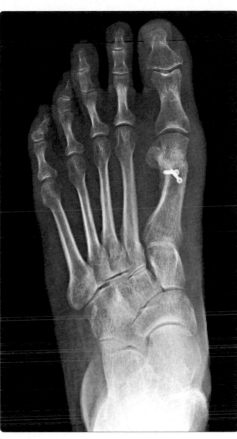

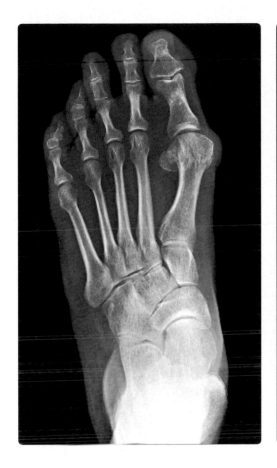

(Left) This patient has an increased distal metatarsal articular angle in addition to an increased intermetatarsal angle. If performing any distal osteotomy, a medial closing wedge component can be added to address the distal metatarsal articular angle. (Right) In this postoperative x-ray, notice the reduction of both the distal metatarsal articular angle and intermetatarsal angle. The articular surface of the metatarsal head is now perpendicular to the long axis of the metatarsal.

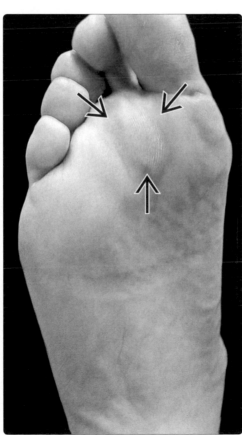

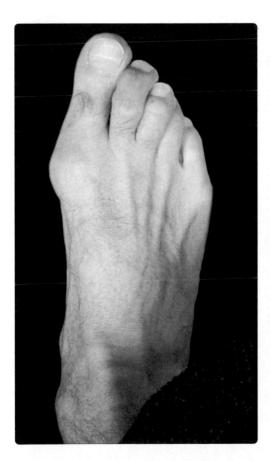

(Left) This non-weight-bearing picture shows a patient with hallux valgus that also has some 2nd toe deformity and pain, as the 2nd toe has a flexion deformity at the proximal interphalangeal joint consistent with a hammer toe. (Right) A callus ➔ is noted underneath the 2nd metatarsal head in this same patient. The patient had pain in this area along with medial bunion pain. A relatively long 2nd ray, as well as a "loose" 1st tarsometatarsal joint, can contribute to this clinical problem.

(Left) *This 60-year-old female patient had medial pain about the big toe as well as pain underneath the 2nd toe. Her 2nd metatarsal was relatively long, but she also had some laxity at the 1st tarsometatarsal joint. A long discussion was had with the patient regarding her options. She ultimately did not want a protracted period of non-weight bearing, and so she elected to have a 1st metatarsal osteotomy and a 2nd metatarsal shortening osteotomy.* (Right) *Patient underwent a distal metatarsal osteotomy with bunion correction as well as a 2nd metatarsal shortening osteotomy and plantar condylectomy.*

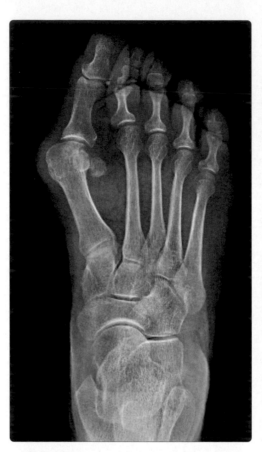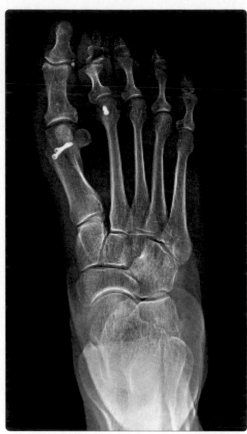

(Left) *An 18-year-old female patient with longstanding pain about the medial big toe desired surgical correction. A Lapidus procedure was ultimately chosen in an effort to get the most durable correction possible in this young patient.* (Right) *Lateral image of the same patient is shown. Although the Lapidus will typically invoke a longer recovery, it makes more sense in younger patients who are possibly at greater risk of recurrence in an effort to mitigate that risk.*

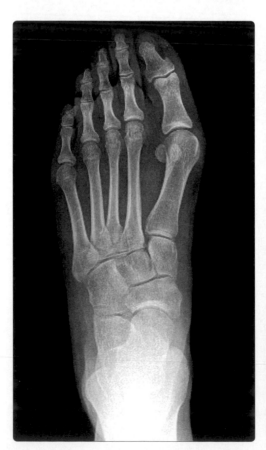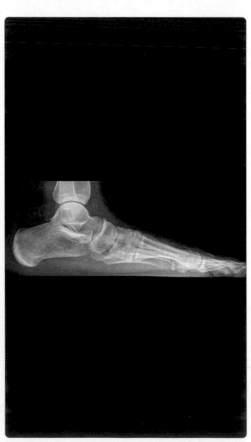

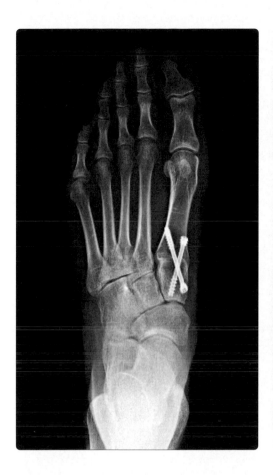

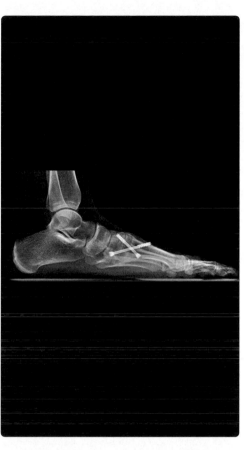

(Left) *Patient had a Lapidus procedure with uneventful healing and returned to full activities without restriction.* **(Right)** *Lateral image of the healed Lapidus is shown. While the risk of recurrence is poorly understood currently, many surgeons feel that laxity of the 1st tarsometatarsal joint has a role in the genesis of the deformity, and so fusing that joint minimizes the risk of recurrence.*

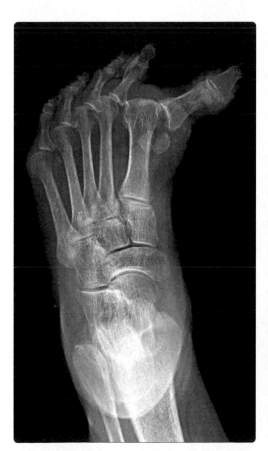

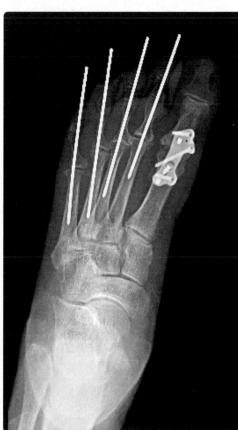

(Left) *A 71-year-old female patient with an incompletely described neuromuscular disorder presented with increasing foot deformity over several years to the point that wearing shoes was nearly impossible.* **(Right)** *Patient had 1st metatarsophalangeal fusion with 2-5 metatarsal head resection and pinning. Upon healing, she was able to wear closed shoes, which she had been unable to do for quite some time.*

HALLUX RIGIDUS

- Hallux rigidus is the most common arthritic condition in the foot.
- Hallux rigidus tends to be bilateral, although it is often not synchronous.
- The 1st metatarsophalangeal (MTP) joint generally becomes stiffer and more painful as the arthritis progresses, although progression is inconsistent. Some patients will progress linearly, while others' symptoms will remain consistent over time.
- Nonoperative treatment is similar to nonoperative treatment for arthritis in any joint with the added component of a stiff insert or shoe to limit 1st MTP motion.

- Operative treatment depends on how advanced the arthritis is, although symptoms are the best indicator of what treatment is most appropriate. Joint-sparing procedures (cheilectomy, Moberg osteotomy) are generally used for less severe arthritis, and fusion has traditionally been the gold standard for more severe arthritis. Implant arthroplasty with a synthetic implant is not inferior to fusion in early data.

SESAMOID PATHOLOGY

- Sesamoiditis is a poorly understood pathology that can cause significant pain and disability. Treatment consists of offloading or sesamoidectomy for refractory cases.
- Turf toe injuries can be devastating injuries to the big toe and typically require surgical reconstruction and repair of the plantar tissues of the 1st MTP joint.

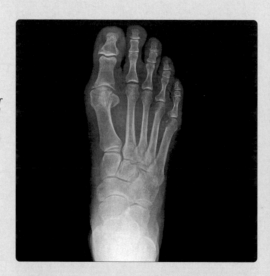

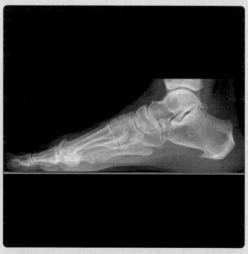

(Left) *A 50-year-old female patient with hallux rigidus symptoms as her primary complaint is shown. She also had some hallux valgus. She had tried shoe modifications without much decrease in her symptoms.* (Right) *The dorsal osteophyte is seen at the 1st metatarsophalangeal joint in the same patient. The osteophyte was rubbing on her shoe, which made shoewear difficult.*

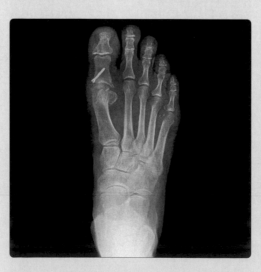

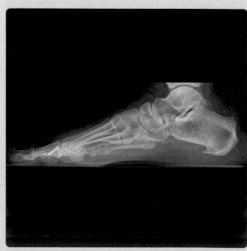

(Left) *A cheilectomy was performed with a median eminence resection and a combination of a Moberg and Akin osteotomy taking out a dorsomedial wedge to allow for some effective increase in dorsiflexion, while also correcting the bunion to some degree.* (Right) *The lateral view shows the degree to which the dorsal osteophyte was resected, while also showing the fixation for the phalangeal osteotomy. The patient reported an improvement both in pain and function after surgery.*

TERMINOLOGY

- Osteoarthritis of the 1st metatarsophalangeal (MTP) joint is termed hallux rigidus. Hallux refers to the 1st ray, while the term rigidus is applied since the 1st MTP generally becomes stiff as the disease progresses.

- The inciting cause is not entirely clear in this pathology, although the arthritis typically affects the dorsal aspect of the joint first.

EPIDEMIOLOGY

- In 1 epidemiologic study of hallux rigidus, 70% of patients had bilateral disease.
  - Indeed, hallux rigidus is often bilateral, although not always synchronous.

- 66% of affected individuals were female.
  - An older study had noted hallux rigidus to be much more common in men, although another more recent study had 63% female patients.

- The mean age at onset was 44 years (range: 14-68 years), and the duration of symptoms prior to treatment was 6 years.

- 22% of patients recalled some trauma to the hallux; 74% of these patients had unilateral disease.

ETIOLOGY

- This is not entirely clear and may represent a group of pathologies that have a similar endpoint.

Theorized Predisposing Factors

- Hindfoot valgus has been theorized to cause increased strain on the MTP joint and was associated with a 23% increased risk of hallux rigidus in 1 study.
- The relative length of the 1st metatarsal has also been theorized as a potentially causative factor in hallux rigidus.
  - A few radiographic studies have noted relatively longer 1st rays in those patients with hallux rigidus, although others have noted no correlation.
  - Metatarsus primus elevatus, or an elevation of the 1st metatarsal in the sagittal plane, has been theorized as a cause of hallux rigidus. The theory goes that dorsiflexion at the great toe is limited due to tightening of the plantar fascia caused by elevation of the great toe, which leads to dorsal impingement at the joint and subsequent arthritis.
    - Numerous studies have largely debunked this theory, as metatarsal elevation has been found in patients both ± hallux rigidus. Further, in those patients with elevation and hallux rigidus, the degree of arthrosis did not linearly correlate with the degree of elevation. It is ultimately unclear whether the elevation is a cause or an effect of hallux rigidus.
- Trauma to the 1st MTP joint can certainly be a cause of subsequent arthritis, although articular injuries of the 1st MTP joint are generally uncommon.

- Osteochondral lesions of the metatarsal head are increasingly recognized as a potential cause of pain in the 1st MTP joint as well as possibly being a precursor to hallux rigidus.
- Inflammatory arthropathies can certainly affect the 1st MTP joint, although this pathology typically involves more than just the 1st MTP. Also, with the advent of disease-modifying antirheumatic drugs, the incidence of severe forefoot pathology in these patients appears to be decreasing.

HISTORY AND PHYSICAL EXAM FINDINGS

History

- Patients will typically complain of pain in the big toe, especially with push off. Essentially, any movement that requires dorsiflexion of the big toe will be painful.
- The time course of symptoms can be variable. Not uncommonly, patients can have mild symptoms for years and then have sudden exacerbations of unclear origin.
- People's ability to adapt to pain can be manifested in this condition in the following way. Since push off or toe off requires dorsiflexion and is painful, patients will often "roll out," i.e., disengage the big toe when they push off or "roll" their foot to the outside so that the push off comes through the lesser toe joints and involves the big toe less. Rarely, patients will present with lateral (e.g., 4th) metatarsal stress fractures that are otherwise uncommon due to this mechanical adaptation.
- Interestingly, unilateral hallux rigidus has been found to produce calf asymmetry due to a lack of fully engaging the calf musculature at push off. The atrophy develops over a long period of time and, thus, may not be noticed until it is quite pronounced. In this setting, this calf asymmetry has occasionally been thought to represent abnormal swelling on what is ostensibly the normal side, leading to an expensive, and at times invasive, work-up.

Physical Examination

- Patients will often have a dorsal osteophyte that is variably prominent emanating from the 1st metatarsal head. Generally speaking, patients can have pain from this osteophyte alone, in which case, the pain will be with dorsal palpation; they can have pain from the arthritis, in which case, pain will occur with motion of the 1st MTP; or the patients can have some degree of both.
- Range of motion of the 1st MTP joint will often be restricted to some degree, although it must be noted that "normal" motion at the 1st MTP joint can be incredibly variable and is very much a moving target. As an example, normal total 1st MTP motion for a large, burly man may be only ~ 50-60°, while a lithe female dancer may have close to 180° of motion. In this setting, the contralateral side can be used as an internal control, although only in those situations in which it is unaffected.
- Early in the course of the disease, pain typically occurs dorsally and with dorsiflexion as above. As the arthritis progresses in later stages, pain can occur throughout the joint and with any motion of the joint
- Patients can have some evidence of lesser metatarsalgia due to lack of engagement of the big toe as above.

IMAGING

Radiographs

- Weight-bearing AP, oblique, and lateral radiographs are warranted.
  - General radiographic signs of arthritis, such as joint space narrowing, subchondral sclerosis, subchondral cysts, and osteophyte formation, prevail.
  - While the progression of the symptoms of the disease generally parallels the severity of the radiographic findings, this statement is not universally true, as there are plenty of patients whose radiographic disease is worse than their clinical disease.

Advanced Imaging

- Advanced imaging is seldom necessary in the setting of hallux rigidus. However, in those patients that may have an osteochondral lesion of the metatarsal head without clear arthritis, an MR can be beneficial to identify and characterize such a lesion.

CLASSIFICATION

- Coughlin and Shurnas developed the most widely used grading system for severity of hallux rigidus, utilizing both clinical and radiographic parameters.
  - Grade 0
    - 10-20% loss of motion of contralateral side, 40-60° motion, normal radiographs, no pain
  - Grade 1
    - Loss of 20-50% of motion of normal side, 30-40° motion
    - Radiographs show dorsal osteophyte mainly with minimal other findings; mild, occasional pain; pain at extremes of motion (i.e., maximal dorsiflexion or plantarflexion).
  - Grade 2
    - Loss of 50-75% of motion of normal side, 10-30° motion
    - Radiographs show dorsal, lateral, medial osteophytes, which may make metatarsal head appear flattened; up to 25% of dorsal joint space involved; mild to moderate joint space narrowing; sesamoids not involved.
    - Moderate to severe pain and stiffness, maximal pain just before maximal dorsiflexion or plantarflexion on exam
  - Grade 3
    - Almost complete loss of motion with < 10° arc
    - Radiographs are similar to grade 2 with notable exceptions that entire joint is involved, and sesamoids may be involved.
    - Nearly constant pain and stiffness, pain still at extremes but not in mid range of motion
  - Grade 4
    - Motion and radiographic findings similar to grade 3; primary difference is that pain is throughout range of motion.

TREATMENT

Nonoperative Treatment

- If the pain is somewhat acute in onset, a brief period of time in a CAM Walker boot with oral antiinflammatories may be appropriate in an effort to quell inflammation and decrease pain.
- The basic concept behind nonoperative treatment essentially follows the same logic, i.e., minimize motion and inflammation at the 1st MTP joint. A deep toe box shoe can be beneficial as well in an effort to decrease pain from rubbing on dorsal osteophytes.
- Motion at the 1st MTP joint can be restricted using any of a number of different types of shoe inserts. In general, stiff inserts of some description are used to restrict primarily 1st MTP dorsiflexion. What individual type of insert is used depends on surgeon preference and cost.
  - Options include full-length carbon fiber foot plates or an orthotic with a Morton extension. On occasion, simply a stiff-soled shoe, such as a clog, may be sufficient.
- As with arthritis in any joint, antiinflammatories may be of some benefit and are certainly worth trying.
- Steroid injections can be used judiciously, although some surgeons worry about potential effects to the soft tissue envelope in patients who may ultimately need surgery, given the subcutaneous nature of the joint.
- There are few studies specifically of nonoperative treatment, although 1 study of 24 feet noted that surgery could be avoided with little progression of disease over a 12-year period.

Operative Treatment

- Operative treatment is generally broken down into 2 basic types of options. Either an effort is made to retain the joint in those patients with milder disease, or the joint is eliminated in more severe disease.
  - For milder disease (grades 1 and 2), joint preservation is preferred.
    - A cheilectomy, or dorsal exostectomy, is the procedure of choice. In this procedure, the joint is approached dorsally, and 20-30% of the dorsal metatarsal head is excised with the dorsal osteophyte. The goal at the time of surgery is to get at least 60° of dorsiflexion. Cheilectomy had shown good results both in the short term and in the long term, although surgeons must counsel patients that it is not a curative operation, and the arthritis and symptoms may return at some point in the future.
    - Phalangeal osteotomies have been added to try to allow for better effective dorsiflexion by "stealing" some plantarflexion motion. The Moberg osteotomy, a dorsal closing wedge osteotomy, makes it so that the toe engages the ground later in push off, which effectively increases dorsiflexion of the big toe. This osteotomy generally works well for hallux rigidus, and some authors have pushed to use it with cheilectomy even in advanced cases of hallux rigidus, i.e., grade 3.

— While a host of metatarsal osteotomies have been described for hallux rigidus, outcomes have been inconsistent and inconsistently reported. Moreover, many of the osteotomies seek to address issues that are not clearly pathologic, such as metatarsal elevation or relative length. As a result, these osteotomies are not routinely recommended.

- For more severe disease (grades 3 and 4), more ablative procedures are generally recommended.
  - The Keller procedure, a resection arthroplasty of the 1st MTP joint, has been used historically for hallux rigidus. In this procedure, the base of the proximal phalanx is resected. Although this procedure can work reasonably well for pain relief, it diminishes push-off power and thereby negatively impacts patient function. It is therefore rarely used.
  - Another option is the capsular interposition arthroplasty. This option has historically been reserved for those patients with severe hallux rigidus who do not want a fusion, often women who have a desire to wear heels. In this procedure, a cheilectomy is performed as well as a Keller. However, crucially, the proximal phalangeal base is retained and with it the capsular and flexor hallucis brevis insertions, thereby allowing retention of push-off power.
    - Results from this procedure were generally good with ~ a 10% rate of subsequent conversion to arthrodesis.
  - Metatarsophalangeal arthrodesis has been and remains the gold standard or treatment for end-stage hallux rigidus. It has long been a reliable option for providing pain relief in this group of patients.
    - There are a variety of techniques of fixation without any clear hierarchy as to which is best. Most surgeons either use a lag screw and plate construct or crossed screws.
    - Patients are generally kept non-weight bearing for 4 weeks after surgery.
    - Results are uniformly good; patients often have a somewhat unfounded dislike of fusion operations, as they feel they will be unable to walk appropriately. However, clinical studies and gait studies show uniform improvement in many parameters after 1st MTP fusion, and patients are often able to be active at a level that was not possible prior to fusion.
    - Total joint arthroplasty can work for hallux rigidus, but, when it fails, it tends to fail catastrophically, with significant bone loss, leaving a difficult reconstructive situation. Many surgeons view total joint arthroplasty as an inappropriate treatment for hallux rigidus at this point.
  - More recently, a synthetic cartilage implant has been developed for those patients with end-stage disease who would like to avoid fusion.
    - The implant works by distracting the joint to some degree, thereby hopefully increasing motion to some degree and decreasing pain.
    - An initial noninferiority study showed that it was not overtly inferior to arthrodesis. Moreover, if it does fail, surgical revision to arthrodesis is easily accomplished.

SESAMOID PATHOLOGY

Sesamoiditis

- Sesamoiditis is a poorly understood process, whereby the patient develops pain in the sesamoid bones without a clear cause. Many primary causes, including osteonecrosis, have been postulated to lead to sesamoiditis, although the pathogenesis remains unexplained.
  - Clinically, sesamoiditis can be a significant problem, simply due to the fact that the sesamoid bones see significant stress with any amount of walking. Severe sesamoiditis can make any amount of walking a significant chore for these patients and thereby limit them.
  - Treatment often consists of attempting to offload the affected area. In the acute phase, a CAM Walker boot may be most appropriate in an effort to decrease pain. Subsequently, a metatarsal pad either in isolation or as part of an orthotic can be fashioned to try to more formally offload the affected area.
  - Surgical treatment consists of sesamoidectomy, which is often curative. The sesamoid bones act as a pulley for the flexor hallucis brevis. Removal of 1 sesamoid does not greatly affect this setup in a negative way, but removal of both sesamoids is ill advised.
    - Prior to proceeding with a sesamoidectomy, an MR should be obtained to confirm sesamoid abnormality. Rarely, an osteochondral lesion of the underside of the metatarsal head can mimic sesamoiditis. In that setting, addressing the chondral lesion without sesamoidectomy can diminish the symptoms.

Sesamoid Fracture/Turf Toe Injury

- Sesamoid fractures are rare injuries that must be differentiated from a bipartite sesamoid.
  - The rate of bipartite sesamoids is ~ 15% in the general population, and they will often look different than an acute injury radiographically. Bipartite sesamoids are more common in the medial sesamoid.
  - Clinically, a sesamoid fracture is often a relatively high-energy injury and will typically not be subtle. Patients will have an acute inability to walk and severe pain.
  - Turf toe injury is an injury to the plantar stabilizing structures of the 1st MTP joint. Sesamoid fractures will often occur with turf toe injuries.
    - Despite the relatively small anatomic area in which these injuries are manifested, they can lead to significant functional deficits in some cases making it very difficult to walk, much less run or play sports. Turf toe injuries have ended professional athletes' careers.
    - Turf toe injuries will typically require surgical treatment; what is done depends on what is injured. In general, although not always, the plantar plate is torn off the phalanx. Surgery thus consists of repair with possible augmentation with the abductor tendon.
    - Traumatic hallux valgus is a similar injury in which the capsular insufficiency is more medial than plantar. In this setting, a median eminence resection and adductor tenotomy can accompany soft tissue repair.

SELECTED REFERENCES

1. Vulcano E et al: Long-term follow-up of capsular interposition arthroplasty for hallux rigidus. Foot Ankle Int. 39(1):1-5, 2018

2. Baumhauer JF et al: Correlation of hallux rigidus grade with motion, VAS pain, intraoperative cartilage loss, and treatment success for first MTP joint arthrodesis and synthetic cartilage implant. Foot Ankle Int. 38(11):1175-1182, 2017

3. Covell DJ et al: Operative treatment of traumatic hallux valgus in elite athletes. Foot Ankle Int. 38(6):590-595, 2017

4. Daniels TR et al: Midterm outcomes of polyvinyl alcohol hydrogel hemiarthroplasty of the first metatarsophalangeal joint in advanced hallux rigidus. Foot Ankle Int. 38(3):243-247, 2017

5. Glazebrook M et al: Treatment of first metatarsophalangeal joint arthritis using hemiarthroplasty with a synthetic cartilage implant or arthrodesis: a comparison of operative and recovery time. Foot Ankle Surg. ePub, 2017

6. Goldberg A et al: Association between patient factors and outcome of synthetic cartilage implant hemiarthroplasty vs. first metatarsophalangeal joint arthrodesis in advanced hallux rigidus. Foot Ankle Int. 38(11):1199-1206, 2017

7. Nixon DC et al: Hallux rigidus grade does not correlate with foot and ankle ability measure score. J Am Acad Orthop Surg. 25(9):648-653, 2017

8. Baumhauer JF et al: Prospective, randomized, multi-centered clinical trial assessing safety and efficacy of a synthetic cartilage implant versus first metatarsophalangeal arthrodesis in advanced hallux rigidus. Foot Ankle Int. 37(5):457-69, 2016

9. Chraim M et al: Long-term outcome of first metatarsophalangeal joint fusion in the treatment of severe hallux rigidus. Int Orthop. 40(11):2401-2408, 2016

10. Kim PH et al: Moberg osteotomy shifts contact pressure plantarly in the first metatarsophalangeal joint in a biomechanical model. Foot Ankle Int. 37(1):96-101, 2016

11. Korim MT et al: Effect of pathology on union of first metatarsophalangeal joint arthrodesis. Foot Ankle Int. 36(1):51-4, 2015

12. Perez-Aznar A et al: Dorsal wedge phalangeal osteotomy for grade II-III hallux rigidus in active adult patients. Foot Ankle Int. 36(2):188-96, 2015

13. Greisberg J: The failed first metatarsophalangeal joint implant arthroplasty. Foot Ankle Clin. 19(3):343-8, 2014

14. Bussewitz BW et al: Intermediate-term results following first metatarsal cheilectomy. Foot Ankle Spec. 6(3):191-5, 2013

15. McNeil DS et al: Evidence-based analysis of the efficacy for operative treatment of hallux rigidus. Foot Ankle Int. 34(1):15-32, 2013

16. O'Malley MJ et al: Treatment of advanced stages of hallux rigidus with cheilectomy and phalangeal osteotomy. J Bone Joint Surg Am. 95(7):606-10, 2013

17. Deland JT et al: Surgical management of hallux rigidus. J Am Acad Orthop Surg. 20(6):347-58, 2012

18. Kim YS et al: Clinical comparison of the osteochondral autograft transfer system and subchondral drilling in osteochondral defects of the first metatarsal head. Am J Sports Med. 40(8):1824-33, 2012

19. McCormick JJ et al: Turf toe: anatomy, diagnosis, and treatment. Sports Health. 2(6):487-94, 2010

20. van Doeselaar DJ et al: Foot function after fusion of the first metatarsophalangeal joint. Foot Ankle Int. 31(8):670-5, 2010

21. Beeson P et al: Hallux rigidus: a cross-sectional study to evaluate clinical parameters. Foot (Edinb). 19(2):80-92, 2009

22. Calvo A et al: The importance of the length of the first metatarsal and the proximal phalanx of hallux in the etiopathogeny of the hallux rigidus. Foot Ankle Surg. 15(2):69-74, 2009

23. Brodsky JW et al: Prospective gait analysis in patients with first metatarsophalangeal joint arthrodesis for hallux rigidus. Foot Ankle Int. 28(2):162-5, 2007

24. Mahiquez MY et al: Positive hindfoot valgus and osteoarthritis of the first metatarsophalangeal joint. Foot Ankle Int. 27(12):1055-9, 2006

25. Coughlin MJ et al: Hallux rigidus: demographics, etiology, and radiographic assessment. Foot Ankle Int. 24(10):731-43, 2003

26. Smith RW et al: Outcomes in hallux rigidus patients treated nonoperatively: a long-term follow-up study. Foot Ankle Int. 21(11):906-13, 2000

27. Anderson RJ: Hallux rigidus and atrophy of calf muscles. N Engl J Med. 340(14):1123, 1999

28. Horton GA et al: Role of metatarsus primus elevatus in the pathogenesis of hallux rigidus. Foot Ankle Int. 20(12):777-80, 1999

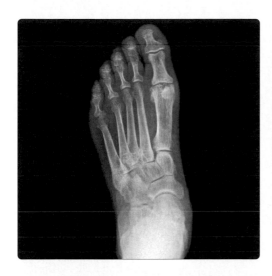

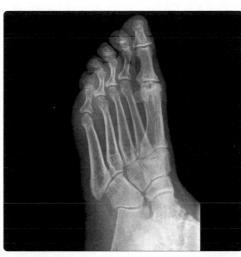

(Left) *Radiograph shows an atypical hallux rigidus with loss of bony integrity in the central aspect of the joint as seen on preoperative images. This patient had collapse of the subchondral bone in the central metatarsal.* **(Right)** *The collapse of the subchondral bone is seen clearly here. The patient's onset of symptoms was somewhat acute, and the pain was debilitating for him.*

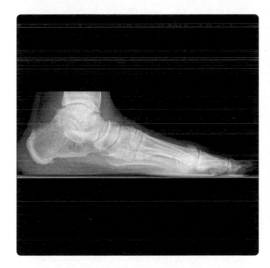

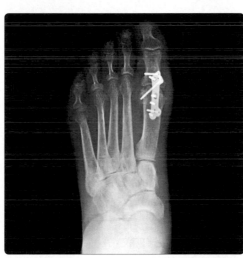

(Left) *The dorsal osteophyte in this case is relatively underwhelming. This patient had only minimal complaints of pain from rubbing of the osteophyte. He did, however, have pain with virtually any motion of the metatarsophalangeal joint.* **(Right)** *The patient underwent successful 1st metatarsophalangeal fusion. Cup and cone reamers were used to denude any remaining cartilage. Compression was achieved through the plate.*

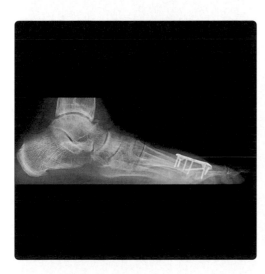

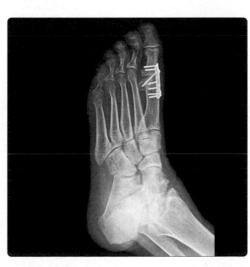

(Left) *Lateral view shows optimal positioning of the 1st metatarsophalangeal fusion with ~ 20-30° of the dorsiflexion of the phalanx on the metatarsal head. The patient's fusion healed uneventfully.* **(Right)** *This oblique image shows healing of the arthrodesis site. The patient had complete resolution of his pain, and he has been able to get back into baseline activities without limitation.*

(Left) *A 62-year-old female patient with severe hallux rigidus is shown, although the principle feature that bothered her was her large dorsal osteophyte. Severe loss of joint space is seen.*
(Right) *Large dorsal osteophyte at the 1st metatarsophalangeal joint is shown; the patient's pain was much more related to that than any arthritic pain, and her pain had progressed to the point that she felt limited in terms of activity.*

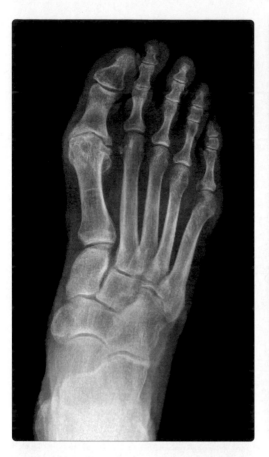
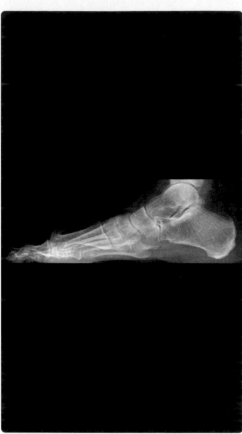

(Left) *Six months out from surgery, it appears that the radiographic arthritis has, if anything, progressed, although the patient's symptoms were much improved after surgery.*
(Right) *The dorsal osteophyte has been resected. Despite the possible radiographic progression of the disease, the patient was symptomatically much improved.*

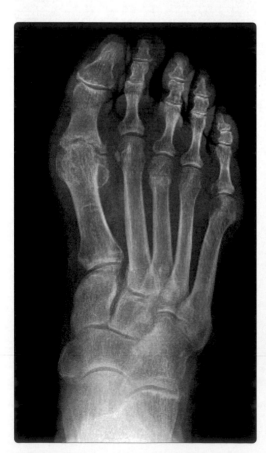
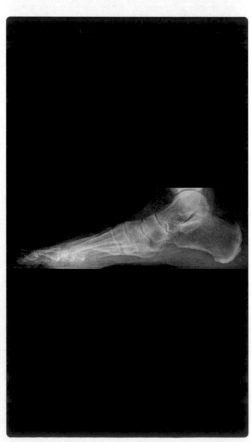

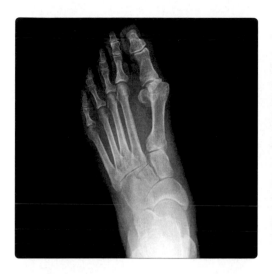

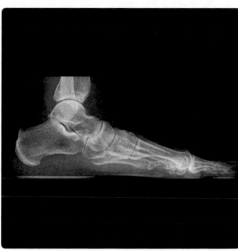

(Left) *A 52-year-old female patient with an arthritic bunion whose symptoms were much more referable to her hallux valgus than the rigidus is shown. We went over fusion as a potentially more predictable option, although she did not want a fusion. She elected to have more of a hallux valgus procedure coupled with a cheilectomy.* **(Right)** *Note the dorsal osteophyte at the 1st metatarsophalangeal joint, consistent with her hallux rigidus. The dorsal osteophyte only gave her mild pain.*

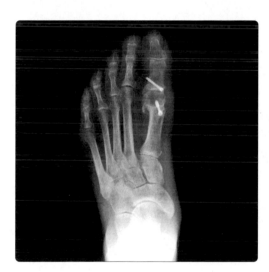

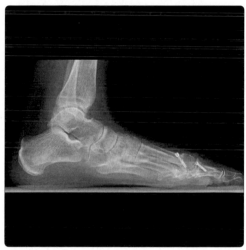

(Left) *Eight months status post distal metatarsal osteotomy, Akin, and cheilectomy, patient was much improved from a pain perspective and able to be more active.* **(Right)** *A thorough understanding of a patient's pain generators will help in surgical decision-making. The patient needs to understand what can be made better with an operation, and, if a definitive procedure is not chosen, the patient must understand the possible risk of progression.*

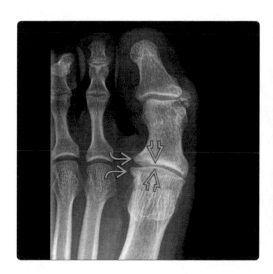

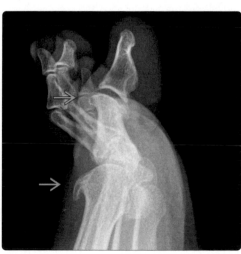

(Left) *Early hallux rigidus with some posttraumatic changes at the interphalangeal joint is shown. Note the joint space narrowing ⇨ and osteophytes ⇨ with some mild subchondral sclerosis.* **(Right)** *Dorsal osteophytes ⇨ at both the metatarsophalangeal and interphalangeal joints are shown. The metatarsophalangeal joint pathology was hallux rigidus, while the interphalangeal joint pathology was posttraumatic.*

(Left) *A 67-year-old female patient with longstanding big toe and 2nd toe pain is shown. She had arthritic pain in the 1st metatarsophalangeal joint and pain at the 2nd metatarsophalangeal joint as well as where the 1st and 2nd toes overlap.* **(Right)** *Patient underwent implant arthroplasty of the 1st metatarsophalangeal with Akin osteotomy and 2nd toe plantar condylectomy with hammer toe correction.*

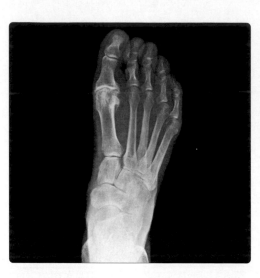 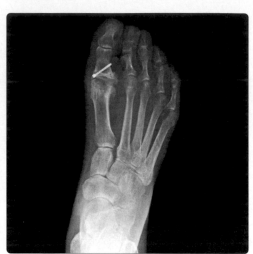

(Left) *The dorsal osteophyte is seen at the 1st metatarsophalangeal, as is the 2nd hammer toe. The patient had pain in both areas, and neither was dominant.* **(Right)** *The patient's pain was much improved at both the 1st and 2nd toes. Moreover, she was able to retain some motion at the 1st metatarsophalangeal joint.*

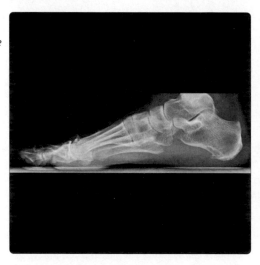 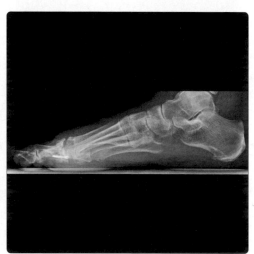

(Left) *Oblique image allows for a further look at the degree of arthrosis in the 1st metatarsophalangeal joint, while the lesser metatarsals appear ostensibly normal.* **(Right)** *Postoperative oblique image does show the implant a little more thoroughly at the 1st metatarsophalangeal joint. This non-weight-bearing image is less helpful for assessment of alignment and toe position.*

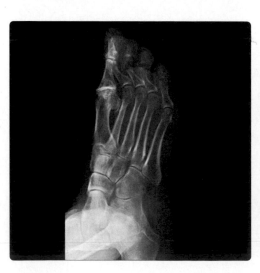 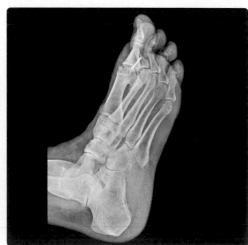

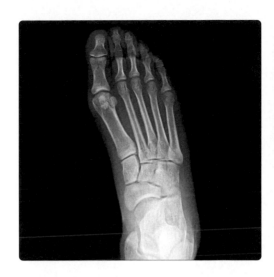

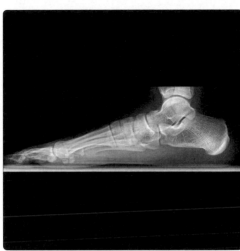

(Left) *A 20-year-old collegiate track athlete with plantar pain about the 1st metatarsophalangeal joint refractory to nonoperative treatment is shown.* **(Right)** *Note the bipartite medial sesamoid. Bipartite sesamoids tend to have well-corticated edges, as opposed to acute injuries, which are often more jagged. Sesamoiditis can occur in radiographically normal or bipartite sesamoids.*

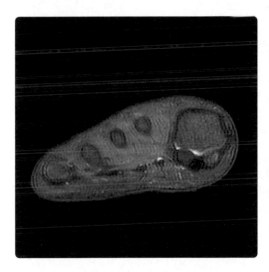

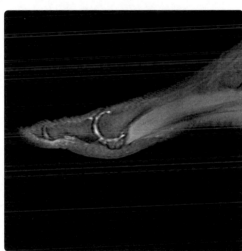

(Left) *Moderate signal in the medial sesamoid is shown on this coronal image. The patient had tried months of nonoperative treatment without success, and she ultimately elected to have sesamoidectomy.* **(Right)** *Mild signal in the medial sesamoid is shown once again.*

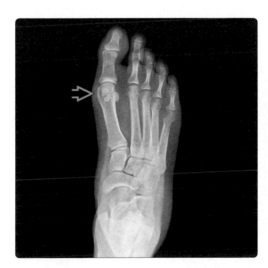

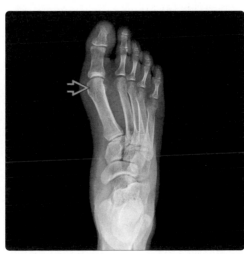

(Left) *A 69-year-old male patient that had no history of trauma to the big toe presented with several months of big toe pain refractory to nonoperative treatment. Radiograph shows a bipartite medial sesamoid ⬅. He elected to undergo sesamoidectomy with resolution of symptoms.* **(Right)** *The medial sesamoid has been removed ⬅. After the sesamoid is removed, the surgeon should be careful to find and assess the flexor hallucis longus tendon to make sure that it has not been injured during the surgery.*

(Left) *Severe forefoot deformity in a 73-year-old patient with rheumatoid arthritis is shown. Given the relatively new disease-modifying antirheumatic drugs, the rheumatoid forefoot is generally less common than it has been historically.* **(Right)** *The deformity in these feet can be dramatic with severe hammer toes and overlapping of toes, along with severe hallux valgus. Patients are often very limited in shoewear as a result.*

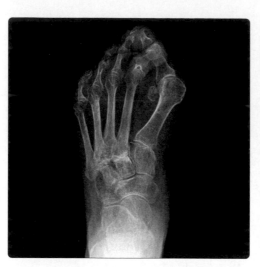
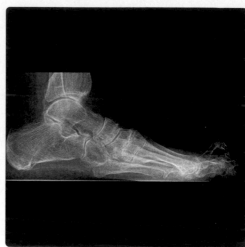

(Left) *Patient underwent 1st metatarsophalangeal fusion with lesser metatarsal head resections, seen here at 6 months doing clinically well. Patients are often very happy with the clinical results, as a very abnormal foot preoperatively often looks much more normal postoperatively.* **(Right)** *The hammer toes have been straightened out, and the foot appears much more normal.*

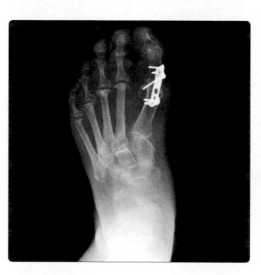
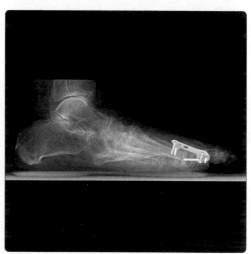

(Left) *A 68-year-old female patient with rheumatoid arthritis with longstanding foot deformity and pain is shown. Once again, note the hallux valgus with arthritis in the great toe. Moreover, the lesser toes are all crossing over.* **(Right)** *Patient 6 months out from rheumatoid forefoot correction is shown. Patient was comfortably able to wear shoes that had been difficult for her prior to surgery, and she was very pleased with the appearance of her foot.*

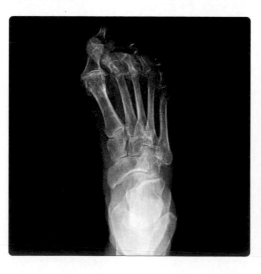
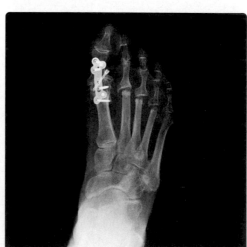

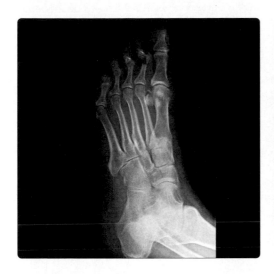

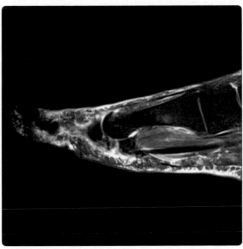

(Left) *Turf toe injury is shown. Note the medial and lateral sesamoid fracture. These are devastating injuries that seem trivial but can lead to significant functional limitation, as the toe often ends up quite stiff.* **(Right)** *Medial sesamoid fracture is shown. Often, the entire plantar stabilizing mechanism of the toe is disrupted. Most often, the disruption is off the phalanx, although in this case, the sesamoids were fractured.*

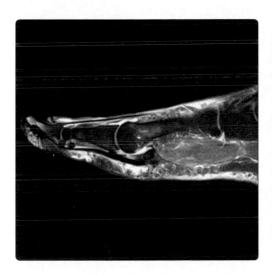

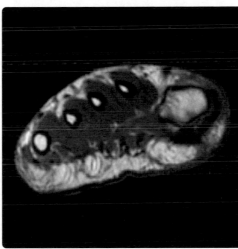

(Left) *Soft tissue disruption of the lateral plantar capsule is shown. Once again, the severe degree of injury to the plantar structures is apparent here.* **(Right)** *A 45-year-old female patient presented with pain that mimicked sesamoiditis, although MR was concerning for an osteochondral defect of the plantar surface of the 1st metatarsal head.*

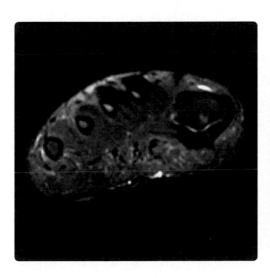

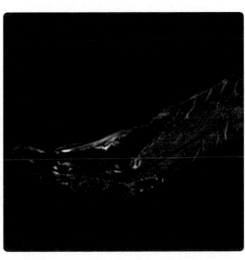

(Left) *T2 MR shows some bony edema in the area of abnormality on the T1, possibly consistent with an osteochondral lesion of the inferior metatarsal head.* **(Right)** *At the time of surgery, the osteochondral defect was confirmed, and a debridement with microfracture was performed. These lesions can mimic the symptoms of sesamoiditis, although they are a distinct pathology.*

KEY FACTS

- An interdependent system of dynamic, static, and bony restraints is responsible for the maintenance of normal toe alignment and stability.
- Given the relatively small size of the lesser toes in proportion to the relatively large repetitive stresses they experience during normal gait, failure of 1 of these restraints can lead to a domino-like failure of the others, leading to deformity and dysfunction.
- Optimal treatment of lesser toe deformities necessitates not only examining the presenting deformities but also understanding the problems of etiology and contributing mechanical factors to determine the most appropriate nonoperative or operative treatment.
- To further complicate treatment of toe problems, many systemic conditions, most notably peripheral vascular disease and peripheral neuropathy, will often first manifest themselves in the feet and toes, adding the consideration of nonmechanical sources of foot pain to the physician's differential diagnosis.

- These systemic conditions, as well as the foot's dependent nature, can produce challenges in treatment of these disorders, in that vascular embarrassment and healing difficulties can accompany toe surgery, adding importance to understanding optimal nonoperative treatment modalities.
- Toe surgery, while often correcting the underlying deformity, has limitations and can lead to stiffness, prolonged and sometimes permanent swelling, and scar formation.
- These complications, while usually well tolerated by patients, necessitate thorough understanding and realistic expectations by both the physician and the patient in order to maximize both the perceived and objective surgical outcomes.

(Left) *This is a cartoon of a mallet toe; note that the distal interphalangeal (DIP) joint is the only joint with deformity, while the proximal interphalangeal (PIP) and metatarsophalangeal (MTP) joints are relatively normal.* **(Right)** *A hammer toe deformity is shown. Note the flexion deformity of the PIP joint with relative extension at the DIP joint and some extension at the MTP joint.*

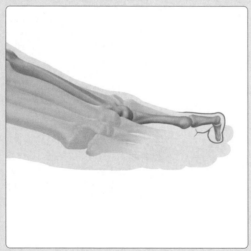 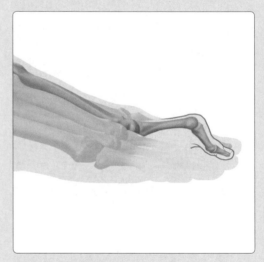

(Left) *A claw toe deformity can sometimes be difficult to differentiate from a hammer toe deformity. Both involve flexion at the PIP joint with some MTP joint extension, although a claw toe has flexion at the DIP joint.* **(Right)** *A crossover toe usually results from an MTP joint overload with failure of the plantar plate and the lateral collateral ligament, allowing dorsiflexion and medial drift of the toe. A hammer toe often accompanies the deformity.*

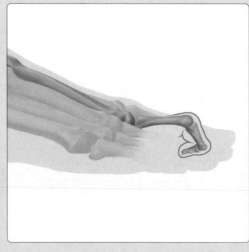 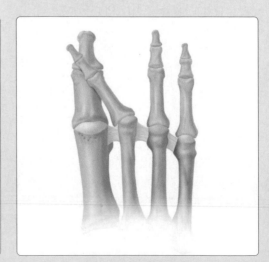

HAMMER TOES, MALLET TOES, AND CLAW TOES

Introduction

- **Hammer toes, mallet toes**, and **claw toes** are sagittal plane deformities of the lesser toes. They are common and vary from asymptomatic minor deformities to painful disabling ones. Consultation is generally sought because of shoewear difficulties or pain.

Definitions

- There is some overlap in aspects of these deformities, although currently agreed definitions for these deformities is discussed in this chapter. The terms **hammer toe** and **claw toe** are used somewhat interchangeably.
- **Mallet toe deformity** is generally defined as a flexion deformity at the distal interphalangeal (DIP) joint of the toe. Mallet toes often involve the longest lesser toe.
- **Hammer toe deformity** is defined as primarily a flexion deformity at the proximal interphalangeal (PIP) joint sometimes accompanied by a metatarsophalangeal (MTP) joint extension deformity. A hammer toe may involve several toes or just 1 toe and most commonly has a mechanical cause.
- **A crossover toe deformity** is likely an extension of a hammer toe deformity. However, a hammer toe is a purely sagittal plane deformity, while a crossover toe has a sagittal plane deformity as well as an axial plane deformity.
- **A claw toe deformity** is defined as a toe where the primary deformity is a hyperextension deformity at the MTP joint. There is often a PIP joint flexion deformity as in hammer toes, although claw toes commonly will have a DIP joint flexion deformity. Claw toes will more commonly be neurologic in nature (e.g., Charcot-Marie Tooth) and more commonly involve several toes.
- All the toe deformities are further classified as "rigid" or "flexible" deformities, depending on whether the deformity is passively correctable.

Anatomy

- The primary static restraints of the toe are the thick plantar plate, plantar aponeurosis, joint capsule, and collateral ligaments. These structures allow the DIP joint and PIP joint to flex but block extension past neutral while they allow the MTP joint to flex and extend during the normal gait cycle.
- The dynamic stabilizers of the toes can be divided into intrinsic (originating in the foot) and extrinsic (originating in the leg) muscles. The tibial nerve innervates all the intrinsic muscles as well as the extrinsic flexor muscles, while the peroneal nerve innervates the extrinsic extensor muscles.
- The extrinsic muscles terminating at the lesser toes are the extensor digitorum longus (EDL) and flexor digitorum longus (FDL). The intrinsic muscles terminating at the lesser toes comprise the 7 interosseus muscles, 4 lumbricals, and abductor digiti minimi as well as the extensor digitorum brevis (EDB) and flexor digitorum brevis (FDB).

Extrinsic Muscles

- The EDL runs over the dorsal aspect of the MTP joint and invests the extensor hood over the proximal phalanx before inserting on both the middle and distal phalanx.
- The EDL is a strong extensor at the MTP joint through its attachments at the extensor hood. However, it can extend the PIP and DIP joints only when the intrinsic muscles hold the proximal phalanx in a neutral or flexed position at the MTP joint.
- The FDL runs under the metatarsal head dorsal to the FDB and inserts on the distal phalanx. As a result of having no direct connection to the proximal phalanx, the FDL serves as a strong flexor of the DIP joint but is a weak flexor of the MTP joint.

Intrinsic Muscles

- The EDB is an intrinsic muscle that sends a slip to the 2nd, 3rd, and 4th toes. The EDB tendon inserts into the lateral aspect of the EDL tendon and weakly extends the PIP joint.
- The FDB runs plantar to the FDL tendon through most of its course, splitting into 2 terminal slips at the level of the proximal phalanx, and traveling over either side of the FDL before inserting on the middle phalanx. The FDB is a weak flexor of the MTP joint.
- The 4 lumbricals originate from the FDL tendon, run under the intermetatarsal ligament, and insert on the tibial side of the plantar plate and the extensor hood at the level of the MTP joint. They are strong flexors of the MTP joint when the joint is in neutral but quickly lose their mechanical advantage as the joint is extended.
- Prior to inserting on the extensor hood, the 7 interosseus muscles of the foot, 4 dorsal and 3 plantar, run dorsal to the intermetatarsal ligament but plantar to the axis of rotation of the metatarsal head when the toe is in a neutral position. As the MTP joint dorsiflexes, the tendons of the interossei will travel dorsally with the extensor hood closer to the axis of rotation of the joint and then eventually dorsal to the axis of rotation, converting them from flexors to extensors of the joint.

Flexion and Extension Forces at Joints

- At the DIP joint, the FDL provides a strong flexion force, while the EDL provides a relatively weak extension force, and then only if the intrinsic muscles are able to hold the proximal phalanx in a neutral alignment.
- At the PIP joint, the FDL provides weak flexion, while the FDB provides strong flexion through its direct insertion on the middle phalanx. As at the DIP joint, the EDL provides a relatively weak extension force if the intrinsic muscles are able to hold the proximal phalanx in a neutral alignment.
- At the MTP joint, the EDL is a strong extensor. The FDL and FDB, with no direct insertions on the proximal phalanx, provide weak flexion power, while the lumbricals and the interossei provide the majority of the flexion power to oppose the EDL.
- The strong pull of the intrinsic muscles is dependent on the position of the proximal phalanx. With MTP joint extension, the flexion power is greatly diminished, as the interossei muscles become extensors of the joint, as their mobile tendons travel dorsally, and the lumbrical muscles lose their mechanical advantage.

Pathophysiology

- A **mallet toe** is a flexion deformity at the DIP joint. Through trauma or impingement of tight shoes, the EDL tendon at the DIP joint attenuates or ruptures, creating a strong unopposed flexion by the FDL tendon at the DIP joint.

- A **hammer toe** (a flexion deformity at the PIP joint) is thought to occur as the result of impingement of the end of the toe against the shoe or MTP joint synovitis causing the MTP joint to dorsiflex. This results in the FDB and FDL strongly flexing the PIP joint without the EDL being able to oppose the flexion, as it can extend the joint only when the proximal phalanx is neutrally aligned.
- A **claw toe** is notable for dorsiflexion deformity at the MTP joint and flexion deformity at the PIP joint and DIP joint. It often involves more than 1 toe and has a neurologic origin. It develops as the extrinsic muscles overpower the intrinsic muscles of the foot; the EDL overpowers the lumbrical and interossei muscles, creating dorsiflexion at the MTP joint. As the dorsiflexion deformity increases, the lumbricals lose their ability to flex the MTP joint. The interossei tendons pass dorsal to the axis of rotation of the MTP joint and function as extensors, leaving the FDL and FDB overwhelmed by the EDL extension force at the MTP joint, resulting in MTP joint extension deformity. With the resultant MTP dorsiflexion deformity, the FDL and FDB flex the PIP joint, and the FDL flexes the DIP joint without the counterbalancing extension by the EDL, which cannot extend these joints with the MTP joint dorsiflexed.

Evaluation

- A history should elicit as precisely as possible the patients' problem, as they see it. If they are complaining primarily of pain, the exact location as well as the degree and frequency of discomfort should be recorded.
- The shoewear requirements for the patient's occupation as well as the patient's shoewear desires are important to understand, as successful nonoperative treatment will usually require shoewear modification.
- Lesser toe deformities usually present with toe complaints in 1 of 3 areas: The tip of the toe, the dorsal aspect of the PIP joint, or under the foot at the MTP joint. These areas should be evaluated for evidence of callus or corn formation.
  - The pain at the tip of the toe results from the shoe rubbing on the toe or the relatively unpadded toe tip resting on the ground or grabbing the ground as the patients walk.
  - The PIP joint pain occurs from the shoes rubbing on the toe box.
  - Pain at the metatarsal head occurs as the proximal phalanx dorsiflexes on the metatarsal head, increasing the plantar pressures on the metatarsal head. In addition, as the proximal phalanx dorsiflexes, it takes the plantar fat pad with it, relatively uncovering the metatarsal head.
- Checking the ankle range of motion and strength is an important part of the examination. Equinus deformity or weakness of the anterior tibial muscle will result in the recruitment and compensatory overpull of the EDL tendon, potentially leading to a claw toe deformity.
- The **push-up test** involves passively pushing up under the metatarsal heads on the non-weight-bearing foot until the ankle is brought to neutral. In the case of a flexible toe deformity, the toes should correct to a neutral alignment, whereas in a rigid deformity, they will not.

Nonoperative Treatment

- Most lesser toe deformity problems will improve with the general recommendation of shoewear modification, specifically switching to a shoe with a wider &/or higher toe box.
- Other nonoperative treatments target the specific area of discomfort. Pain under the metatarsal heads can be improved with a metatarsal pad.
- PIP joint discomfort can be treated with various toe pads or a Budin splint to try to hold the dorsally prominent PIP joint down.
- Discomfort at the tip of the toe can often be improved with a soft toe cap or a toe crest that fits under the toes and helps relieve the pressure on the tip of the toe.
- As a rule, most flexible toe deformities tend to respond much better to conservative care than do rigid deformities.

Operative Treatment

- The number 1 predictor of patient satisfaction **after** toe surgery is realistic **preoperative** expectations. Toe surgery will generally lead to a toe that is shorter and more swollen with less motion and less volitional control. This is the surgical trade-off for a toe that is less painful, straighter, and "shoeable." The toe is not "normal."
- Toe surgery also carries significant neurovascular risk, especially if the patient has peripheral vascular disease, has had previous toe surgery, or is in need of an extensive toe procedure. A common complication of surgery is some recurrence of deformity.
- **Mallet toe**
  - A **flexible mallet toe** is generally treated with a simple flexor tenotomy from a plantar approach with pinning of the DIP joint for 3 weeks.
  - A **fixed mallet toe deformity** is generally treated with a DIP joint resection followed by pinning of the DIP joint for 6 weeks ± a flexor tenotomy, depending on the degree of correction obtained with the bony resection.
- **Hammer toe**
  - A **flexible hammer toe deformity** can be treated with a flexor to extensor tendon transfer. The FDL tendon is released from its insertion at the distal phalanx through a plantar approach. The tendon is then split in 2 and passed dorsally at the level of the proximal phalanx. The 2 limbs are reunited on the dorsal aspect of the toe and secured to the EDL. This FDL transfer removes the deforming flexion force of the FDL tendon at the DIP joint and PIP joint and establishes a secure attachment of the FDL to the proximal phalanx, making the FDL a strong flexor at the MTP joint.
  - A **fixed hammer toe deformity** is treated with a dorsal approach to the PIP joint with resection of the PIP joint and pinning of the toe for 6 weeks.
- **Claw toe**
  - A **flexible claw toe deformity** is generally treated similarly to a flexible hammer toe deformity with a flexor to extensor tendon transfer.

- o A **fixed claw toe deformity** is generally treated in a stepwise fashion from proximal to distal, attempting to correct the deformity. The MTP deformity is addressed with an EDL Z-lengthening and EDB tenotomy. If the deformity remains, sequentially the MTP joint capsule is released, followed by the dorsal 1/3 of the medial and lateral collateral ligaments. Further correction may necessitate a metatarsal shortening osteotomy. The **fixed claw toe deformity** at the PIP joint is treated with a PIP joint resection similar to a fixed hammer toe deformity.

2ND METATARSOPHALANGEAL JOINT INSTABILITY

Introduction

- Second MTP joint instability is a painful condition typically arising from a progressive failure of the restraints to dorsal translation of the phalanx on the metatarsal at the MTP joint.
- Although acute rupture of the plantar plate can cause spontaneous 2nd MTP joint instability, the more common situation is gradual attenuation of the plantar plate as the result of mechanical overload. This subluxation during the toe-off portion of gait causes synovitis, which can lead to significant pain and functional limitation.
- Predisposing factors include a relatively long 2nd metatarsal, hypermobile 1st ray, equinus deformity, hallux rigidus, and hammer and claw toe deformities, which can all lead to increases in 2nd MTP joint pressure and begin the cycle of synovitis, static restraint compromise, and joint subluxation.

Anatomy and Pathophysiology

- The 2nd proximal phalanx is firmly attached to the metatarsal through a thick plantar plate as well as medial and lateral collateral ligaments. The plantar plate, along with the collateral ligaments, acts to block dorsal translation of the MTP joint as it is loaded.
- As the 2nd MTP joint is mechanically stressed, the synovium of the joint becomes inflamed. The synovitis erodes the collateral ligaments and plantar plate. As the static restraints of the toe are weakened, the toe will begin to sublux to a greater degree with less force exerted on it. At the MTP joint, the increased subluxation will mechanically make it difficult for the dynamic restraints (FDL, FDB, intrinsic muscles, and lumbricals) to resist subluxation of the toe.
- As the toe continues to sublux with gait, the synovitis within the joint will increase, and the static supports will be further compromised, causing the toe to drift up with the subsequent development of a flexible and then fixed hammer toe deformity. As the collateral ligaments attenuate, medial deviation may develop as well (crossover toe deformity).

Evaluation

- Pain is typically activity related and can be significant. A history of shooting pain into the toes or burning in the forefoot may indicate a traction neuritis but may also indicate the existence of a neuroma, which can accompany this condition.
- Acute 2nd MTP joint instability will present with a patient giving the history of a "pop" in their foot. The pop will be accompanied by swelling and pain in the area of the 2nd MTP joint.
- Inspection should focus on the presence of any deformity, swelling, and bruising. Occasionally, a separation of the 2nd and 3rd toes can be seen, indicating 2nd MTP joint synovitis and chronic forefoot overload.
- The areas of maximal tenderness should be sought; metatarsalgia pain will often be directly underneath the metatarsal head, whereas neuroma pain will typically be a little more distal and in the webspace. It can sometimes be difficult to clinically differentiate these 2 pathologies on clinical exam. Range of motion of the MTP joints, ankle joint, and 1st MTP joint is important. Restricted range of motion of the ankle joint will lead to increased forefoot pressures, most commonly in the 2nd MTP joint. The presence of an equinus contracture should be sought.
- The drawer test is specific for metatarsalgia; the foot is held stable with one hand, while the other exerts a dorsal pressure on the phalanx. A positive test will typically have increased superior translation as well as causing the patient significant pain.
- Radiographs should be reviewed for predisposing causes of 2nd MTP joint overload: Hallux valgus, hallux rigidus, or a relatively long 2nd metatarsal.
- An MR can sometimes, but not always, differentiate metatarsalgia from an interdigital neuroma. Occasionally, a selective anesthetic injection into the MTP joint can help to differentiate the 2, although most surgeons will simply start with empiric nonoperative treatment.

Nonoperative Treatment

- Nonoperative treatment involves 2 parts: Alleviating the patient's pain and then addressing the predisposing factors that may lead to recurrence. The nonoperative treatment course is based on the severity of the symptoms. The patient should be counseled that the treatment goal is to decrease pain and that any toe deformity that has occurred to this point most likely will remain without operative care.
- Mild discomfort can be treated with splinting or taping of the toe with unloading of the metatarsal head with a metatarsal pad. Addressing the patient's equinus deformity with a daily stretching program can be initiated after the initial acute phase has resolved.

Operative Treatment

- A variety of procedures have been described, including plantar condylectomy and pinning, metatarsal osteotomy, plantar plate repair, or some combination of all these options.
- Plantar condylectomy involves removing 25-33% of the plantar metatarsal head and is often performed with extensor lengthening and possible release of the dorsal capsule and portion of the collateral ligaments. The toe is pinned for 3 weeks followed by a course of taping for another 3 weeks.

- A shortening metatarsal osteotomy is meant to take pressure off the plantar metatarsal head. A Weil-type osteotomy is made parallel to the plantar surface of the foot through the dorsal aspect of the metatarsal head or just superior to the cartilage of the metatarsal head. The toe is shortened until it falls into the normal cascade between the 1st and 3rd metatarsal heads. Pinning of the MTP joint is optional.
  - Because the plane of the osteotomy is not parallel to the plantar surface of the foot, shortening with a horizontal (Weil) osteotomy displaces the metatarsal head plantarly, and surgeons will often make a 2nd cut, taking out a wafer of bone so as to counteract this declination of the metatarsal head.
  - A metatarsal osteotomy can lead to a floating toe deformity, whereby the toe sits in a relatively elevated position. Care should be taken not to shorten the metatarsal too much.
- While most of these surgical treatments are performed in an effort to address the baseline mechanical defect, the often insufficient plantar plate can also be directly repaired so as to provide an immediate restraint to dorsal subluxation at the MTP joint. Much work has been done recently to better characterize the nature of injuries to the plantar plate and the role of plantar plate repair in the treatment of metatarsalgia.
- It is important to recognize that metatarsalgia does not exist in a vacuum and often exists as a syndrome, whereby a lax 1st tarsometatarsal joint, arthritic 1st MTP joint, or gastrocnemius equinus may play a significant role in the pathology and merit surgical correction to fully address the pathology.

BUNIONETTE DEFORMITY

Introduction

- A bunionette deformity is the rough equivalent of a hallux valgus deformity, but of the 5th toe. The lateral aspect of the 5th metatarsal head with medial drift of the 5th toe proximal phalanx results in a symptomatic protrusion on the lateral aspect of the foot.

Anatomy

- As the most lateral metatarsal, the lateral eminence of the 5th metatarsal is exposed to pressure from ill-fitting shoewear.
- The 5th toe shares similar anatomy with the other lesser toes but with 2 differences: It does not receive a slip from EDB, as do the other toes, and has an additional muscle, abductor digiti minimi, inserting on the lateral aspect of the proximal phalanx of the 5th toe. This muscle is analogous to the abductor hallucis of the great toe.

Pathophysiology

- Widening of the forefoot, secondary to hallux valgus deformity, indirectly increases pressure on the lesser 5th toe, leading to pain. A symptomatic bunionette deformity occurs from pressure on the 5th toe as a result of shoewear.

Evaluation

- A symptomatic bunionette deformity will present with pain with restrictive shoewear.

- The foot should be examined for a concomitant hallux valgus deformity. The widening of the forefoot that accompanies a hallux valgus deformity will result in an exacerbation of lateral eminence pressure with shoewear.
- Strictly speaking, a bunionette deformity refers to the hyperkeratosis or bursitis that occurs over the lateral eminence of the 5th metatarsal, but occasionally, an intractable plantar keratosis (IPK) may accompany the bunionette deformity, typically in the cavovarus foot.
- There are 2 radiographic parameters that are useful in bunionette evaluation: The 4th-5th intermetatarsal angle (IMA) (abnormal > 8°) and the 5th MTP angle (normal < 10°).

Nonoperative Treatment

- The mainstay of bunionette treatment is shoe modification. A wider toe box should be recommended to help accommodate the bunionette. A metatarsal pad or an orthosis may be helpful to relieve pain from a plantar 5th metatarsal keratosis.

Operative Treatment

- In the author's experience, surgical treatment of bunionette deformities is not commonly needed. Operative treatments for bunionette deformities are generally predicated on the specific deformity of the 5th metatarsal and whether a plantar keratosis accompanies the deformity. Generally speaking, bunionettes with a prominent lateral eminence can be treated with resection of the lateral eminence and capsular repair. If there is lateral bowing of the metatarsal or an increased 4-5 IMA, then a metatarsal osteotomy can be considered. Distal and shaft osteotomies have been described, although the proximal metatarsal should be avoided.
- A plantar keratosis under the 5th metatarsal often accompanies bunionette deformity. The keratosis indicates an overly prominent metatarsal head fibular condyle or a varus foot posture. It is recommended that this keratosis be addressed at the time of surgery either with a plantar condylectomy or with an elevation component to the metatarsal osteotomy.
- As with hallux valgus surgery, bunionette surgery complications include recurrence, incomplete relief of pain, painful scars, and MTP joint subluxation. As with hallux valgus surgery, returning to tight or ill-fitting shoewear should be strongly discouraged.

FREIBERG INFRACTION

Introduction

- Freiberg infraction is an osteochondrosis of the lesser metatarsal head. It is thought to result from a vascular insult to the subchondral bone and is most commonly seen in the 2nd metatarsal but can also occur in the 3rd or 4th. It typically occurs in younger females, although it can occur at any age.
- This pathology initially leads to swelling and stiffness of the joint and, in its later stages, leads to various degrees of subchondral collapse and arthritic changes of the MTP joint.

Diagnostic Tests

- Radiographs are reviewed to check for degenerative changes of the MTP joint and evaluate the 2nd metatarsal length, which has been implicated as a predisposing factor in development of this condition.

- A high index of suspicion is necessary to make the diagnosis in its early stages, as Freiberg disease will often present with no significant radiographic findings. MR may be helpful in diagnosis.
- In its later stages, radiographs may demonstrate joint collapse, flattening of the metatarsal head, osteophytes, and joint narrowing.

Nonoperative Treatment

- In the early stages of Freiberg infraction, the patient will present with a stiff, swollen joint, which is painful to move. The initial treatment is centered on restricting the motion at the MTP joint and decreasing pain. During the acute inflammatory period, strapping or taping the toe to restrict dorsiflexion may be useful.
- Based on the degree of symptoms, a carbon fiber plate orthosis, metatarsal pad, rocker bar or a rigid rocker-bottom sole modification to the shoe, or even a walking boot can be used as well.

Operative Intervention

- Surgery needs to be tailored to the patient's particular symptoms, the degree of degeneration of the joint, and the area of joint involvement. The patient should be advised that progression of arthritic change of the joint may continue despite appropriate surgical care.
- If the cartilage injury is limited to the dorsal aspect of the joint, cheilectomy and debridement of the joint will help restore motion and give good symptomatic relief.
- If a larger portion of the metatarsal head is involved, but a significant plantar portion of the head is preserved, a closing wedge osteotomy through the metatarsal head and neck is recommended. This procedure dorsally rotates the portion of the head with intact cartilage so that it can articulate with the proximal phalanx.
- Metatarsal head resection should be reserved for those patients that fail less aggressive surgical options, although it is often a more definitive procedure and does alleviate pain from Frieberg. The mechanical implications for the rest of the foot from metatarsal head resection may lead to pain elsewhere.
- A synthetic cartilage implant used for hallux rigidus has been used for Freiberg. It does make sense for this indication, although there is currently limited data.

INTRACTABLE PLANTAR KERATOSIS

Introduction

- An IPK forms on the sole of the foot under the metatarsal heads as a result of pressure on the underlying skin. The mechanical pressure causes an increase in activity of the skin's keratinocytes, which produces 1 of 2 types of IPK: Discrete and diffuse.
  - **Discrete IPK** appears as small (2- to 3-mm), well-defined areas on the sole of the foot and is the result of plantar pressure exerted on the skin overlying the metatarsal head fibular condyle.
  - **Diffuse IPK** appears as relatively large areas of thickened skin, are rarely symptomatic, and are the result of the skin's response to pressure or shear forces exerted by the entire metatarsal head.

Evaluation

- Diffuse IPK will rarely be symptomatic, but the symptomatic patient will complain of pain under the metatarsal head that is worse in bare feet and better with shoewear. Discrete IPK will present with patients complaining that they feel like they are walking with a pebble in their shoe. The pain is progressive, activity related, and will often seem to be out of proportion to the size of the lesion.
- Discrete IPK can be confused with a plantar wart. A discrete IPK should appear as a 2- to 3-mm area with the skin lines coursing through it. It should be centered over the fibular condyle of a metatarsal head, and it should be painful with direct pressure but not with moderate side-to-side pinching.
- A plantar wart can appear on any area of the foot and can be of any size. After it is pared down, it will have a punctate or stippled appearance secondary to the pattern of the wart's blood vessels as they travel to the surface of the lesion. Generally, it will be tender with direct as well as side-to-side pressure.
- Multiple areas of involvement, areas of involvement other than under the metatarsal heads, and areas in which the skin lines do not travel through the "corn" suggest a wart rather than an IPK. A sesamoid view of the foot can be useful to demonstrate the relative prominence of the metatarsal heads and their corresponding fibular condyles.

Nonoperative Treatment

- Nonoperative treatment for discrete IPK involves trimming the corn and surrounding callus with a scalpel. This should lead to instant improvement in weight-bearing symptoms and will help confirm that the area is not a plantar wart.
- Patients with an IPK can use a pumice stone after showering or bathing to slowly reduce the thickness of the callus. Over-the-counter salicylic acid patches or topical liquid may be useful in softening up the corn so that the patient can more easily manually remove it. A metatarsal pad appropriately placed in the shoe proximal to the area of discomfort may help reduce pressure on the metatarsal head.

Operative Treatment

- Operative treatment is aimed at removing the underlying bony prominence and addressing the mechanical factors leading to the formation of the IPK. A discrete IPK can be treated with a plantar condylectomy. To avoid recurrence, it is important not to leave any residual bony prominences on the plantar aspect of the metatarsal head.
- A diffuse IPK is treated with a metatarsal osteotomy to unload some of the weight-bearing pressure on the metatarsal. The patient should be advised that post correction, a custom orthosis may be necessary to further compensate for pressure variations of the forefoot.

INTERDIGITAL CORNS

Introduction

- Corns are discrete areas of dense hyperkeratinization that form as the result of external pressure on the skin overlying a bony prominence. Two types of corns form on the toes: Hard corns and soft corns.

- o Hard corns commonly occur over the exposed surface of the 5th toe in response to pressure from a shoe box. Hard corns will typically form over the lateral aspect of the PIP or DIP joint of the 5th toe.
- o Soft corns form between the toes and have a unique macerated appearance because they are kept moist from opposition of the neighboring toes. Soft corns most commonly occur between the 4th and 5th toes but can occur between other toes. They are produced by the impingement of the bony prominences of adjacent toes. A tight toe box plays a role in increasing the pressure between the toes, but once the corn forms, it often becomes a self-perpetuating problem, as the hard keratin core of the corn acts as a constant mechanical irritant.

Evaluation

- The patient will often present with other forefoot complaints as well as the interdigital corns. Soft corns should be sought in diabetic patients, as they frequently represent a preulcerative state.
- The key to the physical examination is identifying the area of the corn and the bony prominences responsible for the corns. In the case of interdigital corns, the contributions of both toes to the impingement must be identified.

Nonoperative Treatment

- Nonoperative treatment begins with toe sponge spacers, silicon toe pads, or oval sponge rubber corn pads, but patients need to understand that they need a wider toe box to accommodate the toes.
- Hard corns on the outside of the 5th toe can often be treated by trimming of the corn and application of salicylic acid corn pads combined with routine callus debridement after showering or bathing with a pumice stone.
- Soft corns are best treated with removing the callus with a scalpel and then allowing the toes to dry with a wisp of lamb's wool placed between the toes to allow the moisture to wick out from between the toes. Diabetic patients and other patients who lotion their feet for dry skin should be instructed not to apply lotion between the toes.

Operative Treatment

- The chief principle of operative care for hard and soft corns is to remove the bony prominences responsible for the corn formation without trading the corn for a painful scar.
- In removing bone prominences, an incision is made dorsally, centered over the area of the corn. Full-thickness flaps are made down to the bone, and then the bony prominences are removed. The osteophytes on both adjacent toes need to be removed in line with the shaft of the toe. The goals of surgery are to create a smooth bony surface for the digit and not to overresect an area of prominence and create other areas of impingement.
- A 2nd way to address the soft corn when the corn is located at the skin fold of the web space is to perform a partial syndactylization and eliminate the area of skin irritation altogether. A partial syndactylization to the PIP joint is preferred, because it still allows a space between the toes and is fairly cosmetic.
- Complications of treatment of interdigital corns include persistent swelling (6-9 months) and recurrence, especially if the patient returns to wearing poor-fitting shoes.

SELECTED REFERENCES

1. Federer AE et al: Conservative management of metatarsalgia and lesser toe deformities. Foot Ankle Clin. 23(1):9-20, 2018
2. Frey-Ollivier S et al: Treatment of flexible lesser toe deformities. Foot Ankle Clin. 23(1):69-90, 2018
3. Irwin TA: Management of metatarsalgia and lesser toe deformities. Foot Ankle Clin. 23(1):xv-xvi, 2018
4. Mueller CM et al: Complication rates and short-term outcomes after operative hammertoe correction in older patients. Foot Ankle Int. 1071100718755472, 2018
5. Flint WW et al: Plantar plate repair for lesser metatarsophalangeal joint instability. Foot Ankle Int. 38(3):234-242, 2017
6. Phisitkul P et al: Cadaveric evaluation of dorsal intermetatarsal approach for plantar plate and lateral collateral ligament repair of the lesser metatarsophalangeal joints. Foot Ankle Int. 38(7):791-796, 2017
7. Schrier JC et al: Lesser toe PIP joint resection versus PIP joint fusion: a randomized clinical trial. Foot Ankle Int. 37(6):569-75, 2016
8. Slullitel G et al: Effect of first ray insufficiency and metatarsal index on metatarsalgia in hallux valgus. Foot Ankle Int. 37(3):300-6, 2016
9. Kramer WC et al: Hammertoe correction with k-wire fixation. Foot Ankle Int. 36(5):494-502, 2015
10. Roan LY et al: Why do lesser toes deviate laterally in hallux valgus? A radiographic study. Foot Ankle Int. 36(6):664-72, 2015
11. Dalmau-Pastor M et al: Extensor apparatus of the lesser toes: anatomy with clinical implications—topical review. Foot Ankle Int. 35(10):957-69, 2014
12. Doty JF et al: Metatarsophalangeal joint instability of the lesser toes and plantar plate deficiency. J Am Acad Orthop Surg. 22(4):235-45, 2014
13. Nery C et al: Prospective evaluation of protocol for surgical treatment of lesser MTP joint plantar plate tears. Foot Ankle Int. 35(9):876-85, 2014
14. Chalayon O et al: Role of plantar plate and surgical reconstruction techniques on static stability of lesser metatarsophalangeal joints: a biomechanical study. Foot Ankle Int. 34(10):1436-42, 2013
15. Greisberg J et al: Mobility of the first ray in various foot disorders. Foot Ankle Int. 33(1):44-9, 2012
16. Peck CN et al: Lesser metatarsophalangeal instability: presentation, management, and outcomes. Foot Ankle Int. 33(7):565-70, 2012
17. Myerson MS et al: The role of toe flexor-to-extensor transfer in correcting metatarsophalangeal joint instability of the second toe. Foot Ankle Int. 26(9):675-9, 2005
18. DiGiovanni CW et al: Isolated gastrocnemius tightness. J Bone Joint Surg Am. 84-A(6):962-70, 2002
19. Bhatia D et al: Anatomical restraints to dislocation of the second metatarsophalangeal joint and assessment of a repair technique. J Bone Joint Surg Am. 76(9):1371-5, 1994
20. Katcherian DA: Treatment of Freiberg's disease. Orthop Clin North Am. 25(1):69-81, 1994
21. Thompson FM et al: Problems of the second metatarsophalangeal joint. Orthopedics 10(1):83-9,1987

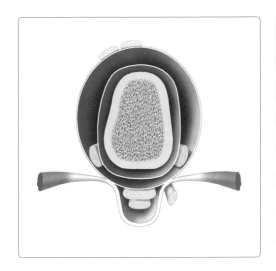

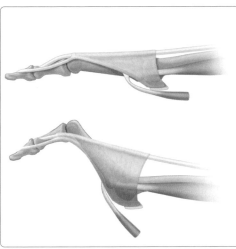

(Left) Cross section through the metatarsal head of the lesser toe is shown. Note the interossei tendons travel dorsal to the transverse metatarsal ligament, whereas the lumbrical tendon travels plantar to it. The plantar plate can be seen as the thickening of the plantar capsule. (Right) Anatomy of the intrinsic and extrinsic musculature of the normal toe (A) and in a claw toe deformity (B) is shown. The intrinsics no longer work effectively as flexors of the MTP joint when the joint is held in a relatively dorsiflexed position.

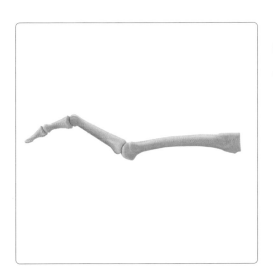

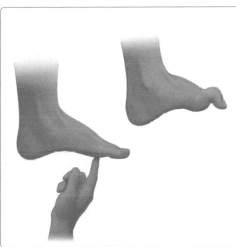

(Left) Intrinsic and extrinsic muscle forces about the lesser toe are shown. The smaller intrinsic muscles working to flex the MTP and extend the interphalangeal (IP) joints are overpowered by the extrinsic muscles, leading to MTP extension and IP flexion and a resultant hammer toe or claw toe deformity. (Right) The push-up test is used to assess the flexibility of the lesser toe deformity. Relative flexibility of the toe can also be assessed by direct palpation and manipulation of the toes themselves.

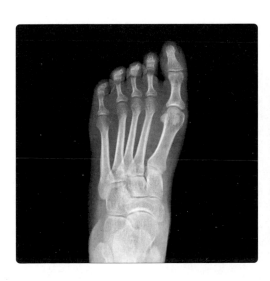

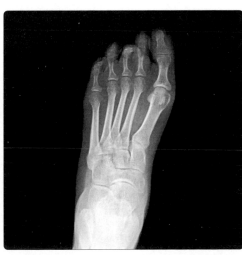

(Left) A 44-year-old female patient with flexible hammer toes at 2, 3, and 4 is shown. She was primarily symptomatic at the 2nd and 4th toes, and so she elected to have flexor-to-extensor transfers at those toes. (Right) The same patient after tendon transfer surgery with correction of deformity at the 2nd and 4th toes is shown. Although the 3rd toe did not initially bother her, she later elected to get that fixed with the same procedure.

(Left) *Treatment of a flexible hammer toe is often accomplished by a flexor-to-extensor transfer in which the flexor is divided plantarly and then sewn on top of the proximal phalanx either to itself or to the extensor.*
(Right) *The drawer test for lesser MTP instability involves holding the toe plantarly and dorsally at the proximal aspect of the proximal phalanx and pushing up on the toe. Some surgeons informally refer to it as the ceiling sign, as patients with severe instability will often have significant pain with the test.*

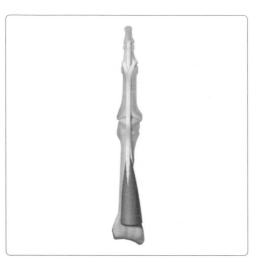
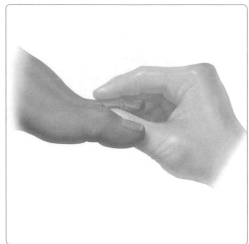

(Left) *A plantar callus in a patient with overload of the 2nd MTP joint is shown. As seen indirectly, the 2nd toe likely has some degree of hammer toe deformity. The plantar callus is indicative of relative overload of the 2nd metatarsal.* **(Right)** *Different options for 2nd metatarsal shortening osteotomies are shown. A Weil-type osteotomy has the advantage of being technically easy with high union rates. A diaphyseal osteotomy may lead to a lower rate of floating toe, although it requires a larger incision and more dissection.*

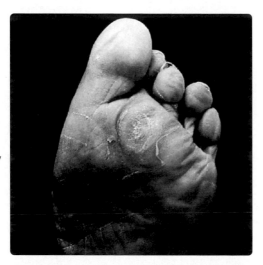
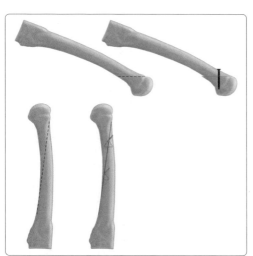

(Left) *Sagittal T2WI FS MR shows full-thickness discontinuity in the distal plantar plate with dorsal displacement of the proximal phalanx. The plantar plate should insert onto the adjacent proximal phalanx base; bone edema is present at this site. (From ExDDx: MSK.)*
(Right) *Sagittal T2WI FS MR shows full-thickness discontinuity in the distal plantar plate; it should insert onto the adjacent proximal phalanx. Plantar plate rupture was confirmed surgically. (From ExDDx: MSK.)*

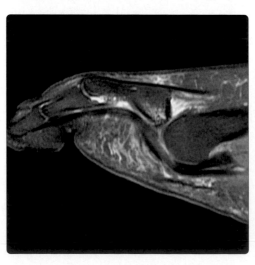
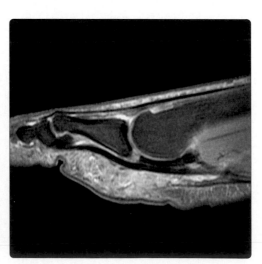

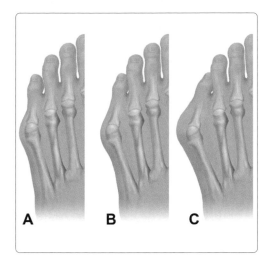

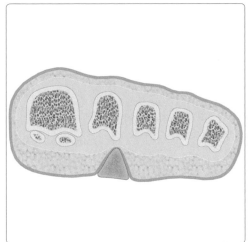

(Left) *The 3 types of bunionette deformities are shown. (A) Type 1 is associated with an enlarged lateral eminence. (B) Type 2 is associated with a lateral bowing of the diaphysis. (C) Type 3 is associated with an increase in the 4th-5th intermetatarsal angle.* **(Right)** *Graphic of a coronal cut through the foot shows a prominent fibular condyle of the metatarsal head resulting in an intractable plantar keratosis (IPK).*

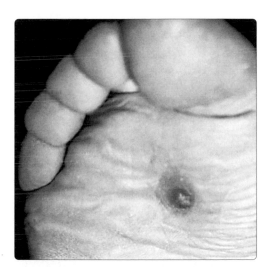

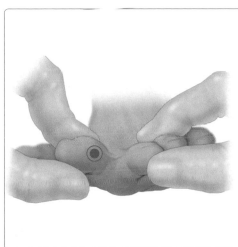

(Left) *An IPK is seen here underneath the 2nd metatarsal head. The patient had tried various means of offloading this area, all with limited success. The patient ultimately underwent excision of a prominent plantar condyle.* **(Right)** *Soft interdigital corn on the medial aspect of the small toe is shown.*

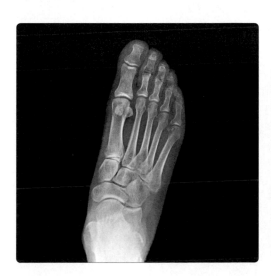

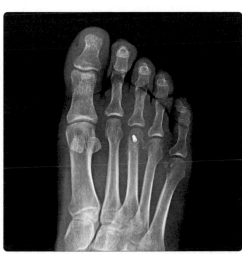

(Left) *This 55-year-old female patient had pain specifically under the 3rd metatarsal head. She had tried multiple inserts and shoe modifications with limited success in terms of alleviating her pain.* **(Right)** *She ultimately elected to undergo 3rd metatarsal plantar condylectomy with metatarsal shortening osteotomy. She ultimately had resolution of her preoperative symptoms.*

KEY FACTS

- The most common etiology of ankle arthritis is posttraumatic.
- The ankle bears the highest load per surface area of any joint in the body, yet has a small surface contact area of only 350 mm².
  - The cartilage in the ankle is thinner than in the hip and knee.
- The ankle joint is highly congruent, and its cartilage is uniform and stiff, allowing it to withstand high forces.
  - Any incongruency or loss of surface area leads to increased contact pressures and the development of arthritis.
- Pain is the most common presenting symptom and is characteristically deep in the anterior ankle or dorsal foot.
- Physical examination should include areas of skin and soft tissue condition (including calluses and scars) tenderness, alignment, range of motion, palpation of pulses, and sensory testing.

- Nonsurgical options for the treatment of ankle arthritis include activity modification, bracing, medications, and injections.
- Many surgical options for the treatment of ankle arthritis exist, including debridement, osteotomies, distraction, partial or total allograft replacement, fusion, total ankle replacement (TAR).
- Ankle fusion is considered the "gold standard" treatment for ankle arthritis.
  - Fusion results in good or excellent results in 90% of patients at long-term follow-up.
  - The late development of adjacent joint arthritis remains a problem and has been the major impetus for the development of motion-preserving techniques for treating ankle arthritis.
- TAR conserves motion at the ankle with potential, though unproven, benefits of improved gait and function and decreased incidence of adjacent joint arthritis.

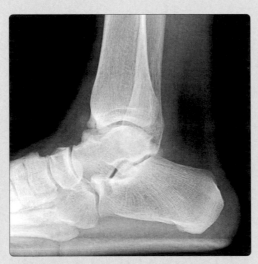
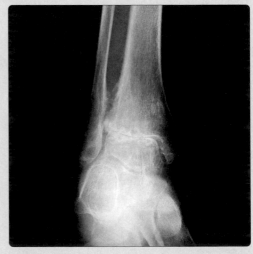

(Left) *Early ankle arthritis is shown. Anterior osteophyte with joint space preservation is a good candidate for anterior debridement.* **(Right)** *AP radiograph of end-stage ankle arthritis with joint space narrowing osteophyte formation and subchondral cysts is shown.*

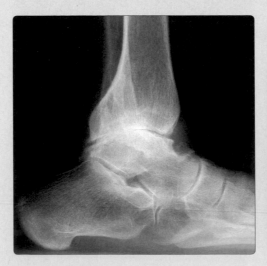
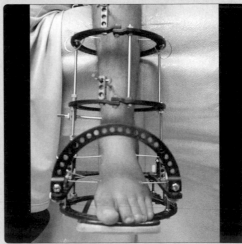

(Left) *Lateral radiograph of end-stage ankle arthritis shows joint space narrowing and anterior and posterior osteophytes and subchondral cysts.* **(Right)** *Distraction arthroplasty is shown. Photograph shows the leg in the Ilizarov external fixator frame.*

POSTTRAUMATIC

- Posttraumatic causes account for ~ 50% of ankle arthritis cases.
  - Arthritis correlates with fracture type, degree of cartilage injury, and incongruity of the articular surface.
- Radiographic evidence of arthritis is usually apparent within 2 years of injury in high-energy injuries.
  - However, in many cases it may be decades before pain becomes severe.
- Arthritis occurs after ~ 14% of ankle (malleolar) fractures.
  - Weber C (proximal) fractures have a higher rate of arthritis (33%), as do trimalleolar fractures.
  - Maintaining fibular length and reduction of the posterior malleolar fragment improve outcome.
  - Larger posterior malleolar fragments involve a greater proportion of the articular surface and accordingly result in a higher rate of arthritis.
- Unreduced syndesmotic injuries are a common cause of posttraumatic arthritis.
  - Because most Weber C injuries include syndesmotic disruption, failure to adequately reduce the syndesmosis may have accounted for the higher rate of arthritis with these injuries in the past.
  - Widening of the syndesmosis by 1 mm increases peak contact pressures in the ankle by 50%.
- Pilon fractures are a higher energy injury and often result in increased rates of cartilage injury.
  - Consequently, there is a higher rate of arthritis, avascular necrosis (AVN), and complications.
  - Soft tissue injury may also be extensive and compromise healing both in the acute setting and following future surgical procedures.
- Early range of motion may decrease the risk of arthritis, but there is little evidence to support this theory.
- Talus fractures are less common but result in rates of posttraumatic arthritis as high as 50-97%.
  - The risk of AVN is also high.
  - AVN is the cause of much of the reported arthritis after talar fractures.
  - The talus is particularly prone to AVN because of its tenuous blood supply and predominately cartilaginous surface.
- Osteochondral lesions of the talus typically do not lead to severe arthritis.
  - Although they can cause pain, they typically involve a small surface area.
  - The natural history of osteochondral lesions, whether small or large, is not well documented.

BIOLOGY OF ANKLE CARTILAGE

- The ankle bears the highest load per surface area of any joint in the body yet has a small surface contact area of only 350 mm².
- The ankle bears up to 5x the body weight with normal walking.
- The cartilage in the ankle is thinner than in the hip and knee.
  - Thickness of ankle cartilage measures 1.0-1.7 mm.
  - Thickness of hip cartilage ranges from 1.4-2.0 mm.
  - Thickness of knee cartilage ranges from 1.7-2.5 mm.
- The ankle joint is highly congruent, and its cartilage is uniform and stiff, allowing it to withstand high forces.
- In the normal situation, this congruency keeps the contact pressures at an acceptable level.
  - But if the surface area of the joint is decreased or the congruency is lost, then the pressures rise quickly, leading to arthritis.
  - This is in contrast to the knee, where slight incongruencies can be compensated for by the menisci.

EVALUATION OF ARTHRITIC ANKLE

History and Physical Examination

- Pain is the most common presenting symptom and is characteristically deep in the anterior ankle or dorsal foot.
- History should include any previous trauma or infection, history of systemic disease, such as diabetes or inflammatory arthritis, previous treatments, shoewear, use of orthotics, and tobacco use.
- Physical examination should include areas of tenderness, alignment, and range of motion.
  - Assessment of alignment of the ankle and hindfoot is particularly important.
    - The presence of severe deformity changes treatment options.
  - Most patients with severe arthritis will have lost the majority of ankle motion.
- The presence and location of calluses may point to underlying deformity or malalignment, while scars are evidence of previous trauma or surgery.
- Observation of the appearance of the soft tissues, palpation of pulses, and monofilament sensory testing provide additional information about healing potential.
  - If pulses are not palpable, vascular assessment is needed.
  - If any signs of neuropathy are found, the source of the neuropathy must be identified.
- Examination of the foot, as well as the ankle, can yield additional useful information.
  - Hindfoot flexibility, stability, and alignment should be noted.
  - Arthritis at adjacent joints may require concurrent treatment to obtain relief of symptoms.
- Gait analysis in patients with ankle arthritis typically shows decreased velocity, stride length, and cadence and more time in double-limb stance.
  - However, a formal gait analysis is generally not required in the work-up of ankle arthritis.

Imaging

- Radiographs should include weight-bearing anteroposterior, lateral, and mortise views of the ankle as well as anteroposterior, lateral, and medial oblique views of the foot.
  - Radiographs should be assessed for joint space narrowing, alignment, and bone quality.
  - The location and size of osteophytes should also be noted, especially when impingement is suspected.
  - Obtaining a weight-bearing film is critical to assess true deformity and joint space narrowing.
- Alignment should be evaluated on both sagittal and coronal views.

- A procurvatum or recurvatum deformity may be noted by examining the relationship of the tibia to the talus, which should be centrally located with its lateral process under the midline of the tibia.
  - In the coronal plane, varus-valgus alignment should be at ~ 0°, measured by the intersection of the midtibial line and the talar dome.
- Specialized views may be useful in certain patients.
  - The weight-bearing hindfoot alignment view shows coronal alignment of the hindfoot.
  - The Harris view shows axial alignment of calcaneus.
  - The Broden view shows the subtalar joint.
- Other imaging modalities are generally not needed for diagnosis and surgical planning unless diagnosis is in doubt.
  - Bone scans may identify occult arthritis, stress fracture, infection, or reflex sympathetic dystrophy.
  - Computed tomography (CT) can be used to identify a subtle syndesmosis injury and for complex fractures.
  - Magnetic resonance imaging is most useful for investigating the soft tissues, such as in cases of infection and tumor.

Other Diagnostic Modalities

- Selective diagnostic injections of local anesthetic, such as lidocaine, may be injected in the ankle and adjacent joints to determine relative contributions to symptomatology.
  - For example, pain from subtalar arthritis may be confused with ankle-related pain and may be clarified with selective injections to aid surgical planning and improve outcome.
- Laboratory data are generally not helpful in diagnosing ankle arthritis.
  - However, if there is concern for infection, complete blood count, erythrocyte sedimentation rate, and C-reactive protein are sensitive indicators.

NONSURGICAL TREATMENT

Activity Modification and Bracing

- Activity modification may minimize the pain of ankle arthritis.
  - Steps include recommending low-impact activities, such as swimming and stationary bicycle, over high-impact exercise, such as example jogging, and sedentary work over occupations that require prolonged standing.
- Weight loss may also alleviate symptoms by decreasing force across the joint and may improve results of future surgical procedures.
- A cane carried in the contralateral hand may partially offload the joint.
- Shoe modifications, orthotics, and braces can also be used to temper the pain of an arthritic ankle.
  - A shoe with a rocker sole may allow more comfortable gait by decreasing the amount of ankle motion needed.
  - A high-top shoe, boot, or lace-up ankle brace can provide some support and immobilization of the ankle.
  - An ankle-foot orthosis also immobilizes the ankle joint, improves axial alignment, and can improve gait.
  - An offloading brace that transfers load away from the ankle and to the patellar tendon and proximal tibia can be used in extreme situations.
    - However, these braces are bulky and cumbersome.

- Casting may be viewed as the ultimate brace for the ankle and offers pain relief by immobilizing the ankle joint.
  - A short leg walking cast can be used for 6 weeks to reduce inflammation and pain, although postimmobilization stiffness should be expected.

Medications

- Medications may also be used to relieve the pain and inflammation of ankle arthritis.
  - Nonsteroidal antiinflammatory drugs act by blocking cyclooxygenase to limit prostaglandin production and thus inflammation.
    - They also have a central effect, which is responsible for their analgesic action.
- Glucosamine is a building block of proteoglycans, the primary component of cartilage matrix.
  - Although data are limited and primarily addresses osteoarthritis of the knee, it has been shown to offer some pain relief to patients and result in decreased inflammation in arthritic joints.
- Glucosamine is commonly coupled with chondroitin, another cartilage matrix protein, and sold as an over-the-counter supplement in a largely unregulated fashion.
  - Quantity and bioavailability of the active agents in these preparations is largely unknown.
- Steroid injections may be used in the ankle and adjacent joints to decrease inflammation and alleviate pain.
  - The ankle joint is injected via the medial or lateral gutter with the needle directed posteriorly.
- Steroid injections have been shown to be beneficial for short-term pain reduction but are no different from placebo in the long term.
  - Repeated injections separated by several months continue to be effective in some patients but often show diminishing returns.
  - Complications include a low risk of infection and skin depigmentation.
  - There is evidence from hip and knee arthroplasty that recent steroid injection can increase the risk of infection during subsequent joint arthroplasty.
- Hyaluronic acid injections in the ankle may be helpful for pain relief, although the evidence is not strong.
- There is no clinical evidence to support the use of platelet-rich plasma injections for ankle arthritis, although that is being explored by some physicians.

SURGICAL TREATMENT

Debridement

- Debridement of the ankle, either open or arthroscopically, has been advocated for treatment of ankle arthritis in certain cases.
  - The ideal patient has a specific indication, such as hypertrophic synovium, loose body, or impinging osteophytes, with relatively preserved joint space.
  - Small chondral lesions, < 1 cm, may also be treated effectively with debridement and drilling.
  - Results of debridement in generalized arthritis with joint space narrowing or deformity are poor.
- For arthroscopic debridement, the anteromedial and anterolateral portals are used as the working portals.

- Care must be taken to avoid injuring neurovascular structures near the portal sites, particularly branches of the superficial peroneal nerve.
- Arthroscopy allows removal of loose bodies, debridement of hypertrophic synovium, drilling of osteochondral defects, and removal of impinging osteophytes.
  - However, treatment of extensive osteophyte complexes may not be possible through an arthroscopic approach and may require an anterior approach to the ankle joint.
  - Impinging bone should be removed to provide an anterior tibia to talar neck angle of > 60°.
- In one older series of 57 patients, 70% good or excellent results were achieved with arthroscopic treatment of synovitis, loose bodies, or osteophytes, compared with only 12% in patients with generalized arthritis.
  - Furthermore, 75% of these arthritic patients went on to fusion or other further surgical treatment after debridement.

Osteotomy

- After fibular fracture, if the distal fibula is not anatomically reduced, instability and resultant arthritis can occur.
  - The fibula is most often shortened and externally rotated, allowing abnormal subluxation of the talus.
  - These patients may present late, after fracture healing, with persistent pain.
- Radiographs may show decreased overlap of the distal fibula and anterior tibia on the anteroposterior view or widening of the tibiofibular clear space on the mortise view.
  - Comparing radiographs with the contralateral ankle or obtaining a CT scan of both ankles may identify subtle injuries.
- Fibular osteotomy may be indicated in these patients with fibular malunion and pain to restore fibular length and ankle stability.
  - The goal of fibular osteotomy is seating of the distal fibula into the incisura fibularis and restoration of a symmetric joint space.
  - Fibular osteotomy as an isolated procedure, however, is contraindicated when there is joint space narrowing of the ankle, indicating that extensive cartilage damage has already taken place.
- Distal tibial osteotomy may be useful in certain circumstances.
  - The tibial osteotomy is usually a medial or lateral closing wedge with internal fixation.
  - It is most useful for angular deformities with loss of joint space on the medial or lateral side of the joint.
  - With realignment, weight-bearing forces are more evenly distributed to the unaffected side of the joint.
- Short-term results of distal tibial osteotomy are generally good for the rare patient with the correct indication.
  - However, as in the knee, the surgeon should expect arthritis to slowly worsen with time.

Distraction

- Distraction arthroplasty is a possibility for a minority of patients with ankle arthritis.
  - The theory is that by distracting and offloading the joint for 3 months, symptoms will reduce, and the cartilage may actually repair itself.

- A thin-wire (Ilizarov) external fixator is placed across the ankle in distraction.
- The technique is based on data from animal studies in which immobilization and distraction reduce mechanical forces across the joint while maintaining intraarticular flow and pressure.
  - Because chondrocytes depend on diffusion for nutrition, maintenance of intraarticular flow without mechanical stress may promote enhanced repair of cartilage.
  - There are, however, no human data showing cartilaginous repair, and animal data show only suggestive evidence.
  - Alternatively, the technique may enhance joint space and relieve symptoms by increasing fibrosis of the joint.
- The technique is generally used in younger patients who prefer an alternative or temporizing measure prior to fusion or arthroplasty.
  - Perhaps the best candidate is a young person with severe arthritis but preserved ankle motion (for whom fusion would not be ideal).
- The technique has been limited to patients with posttraumatic or primary arthritis, as previous reports in patients with inflammatory arthritis of the hip showed poor results.
- Relative contraindications include an infected or a neuropathic joint and inflammatory arthritis.
  - Although deformity may be addressed by Ilizarov technique, simple distraction does not affect alignment and should not be used as an isolated treatment in a severely deformed joint.
- Most importantly, the Ilizarov technique requires a committed and compliant patient and a watchful surgeon.
- The surgical technique for placement of the Ilizarov external fixator and an outline of treatment is provided below.
  - Proximal and distal tibial rings are placed first, followed by a half-ring around the heel with calcaneal wires, a half-ring over the forefoot with metatarsal pins, and a wire through the talus and attached to the foot frame to prevent subtalar distraction.
  - Distraction may be accomplished acutely in the operating room or by distracting 0.5 mm 2x daily until 5 mm total of distraction is achieved.
  - The frame is then worn for up to 3 months with weight bearing generally allowed after the first 1-2 weeks.
  - The frame may be adjusted to concurrently correct equinus deformity.
  - Angular deformity correction with an Ilizarov frame generally requires osteotomies.
- Patients require a special shoe secondary to rigidity of the foot and ankle and must perform careful pin care and skin checks.
- Common complications include pin site infections requiring oral antibiotics and pin breakage.
- The goals of ankle joint distraction are relief of pain through widening of the joint space.
  - A single report did show increased joint space after distraction, but this finding has not been consistent.
- However, even if joint space and range of motion are not improved, a handful of case series show patient satisfaction in 2/3-3/4 of patients with better functional scores over time.

o This implies a progressive improvement of symptoms after completion of the distraction.
- Approximately 1/4 of patients require fusion within 1-2 years.
- One study of 17 patients randomized to arthroscopy or distraction showed improved symptom relief in the distraction group.
  o This study was limited by a small sample size, lack of blinding, and poor control treatment (as arthroscopy has limited benefit in generalized arthritis).
- In summary, distraction arthroplasty shows promising preliminary results in young patients with severe degenerative joint disease.
  o Although it is unclear whether joint space expansion is maintained or whether cartilage repair is actually taking place, patients report improvement in the majority of cases and continue to see improvement with time, at least in 2- to 5-year follow-up.
  o Additionally, distraction does not preclude future arthrodesis or arthroplasty.
  o However, this technique does require a relatively sophisticated patient and committed surgeon to carefully monitor the somewhat difficult and complex Ilizarov frame.
- Distraction arthroplasty remains a viable option because of the lack of good surgical options for the younger patient with arthritis.

Allograft

- Fresh osteochondral allografting is another technique that offers promise to younger patients with severe ankle arthritis who wish to delay or avoid the functional limitations of arthrodesis.
- The technique uses a fresh cadaveric specimen to resurface the tibial plafond and talar dome with full-thickness cartilage and a thin layer of underlying bone that reliably integrates into the host bone.
- Fresh allografts offer a distinct advantage over frozen grafts used in tumor reconstructions in that the damaged articular surface is resurfaced with viable chondrocytes.
  o Limited 2nd-look arthroscopy and retrieved specimen data have shown viable chondrocytes several years after implantation.
- Allografting of the arthritic ankle generally includes resurfacing the entire joint, but smaller allografts may be used for osteochondral lesions or focal AVN.
- Fresh allografts are harvested based on standard tissue procurement guidelines.
  o Tissue is procured within 24-48 hours and stored in enhanced media.
  o Tissue is then matched to a recipient based on size and transplanted within 2-5 weeks.
  o Previously, tissue was transplanted within 7 days, but recent safety concerns have led to a 14-day holding period for microbiologic testing.
  o No tissue matching or postoperative immunosuppressive therapy is currently employed.
- As with distraction, fresh allografts offer promise as a temporizing measure or potential alternative to fusion or implant arthroplasty in young, active patients with severe ankle arthritis.

o Published studies have limited recipients to those under 55 years of age.
o Obesity is also a relative contraindication, as allografts may be unable to tolerate the increased mechanical stress, particularly during early incorporation.
o Osteochondral allografts, like other bone graft materials, should not be placed in the setting of infection.
o Severe bone loss and malalignment are also relative contraindications to allografting.
- The technique of fresh osteochondral allografting of the ankle borrows concepts from total ankle arthroplasty and tumor surgery.
  o A temporary external fixator is first placed to allow joint distraction during allograft placement.
  o An anterior approach to the ankle gives wide exposure of the tibiotalar joint, as in total ankle arthroplasty.
  o The surgeon then resects the distal tibia and talus, adjusting as indicated to correct mild angular deformity.
  o Total ankle allograft cutting jigs may be used to improve precision of the resection.
  o A size-matched allograft is then cut appropriately and fixed into the defect.
- The patient should be assessed preoperatively to determine if an Achilles lengthening or gastrocnemius recession is required as well.
- Patients are generally kept non-weight bearing for 3 months during recovery to allow incorporation of the graft.
- A number of complications of fresh osteochondral allografting have been reported, including graft collapse, fracture, and tissue rejection.
  o Collapse of the subchondral bone may occur, especially with heavier patients or thin grafts.
  o Graft thickness must be balanced between the risk of collapse and a potential infectious or immunogenic risk from thicker grafts.
- No incidence of infection or disease transmission from an osteochondral allograft has been reported, although risk is probably equivalent to that of blood transfusion.
- The majority of allograft recipients show humoral cytotoxic antibodies indicative of an immune response to the foreign tissue, but no immune reaction has been noted in histologic examination of retrieved specimens.
- There is a risk of intraoperative or late fracture of the medial malleolus, which must be carefully preserved when making the tibial cut.
- Case series generally show 2/3-3/4 of the patients will have a good result.
  o Risk factors identified as leading to poor outcome included graft-host mismatch (graft too small) and graft thickness < 7 mm (graft too thin).
- In summary, fresh osteochondral allografting of the ankle represents a promising technique for young, active patients with severe ankle arthritis who are unwilling to accept the functional limitations of arthrodesis.
  o Good results have been reported in long-term follow-up of allografts in the knee, but limited data are available for total resurfacing of the ankle.
  o When compared with implant arthroplasty, allograft replacement of the ankle better preserves bone stock.

ARTHRODESIS

- Arthrodesis or fusion of the ankle is the "gold standard" of treatment for severe ankle arthritis.
- The goal of fusion is to provide a stable, painless, plantigrade ankle.
- General surgical principles of arthrodesis include:
  - Exposure of large bed of cancellous bone for healing
  - Use of stable fixation, usually internal
  - Interfragmentary compression to obtain solid fusion mass
- In contrast to other major joint fusions, ankle arthrodesis can result in a patient with little or no functional limitations.
  - Good results are seen in patients with healthy subtalar and transverse tarsal joints, because these joints provide motion to compensate for the ankle stiffness.
- Patients with arthritis in the hindfoot joints are not ideal candidates for ankle arthrodesis, because the final motion and comfort will not be as good.
- There are other situations in which arthrodesis is not ideal.
  - Smoking carries a 4x greater risk of nonunion.
  - Patients with medical comorbidities also show compromised healing potential.
  - Older literature cites poor outcomes in neuropathic joints, although fusion rates have improved with current techniques.
- The ideal ankle position is neutral dorsiflexion, 5° valgus, and 5° external rotation.
  - Alternatively, the external rotation of the contralateral foot may be matched.
  - Some surgeons advocate translating the talus posteriorly to shorten the lever arm of the foot and provide a biomechanical advantage.
    - Although one downside of this technique is that this may decrease the surface area available for fusion.

Approaches

- Arthrodesis is most commonly approached with an open incision, although some ankles with limited deformity are amenable to an arthroscopic or a mini-open approach.
  - Fixation is not dependent on approach.
- With an arthroscopic approach, a joint distractor is first placed to open the joint, and then anteromedial and anterolateral portals are used to remove the distal tibial and talar cartilage with a burr and curette.
  - Arthroscopic fusion is most appropriate for a joint with little to no deformity.
  - The arthroscopic approach may yield a faster fusion due to limited soft tissue dissection (8.7 vs. 14.5 weeks to fusion) with a similar fusion rate.
  - Other potential advantages are less intraoperative blood loss and no inpatient stay following surgery.
- The mini-open approach uses a similar technique but with enlarged portals for improved exposure.
- The open approach is the standard approach for ankle fusion and maximizes exposure of joint surfaces and ability to correct deformity.
  - The transfibular or lateral approach uses an incision centered over the fibula with an oblique fibular osteotomy just above the joint line.

- There are several options for handling the fibula in a transfibular approach.
  - The fibula can be removed and mulched into bone graft.
    - This option destroys normal ankle morphology after fusion, which might be a problem if converting to a total ankle arthroplasty in the future.
  - The fibula can be removed but preserved.
    - At the end of the procedure, the medial cortex of fibula is removed, and it is lagged back into place alongside the talus.
  - The distal fibula may be left attached to posterior soft tissues and rotated posteriorly on the soft tissue hinge.
    - At the end of the procedure, the medial cortex is removed, and it is replaced into its normal position.
    - In theory, the fibula acts as a vascularized fibular graft.
- With a transfibular approach, an additional smaller incision at the anterior 1/3 of the medial malleolus may improve access to the medial side of the joint.
  - Complete removal of cartilage from the medial gutter may be difficult using a single lateral incision and is aided by this additional medial approach.
  - However, the medial malleolus should be preserved in order to maintain blood supply to the talus through the deep deltoid ligament.
- An anterior approach to the joint in the interval of the extensor hallucis longus and tibialis anterior tendons may also be used for arthrodesis, as for arthroplasty.
- Regardless of approach, the joint space should be distracted with a laminar spreader or other instrument, and all cartilage carefully removed to expose bleeding bone.
  - Articular cartilage should be removed with an osteotome, curette, or burr to maintain the ankle contour.
  - Some surgeons use a large saw, making a transverse or chevron cut across the tibia and talus; these techniques result in more limb shortening.
  - Sclerotic subchondral bone should be drilled to improve healing potential.

Fixation

- Ankle fusion was originally performed with cast immobilization.
  - In 1951, Charnley introduced external fixation as an innovation that greatly improved fusion rates.
  - This was followed by the use of internal fixation, the current standard.
- Internal fixation provides the greatest stability to the fusion construct.
- Numerous techniques for internal fixation have been described and yield reliable fusion rates.
- Traditionally, screws offer greater compression than plates and probably higher fusion rates.
  - Screw placement requires less soft tissue stripping than plating.
- It is possible to provide fixation with a plate, but a lateral plate is limited by the small area for purchase in the talus, therefore requiring a blade or locking plate.
- An anterior T-shaped plate will have good purchase and is cited by some surgeons to work as a tension band, but there are no proven benefits to this technique.
- Newer plate designs incorporate lag screws in some cases, but there are no proven benefits to plates over lag screws.

- When screws are used, 3 yield greater compression than 2 screws, and crossing screws yield greater than parallel.
  - Screws are placed from the tibia and directed laterally, medially, or anteriorly into the talar body or neck.
  - Alternately, some surgeons place 2 screws from the lateral process of the talus back up into the tibia.
- Regardless of location, screws should be placed with all threads past the fusion site and not violate the subtalar joint.
  - Fluoroscopic imaging may be used to ensure screw placement and bony alignment.
- For combined ankle and subtalar fusions, a blade plate or retrograde intramedullary nail may be used.
  - A retrograde nail should not be normally used if the subtalar joint is healthy.
- External fixation may also be used to support the fusion and historically was the 1st type of fixation used in ankle arthrodesis.
  - External fixation is indicated in active infections, open wounds, and severely osteopenic bone that may not support internal fixation.
  - A thin-wire ring fixator (Ilizarov) may be particularly helpful in osteoporosis.
  - Patients may begin to bear weight on an Ilizarov frame shortly after placement.
- The major disadvantage of external fixators is that they offer less interfragmentary compression than internal fixation with perhaps a higher chance for nonunion.
  - Uniplanar external fixators provide less rotational and sagittal stability in biomechanical studies.
  - External fixators also require careful pin care, excellent patient compliance, and frequent physician monitoring.
- Bone grafting should generally be considered to augment the biology of healing.
  - Autologous bone graft can be harvested from proximal tibial metaphysis or sometimes just from osteophyte resected during surgery, along with medial cortex of the fibula from a transfibular approach.
  - Allograft, as well as various bone graft substitutes, in general do not add much "biology."
  - Recombinant platelet-derived growth factor has been shown to be as effective as autograft in a large multicenter trial.
- Allograft bone is generally considered an inferior alternative, although a recent series reported the successful use of bulk frozen allograft during revision arthrodesis of ankles with large bony defects.
- Postoperatively, patients are splinted until wound healing is evident.
  - The patient is then placed in a short leg cast or cast boot to maintain alignment and kept non-weight bearing until radiographic signs of fusion are noted.
- Reports of time to healing after arthrodesis are extremely variable but average 3-4 months in most series.
- There is similar variability in terms of when a nonunion is diagnosed.
  - In the setting of delayed healing, patients should be observed with serial examination and radiographs.
  - There is anecdotal evidence in some cases of healing after 6 months and even 1 year with conservative treatment.

Complications

- The most common serious complications of arthrodesis include nonunion, malunion, and infection.
- Infection rates of 0-28% have been reported after ankle arthrodesis.
  - The risk may be reduced with perioperative antibiotics and prevention of wound hematomas.
  - Certain patients are at higher risk for infection, including diabetics and those with renal and hepatic disease.
- Nonunion is defined as a failure of bony healing or union.
- The rate of nonunion using current techniques for ankle arthrodesis is generally < 10%, but reported rates vary from 0-40%.
  - Certain patient groups are particularly high risk, including smokers and those with impaired vascularity.
  - Other risk factors for impaired healing are previous open fracture, pilon or talus fracture, AVN of the talus, local infection, and patient noncompliance.
  - Age is not associated with nonunion.
- Some surgeons feel it is more difficult to obtain ankle fusion in the patient with previous subtalar fusion, but a few studies have failed to find this to be a significant risk factor.
- Nonunion of an ankle arthrodesis generally presents with persistent pain.
  - Radiographs may show a clear lucency at the bony interface or more subtle signs.
  - Lucency around the screws or shifting of the screws indicates motion at the fusion site.
  - If radiographs are unclear, a CT scan offers a more detailed view of the fusion and may aid detection of a nonunion.
  - Once a nonunion is diagnosed, identification of its cause is critical to treatment.
- Some nonunions are asymptomatic and require no further treatment.
- Malunion may occur as a result of errors in intraoperative positioning, poor bone quality, or deformity at adjacent joints.
  - Pain and increasing deformity may follow, at times leading to revision arthrodesis.
- Tibial stress fracture can occur months to years after fusion and presents with acute onset of pain.
  - These fractures predictably occur in the distal 1/2 of the tibia at a stress riser caused by the internal fixation.
  - Treatment of tibial stress fractures is generally nonoperative, consisting of casting and non-weight bearing.
- Soft tissue breakdown and skin slough may also occur after ankle arthrodesis.
  - The ankle has a relatively thin soft tissue envelope that may be further compromised by previous injury, impaired vascularity, or systemic disease.
  - Recognition and careful observation of patients with risk factors for wound-healing problems, as well as careful surgical technique, may reduce soft tissue problems.
- Wound breakdown may be treated conservatively with local wound care and dressing changes or may require operative debridement.
  - Rarely, a severe skin slough may require treatment with a vascularized free muscle flap.

Results

- Arthrodesis predictably alleviates pain, improves function, and allows acceptable gait.
  - Several large series in patients with posttraumatic arthritis, rheumatoid arthritis, and osteoarthritis have shown good or excellent results in 90% of patients at long-term follow-up.
- Gait can be normal after ankle arthrodesis.
  - If the contralateral limb is normal and there is uncompromised motion of the hindfoot joints, gait efficiency is decreased only 10%, and energy requirement increases 3%.
  - However, activities requiring more motion and energy than normal walking will be compromised after arthrodesis, such as walking on uneven ground or stairs.
- Many patients undergoing ankle arthrodesis have poor preoperative motion.
  - Successful arthrodesis converts a stiff, painful, and sometimes deformed ankle into a stiff, straight, comfortable one.
- Although some studies have shown no change in hindfoot motion after ankle fusion, others have shown increased motion at the transverse tarsal joints.
  - This hindfoot hypermobility partially compensates for the stiff ankle.
- The late development of adjacent joint arthritis remains a problem.
  - Long-term follow-up of ankle arthrodesis shows a high rate of progressive subtalar and talonavicular arthritis.
    - Eight years after fusion, ~ 1/2 of patients have adjacent joint arthritis.
    - After 22 years, nearly all patients have arthritis in the subtalar or talonavicular joint.
- These adjacent hindfoot joints are subject to increased stress after ankle fusion.
  - It is assumed that the increased stress leads to joint degeneration.
  - However, it is possible that these increased stresses were present prior to fusion, when the ankle was arthritic and stiff.
  - Adjacent joint arthritis may be a result of ankle arthritis, not just ankle arthrodesis.
- The complex issue of secondary adjacent arthritis after fusion has been a major impetus for the development of motion-preserving techniques for treating ankle arthritis.

Revision Arthrodesis

- Symptomatic malunion of an ankle fusion may require osteotomy through the fusion site.
  - In some cases, wedge osteotomy in the distal tibia may be the simplest solution.
- In the case of a nonunion, healing is the primary issue.
- The soft tissues, bone, hardware, and general medical condition of the patient must be carefully assessed to identify the contributors to the failure of healing.
  - Patient noncompliance may also be a factor.
  - Soft tissue healing and vascular sufficiency should be carefully assessed.
  - If there is concern for an infected nonunion, laboratory data, such as complete blood count, C-reactive protein, and sedimentation rate, may be helpful indicators, and cultures should be taken at revision.

- If avascular bone is present, it should be resected and grafted.
- If there is a failure of hardware, it must be removed and a stable construct devised.
  - With osteoporosis or bone loss, lag screws may not be feasible.
  - Fixed angle (blade or locking) plate or an external fixator may be a better option.

ARTHROPLASTY

- The success of arthroplasty in the hip and knee, coupled with the limitations of ankle arthrodesis, has generated interest in the development and implementation of a total ankle arthroplasty.
- However, more than 30 years after the 1st ankle replacement, and after more than 20 implant designs, it has proved difficult to recreate normal ankle kinematics, and long-term clinical results have been inferior to those of the hip or knee.
- The theoretical advantage of arthroplasty over arthrodesis is conservation of motion at the ankle with improved gait and function.
  - The preservation of motion might decrease the incidence of adjacent joint arthritis.

History of Total Ankle Replacement and Implant Design

- First-generation designs were trialed in the 1970s.
  - Most were composed of metallic tibial and talar implants that were cemented into place and separated by a polyethylene insert.
  - These implants showed encouraging short-term results but had high rates of loosening and subsidence in the midterm, leading to high rates of conversion to arthrodesis.
  - Problems cited with these initial designs were a large amount of bone resection, which compromised initial fixation and later salvage procedures, and a failure to reestablish normal joint kinetics.
- Early attempts at arthroplasty also suffered from technical errors.
  - Deformities in the foot, which often coexist with ankle arthritis, must be corrected prior to ankle replacement.
- After this initial round of failures, total ankle arthroplasty slowly regained ground in the 1990s with the use of 2 newer designs, the Agility total ankle replacement (TAR) and the Scandinavian TAR (STAR) prostheses.
  - The Agility design is not used currently.
  - The Salto, Inbone, and Trabecular Metal designs are the most commonly seen in the USA.
- A number of factors intrinsic to the ankle joint have made ankle arthroplasty more difficult than other joints.
  - The ankle bears a very high load over a small surface area, resulting in high mechanical stresses on the arthroplasty components.
  - There are high stresses at the implant/bone interface with the potential for implant loosening and subsidence.
  - The metaphyseal bone of the distal tibia is spongiform and not ideal for stable, secure fixation.

- The talus has a precarious blood supply that is centered in the talar body, the usual location for a keel in the component.
  - Compromise of talus vascularity can impair bone ingrowth into the component.
- The soft tissues around the ankle are thin and prone to scarring.
  - Wound-healing problems can lead to devastating infection.
  - Also, the propensity for scarring leads to ankle stiffness.
- The joint cannot be dislocated during surgery, making implant placement during surgery more difficult.
- Two biomechanical factors that have guided implant design are congruence and constraint.
  - Congruence or conformity is a geometric measure of the closeness of fit of the articulation of the prosthesis to the joint.
  - Constraint is the resistance of an implant to a degree of freedom in a plane of motion.
  - Conformity increases articular contact and generally leads to low polyethylene wear rates.
    - However, high conformity can also result in elevated constraint and shear forces that can lead to loosening.
  - The ideal implant optimizes conformity for low wear while minimizing constraint for decreased loosening.
- An additional design factor is the bearing type: Fixed or mobile.
  - A fixed-bearing implant has a single interface of motion, generally between the polyethylene fixed in the tibial component and the talar component.
  - Alternatively, a mobile bearing sits between the tibial and talar components with motion at each interface.
  - A mobile-bearing implant, e.g., the STAR, potentially decreases constraint while maintaining congruence at each articulation.
    - However, use of a mobile bearing increases design complexity and has a potential for dislocation.
  - Mobile-bearing devices have not proven more successful than fixed-bearing designs.

Indications

- The ideal candidate for TAR is elderly with low physical demands and normal bone, vascularity, and alignment.
  - The patient should be underweight and thin with relatively large bones and no osteoporosis.
  - It is difficult to find the ideal candidate.
- The appropriate age restrictions for patients undergoing ankle replacement are somewhat controversial, but younger patients generally have a higher complication rate, leading some authors to advocate limiting use of TAR to patients 60 years of age and older.
  - Ankle arthroplasty in young patients is a problem both because of a longer life required of the components and an expectation of higher activity level.
- Other patient characteristics associated with poor outcome after TAR include obesity, diabetes, and other medical comorbidities.
- Although mild deformity may be corrected with TAR, malalignment of > 15° of varus or valgus cannot be easily corrected with arthroplasty and may require treatment with arthrodesis or concurrent osteotomy.

- Avascularity in the tibia or talus may compromise ingrowth of components.
- Neuropathy is a contraindication to implant arthroplasty because of the potential for rapid failure (neuropathic joint degeneration).
- Absence of the medial malleolus or deltoid ligament incompetence are both problems, because the ankle replacement requires medial stability to prevent valgus collapse.
- Lack of the fibula is not an absolute contraindication but probably leads to poorer results (early failure).
- Indications do not vary considerably among implant designs.
- Perhaps the best candidates for arthroplasty are those who might not be as good of candidates for fusion.
  - Someone with adjacent hindfoot arthritis may be better for replacement than fusion.
  - Bilateral ankle arthritis possibly might be more appropriate for arthroplasty.
  - Person who is not capable of complying with strict non-weight bearing for 6-8 weeks for fusion might be better suited for replacement, as replacement may be more tolerant of some early noncompliance with those restrictions.
- Relative contraindications to TAR are: Age < 60 years, high activity level, infection (past or present), severe deformity, Charcot joint, poor soft tissue envelope, talar AVN.

Approach and Technique

- The most common approach for ankle replacement is an anterior approach, passing between the anterior tibial and extensor hallucis longus tendons.
  - An external fixator can be placed medially to help with distraction and alignment but is usually not used.
- At least 1 newer design (Trabecular Metal) is placed with a lateral approach through a fibular osteotomy.
- Bone cuts are made with the joint reduced, not dislocated (unlike traditional hip or knee arthroplasty), using cutting jigs or freehand in the case of the experienced surgeon.
  - Because the joint is not dislocatable, exposure of the joint surfaces can be difficult.
  - The components are press-fit into place after the bone is prepared.
  - Although cement can be used, it is not standard technique for any implant.
- Appropriate soft tissue balance in surrounding muscles and ligaments is essential to success.

Complications

- Complications of TAR include wound problems, infection, aseptic loosening, subsidence, and osteolysis.
  - There also are problems related to the surgical approach and joint preparation, including nerve injury and malleolar fracture.
- Wound problems and infection are related to the thin soft tissue envelope.
  - Small wound irritations may need only close follow-up and oral antibiotics.
  - Larger wound problems require surgical debridement with possible component removal and antibiotics similar to other joint replacements.

- o Uncontrollable infection may occasionally be best treated with amputation.
- Patients with aseptic loosening may present with pain and radiographic lucency around components.
  - o It is common to see some loosening on follow-up x-rays.
  - o Loosening is not always symptomatic.
- The talar component is particularly prone to loosening.
  - o This is probably because of less vascularity of talus in general with less ingrowth.
  - o It is perhaps also because of less rigid fixation in talus.
- Subsidence of either component can occur and is more likely with obesity and osteoporosis.
  - o Settling of the joint from component subsidence leads to pain from malleolar impingement on the talus.
- Tilting of the talus in the mortise is a difficult problem stemming from imperfect tissue balance.
  - o Tilting remains a problem even for experienced surgeons.
  - o Because modern components are relatively unconstrained, to limit sheer stresses at the bone-implant interface, tilting can occur.
- Osteolysis is loss of bone around the implant, usually due to polyethylene particulate debris in the joint.
  - o Elective grafting of large osteolysis cysts, ± polyethylene liner or component exchange, is often performed.

2-Component Design: Agility

- Many modern ankle replacements are 2 components with a polyethylene liner that is permanently bonded to the tibial tray.
- The Agility replacement was the most widely used 2-component replacement for years but is not currently used.
- It went through several generations with some incongruence and less constraint between the smaller talar and larger tibial components.
  - o As a result, subsidence of the talar component, and tilting of the talus in the mortise was sometimes seen.
  - o The tibial component, which was inserted along with a fusion between the distal tibia and fibula, was robust and not usually a source of trouble.
- Advantages of the 2-component design include complete resurfacing of the ankle and greater surface area to support the tibial component.
  - o This larger surface area distributes forces well across the ankle.
  - o Subsidence of the tibial component is not a common complication.
- The larger component does require more extensive bone resection and consequently a potentially more difficult salvage.
  - o Custom revision components were available for a time, but the USA government has since prohibited the use of custom implants.
- There have been several midterm reports of the Agility total ankle.
  - o In one study of 126 patients with mean follow-up of 9 years, > 90% of patients reported satisfaction and pain relief.
    - – The revision rate was 15%.
    - – Average arc of range of motion was 18°.
    - – Complications included syndesmotic nonunion in 8%, subsidence in 14%, and periimplant lucency in 76%.

- – Importantly, a significant number of patients developed adjacent joint arthritis in the subtalar and talonavicular joints.
- – Greater than 90% of patients reported satisfaction and pain relief.
- – The patients in this series were selected by the inventor of the Agility Ankle and were probably all ideal candidates.
  - o A series of 306 consecutive ankle arthroplasties with an average 33-month follow-up observed less favorable results.
    - – Five-year survivorship was 80% using the end point of failed TAR and 54% using reoperation.
    - – Younger patients (< 55 years) did significantly worse than older patients.
    - – Failure of syndesmosis fusion, loosening, and subsidence were cited as common complications.
    - – A few patients required below-knee amputation (BKA) as a salvage procedure.
    - – This series had less strict inclusion criteria, including many younger patients, and most patients were not ideal candidates.
- Although data regarding outcomes of the Agility TAR are mixed, several points of agreement exist.
  - o The majority of patients are satisfied in the short term, but long-term results are as yet unknown.
  - o Younger patients tend to have worse implant survival and increased complications.
  - o Range of motion is not fully restored after TAR with an average of ~ 30°.
  - o Syndesmosis fusion is important to success.
  - o Adjacent joint arthritis may occur after TAR, but it is unclear whether the rate of arthritis is lower than after ankle arthrodesis.

3-Component Design: Scandinavian Total Ankle Replacement

- The STAR design is a 2nd-generation, 3-component implant that has been widely used in the USA and Europe for decades.
  - o The components include coated, metal alloy tibial and talar implants with a mobile polyethylene bearing.
- The STAR prosthesis is **congruent**, in that the tibial and talar components are similarly sized, but **unconstrained** in that the polyethylene bearing is mobile, and the entire joint is not resurfaced.
  - o The medial and lateral gutters remain to some degree.
  - o Use of a mobile liner adds freedom to the construct but increases risk of polyethylene displacement or dislocation.
  - o The tibial component is a plate that does not resurface the malleoli.
  - o The syndesmosis is not fused.
    - – This avoids the problem of syndesmotic nonunion but leaves the distal tibiofibular joint, a potential source of pain, unaddressed.
- A series of 55 patients who underwent cemented or uncemented STAR arthroplasty showed good results.
  - o At 5 years, the cemented implants showed a 90% survivorship.
  - o The majority of failures were due to aseptic loosening.

- ○ Careful patient selection was emphasized as a requisite for success.
- Many other surgeons have subsequently published their case series of STAR arthroplasties.
  - ○ There are plenty of reports of excellent survivorship at early (~ 5-year) follow-up.
- Modern surgeons continue to work to minimize early failures from loosening, subsidence, and tilting.
- In the longer term, polyethylene wear and osteolysis are potential problems.

Other 2-Component Implants

- The Salto ankle replacement is similar to the STAR with a smaller tibial baseplate that does not cross to the fibula.
  - ○ The Salto has been widely used for many years with similar survivorship to the STAR.
- The Inbone ankle replacement includes a stem on the tibial implant and requires an osteotomy of the tibial anterior cortex for insertion.
- A newer implant, the Trabecular Metal ankle, is inserted from the lateral approach with a fibular osteotomy.
  - ○ This implant is a thinner resurfacing of the talus and tibia, but middle- and long-term outcomes are not available.

Unresolved Questions

- It is unclear whether current TAR accomplishes the goals of recreating ankle kinematics and addressing the shortcomings of ankle arthrodesis.
- Range of motion after TAR is limited to ~ 30°, and gait studies show protected weight bearing of the replaced ankle and altered kinematics even in asymptomatic TAR.
  - ○ 20° or 30° of motion may be functional in the low-demand patient but is certainly not normal.
- It is unproven whether TAR decreases the development of adjacent joint arthritis.
  - ○ Rates of subtalar and talonavicular arthritis after TAR and arthrodesis are similar at 5-year follow-up.
  - ○ It is unknown whether adjacent joint disease in TAR occurs secondary to reduced range of motion, increased stress caused by abnormal ankle joint kinetics, or underlying disease.
- Osteolysis is often seen, sometimes with well-fixed implants.
  - ○ If the cysts become large enough, catastrophic talus fracture and collapse will result.
  - ○ It is not clear whether it is better to revise the entire ankle once osteolysis is beyond a critical size or simply to graft the cysts (and retain implants).

AMPUTATION

- BKA is a viable reconstructive option for many patients.
- A well-functioning prosthesis will provide better athletic function than ankle arthrodesis or arthroplasty in a healthy, young person.
- A well-functioning BKA requires only a moderate increase in energy consumption.
  - ○ Most patients can be fitted with a prosthesis and ambulate successfully, particularly when comparing gait with a stiff and painful ankle.
- Disadvantages of amputation include cosmesis, psychologic distress, and stump difficulties that can result in more proximal amputation.

- Amputation also may be a salvage for patients who have no reasonable reconstructive option.
  - ○ Posttraumatic patients with impaired vascularity and soft tissue envelope, leading to failure of healing
  - ○ Patients with impaired blood supply secondary to primary vascular disease or diabetes not amenable to revascularization
  - ○ Patients with uncontrolled infection unresponsive to local measures and antibiotic treatment
- Although isolated ankle or hindfoot fusions are well tolerated, the young patient with pantalar disease may be better served by BKA.

SELECTED REFERENCES

1. Amendola, A: Emerging methods for treating ankle arthritis. AAOS Instructional Course Lecture. 2005
2. Myerson MS et al: Fresh-frozen structural allografts in the foot and ankle. J Bone Joint Surg Am. 87(1):113-20, 2005
3. Anderson T et al: Uncemented STAR total ankle prostheses. J Bone Joint Surg Am. 86-A Suppl 1(Pt 2):103-11, 2004
4. Knecht SI et al: The Agility total ankle arthroplasty. Seven to sixteen-year follow-up. J Bone Joint Surg Am. 86-A(6):1161-71, 2004
5. Kofoed H: Scandinavian total ankle replacement (STAR). Clin Orthop Relat Res. 73-9, 2004
6. Mizel MS et al: Evaluation and treatment of chronic ankle pain. Instr Course Lect. 53:311-21, 2004
7. Spirt AA et al: Complications and failure after total ankle arthroplasty. J Bone Joint Surg Am. 86-A(6):1172-8, 2004
8. Marijnissen AC et al: Clinical benefit of joint distraction in the treatment of ankle osteoarthritis. Foot Ankle Clin. 8(2):335-46, 2003
9. Thomas RH et al: Ankle arthritis. J Bone Joint Surg Am. 85-A(5):923-36, 2003
10. Tontz WL Jr et al: Use of allografts in the management of ankle arthritis. Foot Ankle Clin. 8(2):361-73, xi, 2003
11. Easley ME et al: Total ankle arthroplasty. J Am Acad Orthop Surg. 10(3):157-67, 2002
12. Marijnissen AC et al: Clinical benefit of joint distraction in the treatment of severe osteoarthritis of the ankle: proof of concept in an open prospective study and in a randomized controlled study. Arthritis Rheum. 46(11):2893-902, 2002
13. Coester LM et al: Long-term results following ankle arthrodesis for post-traumatic arthritis. J Bone Joint Surg Am. 83-A(2):219-28, 2001
14. Abidi NA et al: Ankle arthrodesis: indications and techniques. J Am Acad Orthop Surg. 8(3):200-9, 2000
15. van Valburg AA et al: Joint distraction in treatment of osteoarthritis: a two-year follow-up of the ankle. Osteoarthritis Cartilage. 7(5):474-9, 1999
16. Cheng JC et al: The role of arthroscopy in ankle and subtalar degenerative joint disease. Clin Orthop Relat Res. 65-72, 1998
17. Demetriades L et al: Osteoarthritis of the ankle. Clin Orthop Relat Res. 28-42, 1998
18. Katcherian DA: Treatment of ankle arthrosis. Clin Orthop Relat Res. 48-57, 1998
19. Martin DF et al: Operative ankle arthroscopy. Long-term followup. Am J Sports Med. 17(1):16-23; discussion 23, 1989

Relative Contraindications to Allograft Arthroplasty

Patient Factors	Local Factors
Age > 55 years	Severe bone loss
Obesity	Severe deformity
Active infection	

Ankle Position for Arthrodesis

Dorsiflexion	Neutral
Valgus	5°
External rotation	Matched to contralateral or 5°

Risk Factors for Nonunion After Ankle Arthrodesis

Patient Factors	Local Factors
Smoking	Previous open fracture
Noncompliance	Previous pilon or talus fracture
Impaired vascular supply	Avascular necrosis of talus
Diabetes	Prior or current infection
Neuropathic joint	

Causes of Ankle Arthritis

Etiology	Features
Posttraumatic	Most common cause Result of intraarticular ankle fractures Can also be late result of tibial shaft or calcaneal malunion
Chronic ligamentous instability	Recurrent ankle sprains may lead to chronic instability of ankle Instability can result in joint incongruence and cartilage damage Often see anterior subluxation of talus
Postinfectious	Cartilage destruction occurs secondary to inflammatory cascade Antibiotics and surgical irrigation and debridement may limit cartilage damage
Inflammatory arthritis	Characterized by thickened synovium or pannus, bony erosions, and osteopenia Generally symmetric Forefoot and midfoot more common than ankle Ankylosing spondylitis, Reiter syndrome, and psoriatic arthritis most common in ankle
Crystalline arthropathy	Gout and calcium pyrophosphate deposition disease cause episodic pain and inflammation Best treated with gout-specific medications Less common in ankle than in other foot joints, such as 1st metatarsophalangeal
Neuropathic arthropathy	Diabetes most common cause, but paralysis, peripheral nerve injury, Charcot-Marie-Tooth also rare causes Characterized by bone loss and deformity
Hemochromatosis	Recurrent hemarthroses are painful and over time lead to cartilage destruction
Tumor	Osteoid osteoma in young patients, pigmented villonodular synovitis, synovial chondromatosis
Idiopathic	Rare

Malunion After Ankle Arthrodesis

Malunion Type	Consequence	Bracing Option
Varus	Lateral foot pain, subtalar instability, pressure over base of 5th metatarsal	Neutralizing shoe modification or orthotic
Valgus	Medial knee strain, secondary foot deformity	Accommodative orthotic
Dorsiflexion	Heel pad pain &/or breakdown	Rocker-bottom shoe
Plantar flexion/equinus	Metatarsalgia, back and knee pain	Solid ankle cushion heel shoe

(Left) *Preoperative AP radiograph of the ankle prior to distraction arthroplasty shows loss of joint space.* (Right) *AP radiograph of the ankle during distraction with the Ilizarov external fixator in place shows improvement in joint space narrowing.*

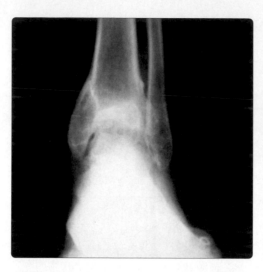
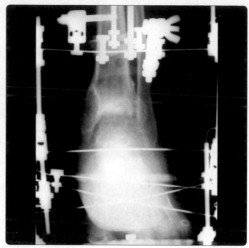

(Left) *One-year follow-up, with suggestion of improved joint space, is shown.* (Right) *Intraoperative photo shows allograft arthroplasty components in place.*

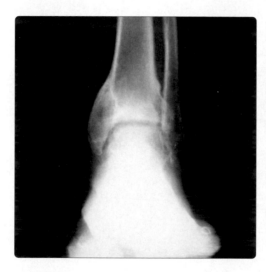
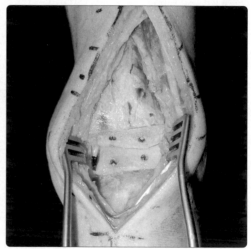

(Left) *Postoperative AP and lateral radiographs show good incorporation of the graft.* (Right) *Screws can be placed in many different locations for ankle arthrodesis. This is one possible configuration. Screws are placed from the tibia and directed laterally, medially, or anteriorly into the talar body or neck.*

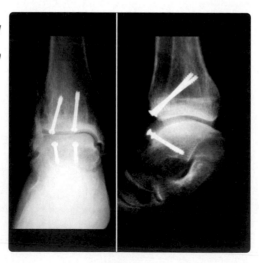
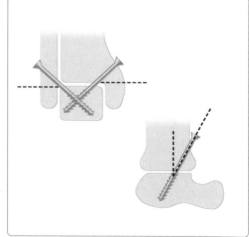

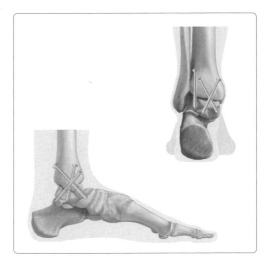

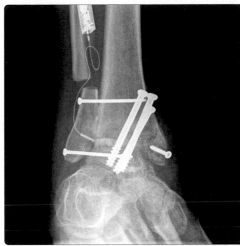

(Left) Another possible screw configuration that can be used for ankle arthrodesis is shown. When screws are used, 3 screws yield greater compression than 2 screws and crossing screws greater than parallel screws. (Right) Postoperative AP radiograph of an ankle arthrodesis shows 3 screws across the joint and 2 screws bridging from the fibula.

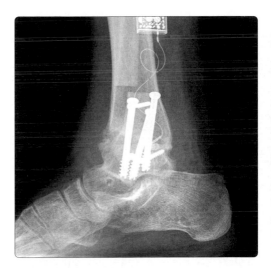

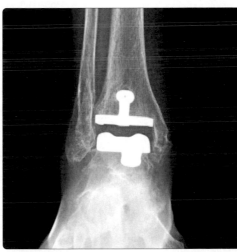

(Left) Postoperative lateral radiograph of an ankle arthrodesis is shown. It is normally best to get screws that are crossing, not parallel, however, parallel screws will work if rigid compression is achieved. (Right) AP radiograph shows a Salto total ankle replacement in the early postoperative stage with good alignment of the talus under the tibia and without any varus or valgus tilt.

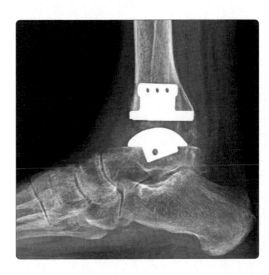

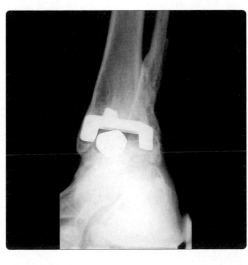

(Left) Lateral radiograph of a Salto total ankle arthroplasty at early postoperative stage shows good alignment of the components with the talus centered under the tibia. (Right) An older total ankle arthroplasty design tilting into valgus due to tissue imbalance is shown. This patient had mild pain from lateral bone impingement, but the potential for catastrophic polyethylene fracture exists (because of edge loading of the talus into the polyethylene).

Heel Pain

- Heel pain results in 1 million medical visits per year and comprises 1% of all visits to orthopaedic surgeons.
- The majority of patients with heel pain will be treated successfully nonoperatively.
- Heel pain can be plantar (subcalcaneal) or posterior.
- Posterior pain is often due to insertional Achilles tendinopathy &/or retrocalcaneal bursitis.
- Etiologies of heel pain include:
  - Plantar fasciitis, most common by far
  - Plantar nerve impingement/entrapment
  - Calcaneal stress fracture
  - Fat pad atrophy
  - Cavus or calcaneus deformity
  - Inflammatory enthesopathy
- Plantar fasciitis is thought to be due to irritation of the proximal plantar fascia.
- Plantar fasciitis has been associated with a tight gastrocnemius and hamstrings.

- Specialized imaging studies are typically not needed in the diagnosis and treatment of plantar fasciitis.
- Initial treatments for plantar fasciitis include rest, antiinflammatories, heel cups, full orthotics, corticosteroid injections, stretching exercises, and immobilization (night splint or cast).
  - Because most patients with plantar fasciitis have a tight gastrocnemius, stretching is a logical treatment choice.
- Treatments for recalcitrant plantar fasciitis include extracorporeal shock wave therapy, radiofrequency ablation, low-level laser therapy, platelet-rich plasma, botulinum toxin injections.
- If plantar fasciitis symptoms have persisted more than 6 months despite appropriate treatment, surgery can be considered. There are several surgical options.

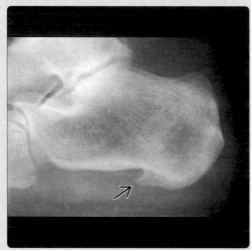

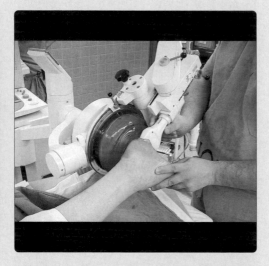

(Left) Heel spurs ➡ are caused by chronic inflammation and are not the primary etiology of heel pain. They are present in ~ 50% of those patients with subcalcaneal pain syndrome and ~ 15% of the general population. (Right) Shock wave therapy is thought to stimulate angiogenesis, promote new bone formation, disrupt calcific deposits, and increase cytokine diffusion. As a 2nd-line treatment for plantar fasciitis, several multicenter trials have found statistically significant success.

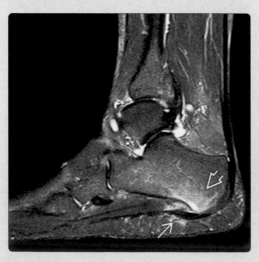

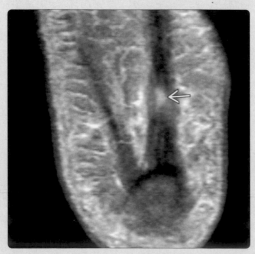

(Left) Thickened fascia ➡ with surrounding edema and edema in the posterior process of the calcaneus ➡ is shown. The absence of cortical erosion distinguishes this case from enthesopathy due to spondyloarthropathy. (From DI: MSK Trauma.) (Right) A focal area of increased signal ➡ in the medial band of the plantar fascia, consistent with plantar fasciitis, is shown. (From DI: MSK Trauma.)

NORMAL HEEL ANATOMY

- The Achilles tendon inserts on the posterior calcaneus.
  - Fibers continue plantarward to merge with the origin of the plantar fascia.
- Between the Achilles tendon and the posterosuperior calcaneal tuberosity lies the retrocalcaneal bursa.
  - This bursa is deep to the Achilles tendon.
- The plantar fascia runs from its origin on the plantar calcaneus to spread out into the plantar aponeurosis.
- The plantar aponeurosis consists of 3 segments:
  - The medial and lateral segments cover the abductor hallucis and abductor digiti quinti.
  - The central portion of the plantar aponeurosis originates from the medial tuberosity of the calcaneus and is referred to as the plantar fascia.
  - The central portion inserts into the plantar plate of the proximal phalanges and through the sesamoids into the great toe.
- Hyperextension of the toes and metatarsophalangeal joints tenses the plantar fascia, raises the longitudinal arch of the foot, inverts the hindfoot, and externally rotates the leg.
  - This apparatus is referred to as the windlass mechanism.
  - The windlass effect provides a passive mechanism for increased foot stability.
- The subcutaneous tissue under the calcaneus is the plantar fat pad.
  - Fibrous septa enclose small "cells" of adipose, giving the entire structure the ability to absorb shock during gait.
- The tibial nerve branches just at or above the medial malleolus into the medial and lateral plantar nerves.
  - The medial calcaneal nerve comes off the medial plantar nerve at this level to supply sensation to the medial, posterior, and inferior heel.
    - When making a posteromedial ankle incision, this nerve can be injured if the incision is carried too far distally.
  - The 1st branch of the lateral plantar nerve runs under the inferomedial calcaneus and deep to the fascia of the abductor hallucis.
    - It provides motor function to the abductor digiti minimi and the flexor digiti brevis as well as innervation to some calcaneal periosteum.

Heel Spurs

- Heel spurs were originally thought to be an etiology of heel pain.
- Epidemiologic studies, however, have improved our understanding of their origin.
- Heel spurs are present in ~ 50% of patients with subcalcaneal pain syndrome and in ~ 15% of the general population.
- Less than 5% of patients with spurs have pain.
- Spurs were assumed to originate in the plantar aponeurosis but are actually located in the origin of the flexor hallucis brevis.
  - This too casts doubt on the spur's role in the etiology of heel pain.
- Spurs are probably caused by chronic inflammation and are not the primary etiology of heel pain.

PLANTAR FASCIITIS

- Many people refer to this condition as a "heel spur," but only 50% of patients with the condition will have a plantar spur, and 15% of normal patients will also have a spur.
  - The exact role of the plantar spur in the condition is not well defined.
    - Treatment probably should not focus on the spur.
- The condition is thought to be due to irritation of the proximal plantar fascia.
  - Although there rarely can be an acute tear, most commonly it is some degree of chronic degeneration.
  - There may or may not be a history of mild trauma.
  - It is bilateral in 15-30% of patients.
  - There probably is not any true inflammation.
- Patients will typically have pain under the plantar heel that is worse on initial weight bearing.
  - The pain may improve as they "walk it off" but then returns with increased time on the feet during the day.
- Plantar fasciitis has been associated with a tight gastrocnemius and hamstrings.
  - The tight gastrocnemius may be the cause of the problem.
- Unlike most muscles, the gastrocnemius has quite a bit of resting tone.
  - This resting tone is the basis for the Silverskold test, where passive ankle dorsiflexion is increased with knee flexion.
- This baseline contracture or tightness of the gastrocnemius is universal in mammals.
  - Extension of the knee leads to plantarflexion of the ankle in quadrupeds.
    - This facilitates ambulation.
- When a human is at rest, the gastrocnemius resumes this natural tension.
- If a person rises from bed or a chair without loosening up the gastrocnemius, the forced dorsiflexion of the ankle from the ground pushing up on the forefoot is opposed by plantarflexion of a tight gastrocnemius.
  - Tension across the plantar fascia is the result.
- On examination, there is usually tenderness at the proximal plantar fascia.
  - Some patients may be tender only under the calcaneal tuberosity.
- Passive dorsiflexion of the toes tightens the fascia and may increase tenderness in the proximal fascia in patients with plantar fasciitis.
- Specialized imaging studies are typically not needed in the diagnosis and treatment of plantar fasciitis.
- In cases where the diagnosis is not clear, bone scans or magnetic resonance imaging (MR) may help differentiate from other pathologies, such as stress fracture.
- Bone scans reveal increased uptake at the inferior aspect of the calcaneus.
  - Patients with this finding may have a better response to local cortisone treatments.
- MR findings are variable and do not always reveal any changes in the plantar fascia.

Treatment of Plantar Fasciitis

- There are many treatment options for plantar fasciitis.

- o Similar to lower back pain, most patients will improve spontaneously with time.
- Initial treatments include rest, antiinflammatories, heel cups, full orthotics, corticosteroid injections, stretching exercises, and immobilization (night splint or cast).
  - o There is probably some value to all these regimens.
- Because most patients with plantar fasciitis have a tight gastrocnemius, stretching is a logical treatment choice.
  - o A prospective study found that regular daily stretching of the plantar fascia and gastrocnemius, combined with an over-the-counter orthotic, was more effective than routine Achilles tendon stretching alone.
  - o Another study found a prefabricated orthotic to be as effective as a custom one for plantar fasciitis.
    - – Correction of a planovalgus foot with orthotics will reduce strain on the origin of the plantar fascia.
- Tisdel and Harper (1996) found that 86% of patients improved after 4 weeks in a weight-bearing short leg cast.
- Although many physicians rely on corticosteroid injections, the evidence for injections is mixed.
  - o Repeat injections can lead to fat pad atrophy, a devastating complication.
  - o Plantar fascial rupture and calcaneal osteomyelitis are other rare complications of injection.
  - o Miller et al (1995) noted recurrence of symptoms in 13 of 24 feet at 5-8 months after injection.
- There are other treatments for recalcitrant plantar fasciitis:
  - o Botulinum toxin injections
  - o Platelet-rich plasma
  - o Radiofrequency ablation
  - o Low-level laser therapy
  - o Extracorporeal shock wave
    - – The literature on these treatments is not conclusive.
- There are trends in the literature:
  - o The natural history for the vast majority of patients is improvement over time, regardless of treatment.
  - o Achilles/gastrocnemius and plantar fascia stretching is probably the most appropriate initial treatment and may be as effective as anything else.
  - o As a whole, 90% of patients will improve by 6 months.

Surgery for Plantar Fasciitis

- If symptoms have persisted more than 6 months despite appropriate treatment, surgery can be considered. There are several surgical options.
- Partial plantar fasciotomy can be done through a medial incision.
  - o The lateral bands of the fascia are left intact to prevent lateral column pain.
- Endoscopic partial plantar fasciotomy can be performed to minimize the skin incision.
  - o Although many assume that endoscopic surgery offers a faster recovery than traditional open technique, this has not been proven.
- In patients with a tight gastrocnemius, gastrocnemius recession may be the best choice.
  - o At least 1 surgeon has proposed plantar fascia release for the patient with a stable or high arch and gastrocnemius lengthening for the patient with a low or collapsed arch.
- In case series, all the above techniques are effective with 70-90% good results.

- The role of heel spur resection is unclear, and most orthopedists do not include it in the surgical procedure.

PLANTAR NERVE IMPINGEMENT

- Compression of the nerve to the abductor digiti minimi (1st branch of the lateral plantar nerve, sometimes referred to as Baxter nerve) is a less common cause of heel pain.
- This may happen through impingement on the edge of the fascia of the abductor hallucis.
- Pain is generally felt more medial on the heel, rather than plantar.
  - o The area of maximal tenderness will be on the medial inferior border of the calcaneus, at the origin of the abductor hallucis.
- For the appropriate patient, surgical release of the medial plantar fascia and the fascia of the abductor hallucis may lead to improvement.

FAT PAD ATROPHY

- The plantar fat pad provides essential shock absorption during gait.
  - o Loss of this function results in chronic heel pain.
- Direct trauma, as seen with a calcaneus fracture, may lead to fat pad atrophy.
- Fat pad atrophy can also result as a side effect of corticosteroid injections.
  - o Although a single injection rarely causes this complication, it can be seen with repeated injections.
- Treatment is focused on providing better padding and shock absorption with padded heel inserts and appropriate (well-padded) shoes.

CALCANEAL STRESS FRACTURE

- Stress fracture of the calcaneus will present with heel pain that is worse with activity and better with rest.
- In contrast to plantar fasciitis, stress fracture pain will usually be mild with the 1st step and increase with further weight bearing.
- Examination will show tenderness at the medial and lateral tuberosity.
  - o This is not seen with plantar fasciitis.
- After a few weeks, plain x-rays may show sclerosis.
  - o MR or bone scan may be useful earlier.
- Treatment should focus on activity modification and rest.
  - o Some patients will need a cast, cast boot, &/or crutches.

CAVUS FOOT PAIN

- The patient with a high-arched foot may have increased loads placed on the heel and metatarsal heads.
  - o This may lead to mechanical heel pain.
- Well-padded shoes or heel pads may provide good relief.
- A custom orthotic with good padding under the heel and a built-up instep to distribute weight-bearing forces away from the heel can also be helpful.
- For recalcitrant cases, osteotomies to lower the arch can be performed, but results may not be good.
  - o Pain in these difficult cases is multifactorial.

Treatment Plan for Plantar Fasciitis

History and Examination Consistent With Plantar Fasciitis
Begin plantar fascia and gastrocnemius stretching multiple times daily
Wear shoes with good support or use prefabricated orthotic
Consider antiinflammatory medication
If No Improvement
Confirm proper performance and frequency of exercises
If Still No Improvement
Consider alternative diagnoses
If still most consistent with plantar fasciitis, consider adding alternative treatment, such as night splint, casting, or corticosteroid injection
If Symptoms Persist More Than 6 Months
Consider alternatives, such as shock wave, platelet-rich plasma, botulinum toxin, radiofrequency, or low-level laser therapy
Consider surgical intervention

- A surgery that makes the foot and the x-ray look better to the surgeon may not improve the pain.

ENTHESOPATHY

- Patients with inflammatory enthesopathies can develop plantar fasciitis as part of systemic disease.
- In cases of refractory or recurrent heel pain, referral to a rheumatologist should be considered.
  - This is especially when other enthesopathies are involved.

SELECTED REFERENCES

1. Babcock MS et al: Treatment of pain attributed to plantar fasciitis with botulinum toxin a: a short-term, randomized, placebo-controlled, double-blind study. Am J Phys Med Rehabil. 84(9):649-54, 2005

2. Thomson CE et al: The effectiveness of extra corporeal shock wave therapy for plantar heel pain: a systematic review and meta-analysis. BMC Musculoskelet Disord. 6:19, 2005

3. Riddle DL et al: Volume of ambulatory care visits and patterns of care for patients diagnosed with plantar fasciitis: a national study of medical doctors. Foot Ankle Int. 25(5):303-10, 2004

4. Theodore GH et al: Extracorporeal shock wave therapy for the treatment of plantar fasciitis. Foot Ankle Int. 25(5):290-7, 2004

5. DiGiovanni BF et al: Tissue-specific plantar fascia-stretching exercise enhances outcomes in patients with chronic heel pain. A prospective, randomized study. J Bone Joint Surg Am. 85-A(7):1270-7, 2003

6. Buchbinder R et al: Ultrasound-guided extracorporeal shock wave therapy for plantar fasciitis: a randomized controlled trial. JAMA. 288(11):1364-72, 2002

7. Pfeffer G et al: Comparison of custom and prefabricated orthoses in the initial treatment of proximal plantar fasciitis. Foot Ankle Int. 20(4):214-21, 1999

8. Tisdel CL et al: Chronic plantar heel pain: treatment with a short leg walking cast. Foot Ankle Int. 17(1):41-2, 1996

9. Miller RA et al: Efficacy of first-time steroid injection for painful heel syndrome. Foot Ankle Int. 16(10):610-2, 1995

10. Baxter DE et al: Treatment of chronic heel pain by surgical release of the first branch of the lateral plantar nerve. Clin Orthop Relat Res. 229-36, 1992

ACHILLES TENDINOSIS

- Achilles tendinosis can be noninsertional or insertional, although it is the same pathology, i.e., degenerative tendinopathy.
- Insertional tendinopathy can be associated with a Haglund deformity, insertional ossification, or both.
- A heel lift and physical therapy are the mainstays of treatment and are often effective, although it tends to be more effective in noninsertional tendinopathy.
- Operative treatment consists of tendon debridement and repair with patients having insertional tendinopathy often requiring resection of any insertional ossification as well as the Haglund deformity. Surgery is often successful in eliminating the patient's symptoms.

ACHILLES TENDON RUPTURE

- Achilles tendon rupture is on the same spectrum as Achilles tendinosis in that a rupture occurs when a tendinotic tendon is subjected to an eccentric contracture of sufficient force to rupture the tendon.
- It often occurs with sporting activity; physical exam is often sufficient diagnostically.
- The goal of treatment is restoration of appropriate tension, which can be accomplished with either nonoperative or operative means.
- There is much debate as to the optimal treatment of Achilles tendon ruptures with the discussion generally framed by the increased risk of wound complications with surgical treatment on the one end and the increased risk of rerupture with nonoperative treatment on the other.

(Left) *Notice the thickening of the tendon in a noninsertional position in this patient with noninsertional Achilles tendinopathy. This thickening is often readily apparent clinically and often tender to palpation.* (Right) *Simply having the patient lay prone with the knees flexed to 90° will often allow for the diagnosis of Achilles tendon rupture, as the resting tension of the injured tendon will show relatively more dorsiflexion.*

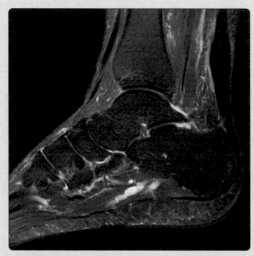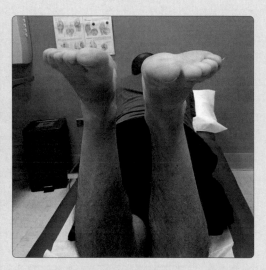

(Left) *An Achilles tendon laceration is more difficult to get right than Achilles tendon ruptures, as the zone of injury is less diffuse. Special attention should be paid to matching the tension of the contralateral side.* (Right) *The proximal stump is very retracted ⇥, and the distal stump is very degenerative ⇥. The tendon is often diffusely degenerative in those patients who rupture their tendons.*

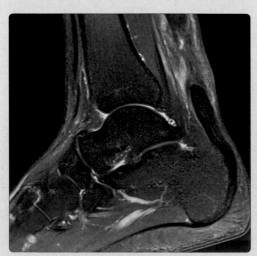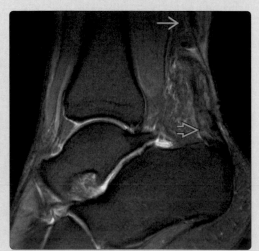

CLINICAL ANATOMY

- The Achilles tendon is formed from the confluence of the gastrocnemius and soleus tendons distally. The gastrocnemius originates from the posterior femoral condyles, while the soleus has its origin from the posterior tibia and fibula.
  - The Achilles tendon is notable for its "twisted" structure with longitudinal rotation from proximal to distal.
    - Right Achilles tendons rotate counterclockwise; left Achilles tendons rotate clockwise.
  - The Achilles inserts in a specific way onto the calcaneus.
    - Soleus and lateral gastrocnemius insert more proximally; medial gastrocnemius inserts more distally.
  - The sural nerve typically runs with the lesser saphenous vein from proximal posterior to more anterior and lateral.
  - Blood supply to the tendon is from the posterior tibial artery proximally and distally and the peroneal artery in its midsection.

PATHOLOGY

Achilles Tendinosis Is (Typically) Focal Degeneration of Achilles Tendon

- The overt cause of Achilles tendinosis remains unclear, although many postulate a gastrocnemius equinus contracture can lead to Achilles degeneration and may be potentiated by activity. In this way, both intrinsic and extrinsic factors likely play a role.
- Achilles tendinosis can be insertional or noninsertional
  - Noninsertional Achilles tendinopathy will often take the appearance of the "snake that swallowed the egg" with a focal swelling in the tendon that is tender to palpation.
  - Insertional Achilles tendinopathy is characterized by swelling in the distal tendon with ossification of the Achilles insertion into the calcaneus.
    - A Haglund deformity, which is a prominent supero-posterior aspect of calcaneus, may be a part of the pathology.

Achilles Tendinosis and Achilles Tendon Rupture Are at Different Ends of Same Spectrum of Disease

- In order for an Achilles tendon to rupture, 2 things generally need to be present: A focus of degeneration in the tendon, or a focus of tendinosis, and an eccentric contracture of the tendon of sufficient force for the tendon to rupture.
  - Kannus and Jozsa noted that no ruptured tendons were healthy, and 97% of the pathological changes were notable for histologic degeneration, i.e., hypoxic degenerative tendinopathy, mucoid degeneration, tendolipomatosis, and calcifying tendinopathy. Also of note was the fact that ~ 1/3 of ostensibly normal tendons showed some evidence of histologic degeneration, implying that these tendons may have been at risk for rupture. Clinically, this fact makes sense given that patients rarely have any symptoms prior to Achilles tendon rupture.
  - Tallon et al histologically graded 3 sets of tendons for degeneration: Those from patients with no known tendon pathology, those from patients having surgery for Achilles tendinopathy, and those having surgery for a ruptured Achilles tendon. These 3 groups formed a clear hierarchy in which the ruptured tendons were significantly more histologically degenerative than the tendinopathic tendons, which were significantly more degenerative than the normal tendons.
- Achilles tendon ruptures are historically much more common in men than women and tended to occur in young patients (mean age: Early 30s). Over the last 15-20 years, the mean age at which patients rupture their Achilles tendons has clearly increased. Moreover, although these tendons still rupture much more commonly in men, there has been a steady increase in the number of women rupturing their Achilles tendons.

Role of Gastrocnemius Contracture

- While some debate the degree to which a gastrocnemius equinus contracture plays a role in some pathologies, most surgeons would agree that a tight gastrocnemius, as evidenced by the Silfverskiöld test, plays a role in the development of Achilles tendinopathy.
- Gastrocnemius stretching is a universally accepted part of physical therapy (PT) protocols for Achilles tendinosis.
- Many surgeons will treat refractory Achilles tendinosis with gastrocnemius recession with good success.
- A related pathology that merits mention is a gastrocnemius tear, sometimes called tennis leg. With this pathology, the muscle belly is injured (most commonly the medial gastrocnemius) and can either partially or wholly rupture. This injury is less severe than an Achilles tendon rupture, as the muscle tendon unit is intact from top to bottom. Treatment is typically supportive; more aggressive treatment is only very rarely necessary.

HISTORY AND PHYSICAL EXAM FINDINGS

Achilles Tendinosis

- History
  - There is some overlap in the symptoms of noninsertional and insertional Achilles tendinosis with the obvious distinction that they typically hurt in different areas.
  - Patients will complain of activity-related pain with both pathologies; shoewear may be more difficult in those patients with insertional Achilles tendinosis.
  - So called "start-up" and early morning pain is common. It will often dissipate once the patient gets mobilized, and the tight Achilles tendon loosens up somewhat.
  - Women will often be more comfortable in heels, as these shoes decrease the pull of the tight gastrocnemius on the degenerative tendon.
- Physical exam
  - As above, patients with noninsertional tendinopathy will have a focal, painful swelling in the tendon, whereas those with insertional tendinopathy will have swelling and fullness at the insertion with pain in that more distal aspect.

Achilles Tendon Rupture

- History

○ Upward of 80% of patients that rupture their Achilles tendons do so as a result of some sporting activity.

○ Patients almost always note an audible and palpable "pop." Often, patients will think that someone kicked them in the back of the leg.

○ Although degeneration of the tendon is necessary for rupture, patients rarely have clinical symptoms prior to rupture.

- Physical exam
  ○ The Thompson test is well described, whereby a positive test occurs when there is a lack of plantarflexion of the ankle with mediolateral squeezing of the calf musculature.
  ○ Another, perhaps easier, test involves just looking at the resting tension of the Achilles tendon. In unilateral tendon ruptures, there will be a clear difference from side to side, whereby the resting tension of the injured side will show significantly more dorsiflexion.

TREATMENT

Noninsertional Achilles Tendinosis

- Nonoperative treatment
  ○ A heel lift (2 cm) is often utilized to decrease the pull from the tight gastrocnemius. In the acutely painful tendinotic tendon, the heel lift is often useful to decrease the acute pain so that PT can be initiated.
  ○ PT is ultimately the mainstay of nonoperative treatment for this condition. PT consists of gastrocnemius stretching and eccentric Achilles exercises. An eccentric muscle contraction, as opposed to a concentric contraction, is one that occurs while the muscle is physically lengthening.
  ○ This treatment paradigm is often very successful with upward of 90% success rates in some studies. It is often worthwhile to pursue at least 2-3 months of PT.
  ○ Injections are another viable option. Steroid injections impede tendon healing and increase the risk of tendon rupture and are therefore contraindicated. However, both platelet-rich plasma and bone marrow concentrate are reasonable alternatives that can augment tendon healing. These treatments are likely best utilized in those patients who fail PT.
  ○ Another viable option is shockwave therapy, which can either be used in isolation or in conjunction with PT. Better results have been found when used in conjunction with PT.

- Operative treatment
  ○ Gastrocnemius recession can be used to minimize the pull from the tight gastrocnemius muscle. Good results have been reported in this setting.
  ○ The most commonly performed surgery for noninsertional Achilles tendinosis is tendon debridement and repair. Generally speaking, a longitudinal split is made in the tendon, and the tendinotic part of the tendon is cut out. The tendon is then repaired side to side.
  ○ If there is a large area of tendon degeneration, a transfer of the flexor hallucis longus tendon can be considered, although this transfer is rarely necessary.

Insertional Achilles Tendinosis

- Nonoperative treatment

○ A heel lift and PT are also the mainstay of treatment for this pathology. The primary difference is that this treatment paradigm in this setting is less successful than it is for noninsertional pathology with success in up to 2/3 of patients.

○ All the other nonoperative treatment modalities, including injections and shockwave, are viable treatments for insertional Achilles tendinopathy.

- Operative treatment
  ○ Since the pathology is in many ways the same, many of the same treatments are described. The principle difference lies in the fact that the posterior prominence at the insertion plays into the pathology. Gastrocnemius recession has also been described for this pathology with some success, although this procedure does not address any distal prominence that may be present.
  ○ The most commonly performed procedure for noninsertional Achilles tendinopathy is Achilles debridement and repair with resection of any tendon ossification and the Haglund deformity. As above, it is not always clear that the Haglund participates in the pathologic process, although it is often resected.
    − Tendon is approached posteriorly with longitudinal split of tendon.
    − Tendon insertion is then horizontally incised, allowing full access to calcaneus anterior to tendon.
    − Flexor hallucis longus transfer was often performed in order to augment Achilles tendon, although recent data has shown that this transfer is likely unnecessary.
    − Tendon is debrided, and any prominent bone is resected.
    − Tendon is then repaired back down calcaneal insertion.

Achilles Tendon Rupture

- Overview
  ○ The goal of treatment of an Achilles tendon rupture is to achieve healing of the tendon with appropriate tension while minimizing the risk of any complications in doing so.
  ○ This subject is the source of significant debate amongst orthopaedic surgeons.
  ○ The argument has been framed as weighing the risk of rerupture, which was thought to be higher with nonoperative treatment, vs. the risk of wound complications, which is clearly higher with operative treatment.
  ○ Advances in rehabilitation protocols have decreased the risk of rerupture, especially with nonoperative treatment. As a result, more Achilles ruptures are being treated nonoperatively now than in the past.
  ○ Willits et al published a hallmark paper in 2010, a multicenter randomized trial looking at operative vs. nonoperative treatment of Achilles tendon rupture, noting that there was no difference in the rerupture rate. It must be noted that they used a very high rerupture rate in doing their power analysis. Further, this paper points to 1 of the difficulties surrounding what treatment is optimal in that operatively treated patients were significantly stronger. Although the authors dismiss this difference as clinically insignificant, it very well could be significant for a host of patients.

- Nonoperative treatment

○ Nonoperative treatment has changed significantly over the years. Traditionally, patients were kept non-weight bearing for protracted periods of time.

○ Today, patients are typically kept non-weight bearing for ~ 2 weeks. This period of time is critical, however, as that initial period after injury is when the tension gets set. Therefore, maintaining non-weight bearing is not the only imperative. It is also imperative that the patient is placed into a splint, cast, or boot and lift that places the tendon ends at appropriate tension. Patients that present beyond 2 weeks that have been weight bearing without any immobilization in plantarflexion are typically disqualified from nonoperative treatment, as the ability to achieve appropriate tension is compromised in those patients.

○ After the initial few weeks of non-weight bearing, patients can begin partial weight bearing in a boot with a heel lift. In this period 3-4 weeks after injury, the patient can move up to weight bearing as tolerated and can begin formal PT.

○ At 6 weeks, the patient takes the lift out of the boot, and at 8 weeks, the boot is discontinued.

○ By the 8-week period, the tendon is more or less healed, rehabilitation then turns to focus solely on strengthening of the tendon, although maximal recovery after this injury can take 6-12 months.

○ Some authors have noted that plantarflexion strength in the affected tendon remains compromised at long-term follow-up despite compensatory flexor hallucis longus hypertrophy.

- Operative treatment
  ○ The basic goal of operative treatment is quite simple: Restore the appropriate tension to the tendon.

  ○ Open repair has been the traditional workhorse of Achilles tendon repair. A variety of suture configurations have been used with no clear difference between them.

  ○ Repair of the paratenon over the repaired tendon is helpful to decrease any friction from suture knots and also to provide a barrier between the skin and the repaired tendon.

  ○ Percutaneous treatment has been devised as means to get the advantage of operative treatment while minimizing the risk by making a smaller incision. Original concerns over potential danger to the sural nerve can be minimized with some technical machinations. It is not clear that the perceived advantages of percutaneous treatment have been fully realized, although it is a viable treatment alternative.

  ○ Chronic Achilles tendon ruptures have had an inconsistent definition in the literature. In general, acute ruptures can be primarily repaired out to 2 months from injury. Injuries outside this window will likely need some sort of supplementation; various means have been described (turn-down flap, flexor hallucis longus transfer, V-Y lengthening, hamstring autograft, etc.).

SELECTED REFERENCES

1. Lightsey HM et al: Online physical therapy protocol quality, variability, and availability in Achilles tendon repair. Foot Ankle Spec. 1938640017751185, 2018

2. Vega J et al: Endoscopic Achilles tendon augmentation with suture anchors after calcaneal exostectomy in haglund syndrome. Foot Ankle Int. 39(5):551-559, 2018

3. Heikkinen J et al: Tendon length, calf muscle atrophy, and strength deficit after acute Achilles tendon rupture: long-term follow-up of patients in a previous study. J Bone Joint Surg Am. 99(18):1509-1515, 2017

4. Ho G et al: Increasing age in Achilles rupture patients over time. Injury. 48(7):1701-1709, 2017

5. Noback PC et al: Risk factors for achilles tendon rupture: a matched case control study. Injury. 48(10):2342-2347, 2017

6. Trofa DP et al: Professional athletes' return to play and performance after operative repair of an Achilles tendon rupture. Am J Sports Med. 45(12):2864-2871, 2017

7. Edama M et al: The twisted structure of the human Achilles tendon. Scand J Med Sci Sports. 25(5):e497-503, 2015

8. Hunt KJ et al: Surgical treatment of insertional Achilles tendinopathy with or without flexor hallucis longus tendon transfer: a prospective, randomized study. Foot Ankle Int. 36(9):998-1005, 2015

9. Nawoczenski DA et al: Isolated gastrocnemius recession for achilles tendinopathy: strength and functional outcomes. J Bone Joint Surg Am. 97(2):99-105, 2015

10. Vosseller JT et al: Achilles tendon rupture in women. Foot Ankle Int. 34(1):49-53, 2013

11. McCoy BW et al: The strength of achilles tendon repair: a comparison of three suture techniques in human cadaver tendons. Foot Ankle Int. 31(8):701-5, 2010

12. Willits K et al: Operative versus nonoperative treatment of acute Achilles tendon ruptures: a multicenter randomized trial using accelerated functional rehabilitation. J Bone Joint Surg Am. 92(17):2767-75, 2010

13. Tallon C et al: Ruptured Achilles tendons are significantly more degenerated than tendinopathic tendons. Med Sci Sports Exerc. 33(12):1983-90, 2001

14. Kannus P et al: Histopathological changes preceding spontaneous rupture of a tendon. A controlled study of 891 patients. J Bone Joint Surg Am. 73(10):1507-25, 1991

(Left) *A 64-year-old male patient with clear tendon swelling and pain refractory to nonoperative treatment is shown. He has severe insertional Achilles tendinopathy without any insertional ossification.* **(Right)** *Moderate insertional ossification is seen at the tendon insertion in this patient. The patient was tender to palpation directly over and just proximal to the Achilles insertion.*

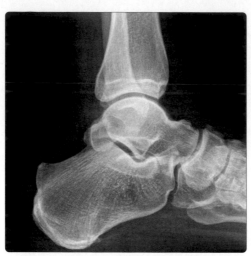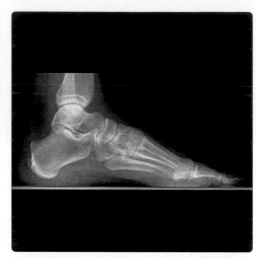

(Left) *Insertional ossification of the Achilles tendon to a much less significant degree is shown; here, it is quite mild. These patients are often a little less successful with nonoperative treatment, as the top of the shoe will often rub in this area.* **(Right)** *As the tendinotic process proceeds, patients will often develop ossification of the tendon insertion, in this case, to a severe degree. This patient failed nonoperative treatment.*

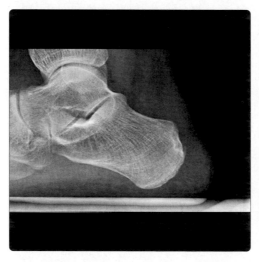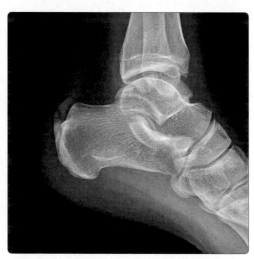

(Left) *The tendon shows thickening and tendinosis, while there is also significant bursitis and inflammation around the tendon with increased signal of the Haglund deformity as well. This patient ultimately had gout of the Achilles enthesis.* **(Right)** *Postoperative image from a patient who had Achilles debridement/repair with Haglund resection is shown. Note the smoothing out of the posterior calcaneus; in this way, the posterior heel is often significantly decompressed.*

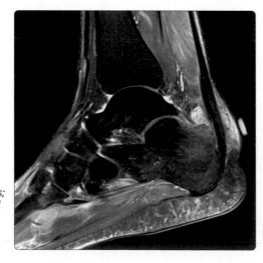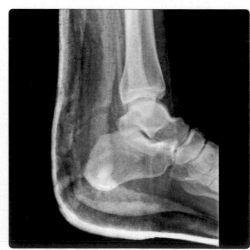

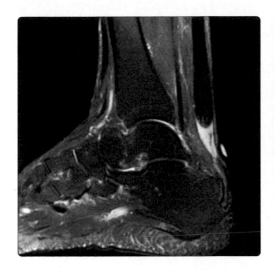

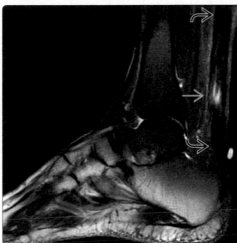

(Left) *A chronic insertional Achilles rupture over 6 months old is shown. The patient was unable to push off and had some plantar heel pain. Surgical treatment required a turn-down flap with flexor hallucis longus transfer, which restored the patient's push-off power and eliminated the heel pain.* **(Right)** *Diffuse and severe noninsertional Achilles tendinopathy with thickening of the tendon* ⟹ *and partial tear of the midsubstance of the tendon* ⟹ *is shown.*

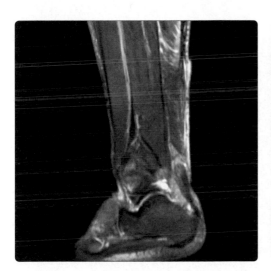

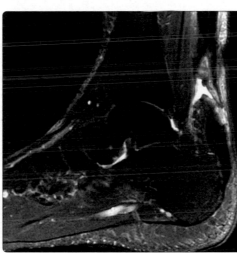

(Left) *Rupture of the Achilles tendon is shown with proximal retraction of the proximal stump. Once again, the distal tendon is degenerative, although it was not directly involved in the rupture.* **(Right)** *Rerupture of the Achilles tendon in a patient initially treated nonoperatively is shown. Note the degree of abnormality in the whole tendon.*

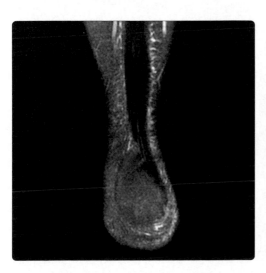

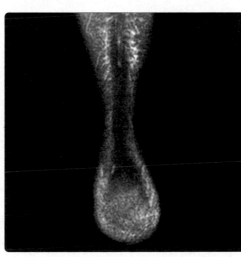

(Left) *The more distal insertion of the medial gastrocnemius can be seen medially, whereas the beginnings of the more proximal insertion of the lateral gastrocnemius and soleus can be seen more laterally.* **(Right)** *The more proximal insertion of the lateral gastrocnemius and soleus can be seen here.*

KEY FACTS

- Tendon pathology is most commonly related to the degenerative process of tendinosis, as is seen in the Achilles and posterior tibial tendons.
- While tendonitis is a more common term colloquially, tendinosis is a much more common problem clinically.
- Predisposing factors should be sought, most notably a cavovarus foot in those patients with peroneal tendon pathology. Predisposing factors for less common tendon pathologies are less clear.
- Anterior tibial tendinopathy is thought to be relatively uncommon, although its incidence has never been objectively sought. It is very possible that the incidence is higher than has been traditionally thought.
- The flexor hallucis longus tendon can become inflamed as it passes posterior to the ankle joint, causing a stenosing tenosynovitis. This pathology is relatively common in dancers, especially ballet dancers.

- Extensor hallucis longus pathology is most commonly related to something being dropped onto the dorsal foot while someone is barefoot, causing a laceration of the tendon.

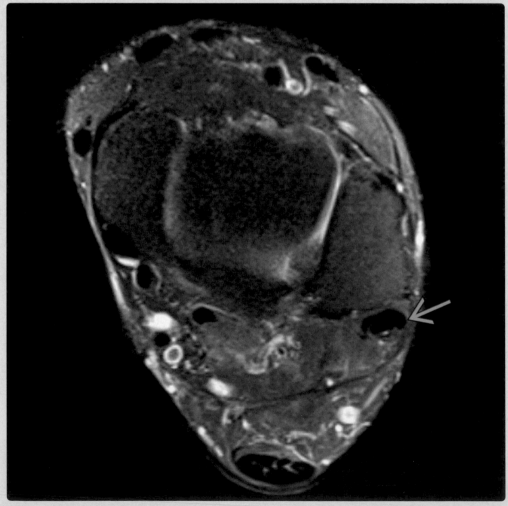

A 39-year-old male patient with lateral ankle pain and a history of ankle sprains is shown. The peroneal tendons can be notoriously difficult to see as they turn about the fibula. However, here, the MR shows a split tear of the peroneus brevis ➡.

TERMINOLOGY

- While the Achilles tendon and the posterior tibial tendon are the most commonly pathologic tendons around the ankle and, as such, rightfully get a lot of attention, other tendon disorders in the foot and ankle are not uncommon and can certainly be just as disabling.

- In general, the most common tendon pathology encountered is the degenerative process known as tendinosis, which is characterized as a failed healing response. This pathology can lead to pain, which can occasionally culminate in rupture.

- In this chapter, the focus will be on the peroneal and anterior tibial tendon (ATT) as well as the extensor and flexor hallucis longus (EHL and FHL, respectively).

PERONEAL TENDONS

Anatomy

- The peroneus brevis and longus muscles, innervated by the superficial peroneal nerve, have their origin off the fibula in the lateral compartment of the leg with the origin of the peroneus longus generally being more proximal.
- The tendons pass through a sheath as they course around the fibula; at the level of the ankle, the peroneus brevis is generally anterior and sometimes medial to the peroneus longus.
- The peroneus brevis inserts at the base of the 5th metatarsal, whereas the peroneus longus courses medial under the cuboid through the cuboid tunnel to attach to the plantar base of the 1st metatarsal/medial cuneiform.

Function

- The peroneus brevis is the primary muscle that provides eversion at the subtalar joint, while the peroneus longus secondarily everts by plantarflexing the 1st ray.
- The primary antagonist of the peroneus brevis is the posterior tibial tendon, while the primary antagonist of the peroneus longus is the ATT.
- The peroneal tendons, and especially the peroneus brevis, are critical for optimal ankle stability. Indeed, rehabilitation from an ankle sprain has a large focus on regaining and maintaining eversion strength.

Pathology

- As previously stated, these tendons can undergo degeneration, which can lead to split tears in the tendon. As a generalization, peroneus brevis issues tend to occur at the distal fibula, whereas peroneus longus issues tend to occur at the cuboid tunnel. This generalization is certainly not universally true but is often the case. A large peroneal tubercle can occasionally cause injury or irritation of the tendons.
- At the distal fibula, a host of potential pathologies can be encountered, which can involve either the tendon itself or something external to the tendon.
  - The tendon can have a single (or multiple) split tear(s). When multiple split tears are present, the structural integrity of the tendon is often compromised such that it is not terribly functional.
  - Generally speaking, the muscle belly of the peroneal tendons should end prior to the sheath through which the tendons travel around the fibula. If this is not the case, this distal muscle belly can cause pain and impair function of the tendons. Also, some patients will have a peroneus quartus or an aberrant "extra" tendon that runs through the sheath around the fibula.
- In the cuboid tunnel, an os peroneum (an accessory ossicle within the tendon) can potentially cause pain or fracture.
- Predisposing factors to peroneal tendon pathology include a cavovarus foot and multiple ankle sprains, factors which are clearly related.
- Peroneal tendon subluxation/dislocation can occur with a forceful dorsiflexion and eversion mechanism, which can cause the superior peroneal retinaculum (SPR) to fail, leading to the tendons sliding out from behind the fibula. This subluxation can lead to direct injury to the tendons in addition to causing pain and disability in and of itself.

HISTORY AND PHYSICAL EXAMINATION

History

- A history of trauma will often be recalled by the patient, although it is not absolutely necessary for tendon pathology. However, ankle trauma is common, and it will sometimes be difficult to draw a direct line between the trauma and the tendon pathology.
- Peroneal pathology should be actively sought in patients with recurrent ankle instability.

Physical Examination

- The station of the foot should be checked with the arch height checked. The subtle cavus foot as noted by the "peek-a-boo" heel sign should be sought.
- Swelling will often be noted about the posterior distal fibula &/or along the posterolateral hindfoot.
- Palpation along the course of the tendons will often elicit pain.
- Pain can also occur with resisted eversion and sometimes with resisted inversion as well.
- Peroneal subluxation can be elicited with dorsiflexion/eversion.

Imaging

- MR is most useful for evaluating the peroneal tendons, although they may be subject to the magic angle phenomenon, whereby it is difficult to achieve adequate visualization of the tendons in the region of the distal fibula.
- Ultrasound can be beneficial as well, especially in its ability to provide a dynamic assessment.

TREATMENT

Peroneal Tendon Tears

- These tears are not tendon tears in the traditional sense that Achilles tendon tears, for example, are. These tears are often longitudinal split tears of the tendon. While the tendons can rupture outright, meaning a discontinuity in the longitudinal course of the tendon, it is not common.

- The surgical options have traditionally been tied to the degree of tendon abnormality. If a single split exists in the tendon, then the split part can be excised. Tendon repair can be attempted, although the tendon has a limited healing capacity. More commonly, surgeons will attempt to tubularize the tendon.
- If multiple splits tears are present with an area of the tendon that is markedly degenerative, then excision of the degenerative segment can be performed with subsequent brevis to longus tenodesis, whereby the peroneus brevis is sutured to the longus proximally and distally.
- More recently, some authors have noted success with allograft tendon repair. Instead of performing tenodesis, surgeons will resect the degenerative tendon segment and suture in a tendon allograft, which substitutes for the degenerative segment.
- If both the peroneus brevis and longus are tendonotic and degenerative, a FHL transfer to the base of the 5th metatarsal can be performed to regain some eversion strength.
- Generally speaking, surgeons will sacrifice peroneus longus function in order to maintain peroneus brevis function in its role as the sole everter of the foot.

Peroneal Tendon Subluxation/Dislocation

- These injuries often result from a failure of the soft tissue restraints that keep the tendons on the posterior border of the fibula, namely the SPR.
- The morphology of the posterior fibula in terms of its relative concavity or lack thereof can certainly play a role in this pathology.
- Treatment is centered on creating a space in the posterior fibula in which the tendons can reside and repairing the soft tissue restraints.
- Some authors have described intrasheath subluxation of the peroneal tendons. In this pathology, there is no injury to the SPR; the tendons switch their positions, causing a painful click. Groove deepening has been found to be effective in these patients for pain relief.

ANTERIOR TIBIAL TENDON

Anatomy

- The anterior tibial muscle has its origin off the lateral aspect of the tibia in the upper 2/3 of the anterior compartment of the leg. It is innervated by the deep peroneal nerve.
- The tendon passes underneath the superior extensor retinaculum on its way to inserting onto the medial cuneiform/base of the 1st metatarsal. It acts in opposition to the peroneus longus.

Function

- The ATT provides the primary dorsiflexion force of the ankle. It also acts to invert the hindfoot.
- Insufficiency of the ATT, whether from direct injury or the after effects of a stroke, will lead to a steppage gait. During gait, the ATT fires to dorsiflex the ankle while the "swing" leg is passing through. An inability to actively dorsiflex will lead to the foot dragging on the ground, often giving the patient the feeling that he or she is going to trip. A steppage gait occurs when a patient flexes the hip and knee in order to clear the leg in swing.

Pathology

- As with any other tendon, patients can develop tendinosis of the ATT, which can cause pain along the course of the tendon. This pain often becomes more significant as the person walks more.
- More rarely, the tendon can rupture if subjected to an eccentric contracture.
- Given the relatively subcutaneous course of the distal tendon, it can occasionally be lacerated by a dropped knife if a person is barefoot, although that is more common with the toe extensors, especially EHL.
- A range of neurologic conditions can cause loss of ATT function, resulting in a foot drop, which, although it is often not a problem inherent to the tendon, does merit mention.

HISTORY AND PHYSICAL EXAMINATION

History

- Predisposing factors for this pathology are not well understood. Patients rarely note trauma prior to the development of symptoms.
- Not unlike Achilles tendon ruptures, patients may rupture the tendon without having much in the way of symptoms prior to rupture.

Physical Examination

- Patients will complain of pain about the anterior ankle or about the dorsal and medial hindfoot.
- A palpable thickening of the tendon can sometimes be noted that is also tender to palpation.
- A gastrocnemius equinus may be noted.
- Patients often note pain with resisted dorsiflexion and inversion.

Imaging

- MR is the test of choice to show both tendinosis and possible rupture.

TREATMENT

Anterior Tibial Tendinosis

- Nonoperative treatment is warranted in those patients that present with tendinosis.
- An ankle-foot-orthosis can be considered depending on the severity of a patient's symptoms. This orthosis decreases the amount of work that the tendon needs to do and can thus decrease symptoms by allowing the tendon to relatively rest.
- The principle issue with an ankle-foot-orthosis is that many, if not most, patients have no desire to wear it for any protracted period of time, as it is bulky and difficult to hide.
- Physical therapy can be effective in healing the tendinotic area.
- Given that the pathology, i.e., tendinosis, is similar to that seen in other tendons of the foot and ankle, other treatments aimed at promoting healing in the tendon are reasonable, including treatments such as shock wave, platelet-rich plasma or bone marrow aspirate concentrate injection, etc. As this pathology is not common, there is little data from which to derive decisions to guide best options.

- Surgical treatment with debridement and repair of the tendon is a last resort. If the tendon is so degenerative that is not salvageable, then tendon transfer with EHL or even allograft tendon are options.

Anterior Tibial Tendon Rupture

- Surgical treatment is often necessary in order to repair or reconstruct the tendon to achieve a maximally functional result.
- The ruptured tendon is often so degenerative and tendinotic that it is not terribly usable for reconstruction.
- The EHL can be harvested distally and either tied into the ATT stump or fixed directly to the bony insertion. Distally, the EHL is tenodesed to the extensor hallucis brevis.
- Reconstruction with allograft tendon has been described in an effort to minimize the morbidity of autograft harvest.

FLEXOR HALLUCIS LONGUS

Anatomy

- The FHL muscle has its origin off the posterior aspect of the middle 1/3 of the fibula. This deep posterior compartment muscle is innervated by the tibial nerve.
- The FHL passes through a fibroosseous tunnel in the posterior ankle on its way to its insertion at the plantar aspect of the distal phalanx of the big toe.
- In the plantar midfoot, the FHL crosses the flexor digitorum longus at the knot of Henry, a site at which there are numerous connections between the 2 tendons.

Function

- The FHL is the primary plantarflexor of the big toe at the interphalangeal joint. It is a secondary plantarflexor of the big toe metatarsophalangeal joint and ankle joint.

Pathology

- The FHL is somewhat unique in its passage through a tight sheath around the ankle; this passage can cause a tenosynovitis with triggering of the big toe.
- Isolated stenosing tenosynovitis is a pathology most commonly seen in dancers.

HISTORY AND PHYSICAL EXAMINATION

History

- Patients complain of posterior ankle pain that can be exacerbated by extreme plantarflexion. Also, extension of the hallux with ankle dorsiflexion can cause posterior ankle pain &/or triggering.

Physical Examination

- Pain is seen with deep palpation in the posterior ankle with big toe motion.
- As previously stated, pain or triggering can be elicited with big toe extension coupled with ankle dorsiflexion.

TREATMENT

Flexor Hallucis Longus Tenosynovitis

- Nonoperative treatment generally consists of NSAIDs and physical therapy with gentle stretching of the big toe.
- The surgical treatment of this pathology is release of the fibroosseous tunnel, allowing the tendon to move freely.

- Debridement of the tendon is sometimes necessary if there has been any fraying of the tendon as it passes through the tunnel.
- Good results have been achieved with resolution of symptoms and return to baseline activity with surgical treatment.

EXTENSOR HALLUCIS LONGUS

Anatomy

- This anterior compartment muscle originates from the anterior aspect of the fibula and interosseous membrane, passing onto the dorsum of the foot and inserting into the dorsal aspect of the distal phalanx of the big toe.
- It runs subcutaneously over the dorsum of the foot.

Function

- Its primary function is to dorsiflex the big toe; it is also a secondary dorsiflexor of the ankle.

Pathology

- The primary way in which the EHL gets injured is from a sharp object falling onto the dorsum of the foot, lacerating the tendon subcutaneously.
- The tendon can sometimes retract back into the leg, beyond the superior extensor retinaculum.

HISTORY AND PHYSICAL EXAMINATION

History

- Most commonly, in the author's experience, this has occurred when a person is cooking barefoot and drops a knife onto his or her foot. The person tends to tense up, making the tendon even more prominent on the dorsum of the foot.

Physical Examination

- The laceration itself may be quite small. An attempt should be made to palpate the tendon.
- Active dorsiflexion of the big toe should be gauged; partial laceration can occur.
- A thorough neurovascular exam should be performed to assess for any concomitant injury.

TREATMENT

Extensor Hallucis Longus Laceration

- Primary repair is warranted to restore normal foot function.
- If the tendon has retracted, an incision may be needed about the anterior ankle to identify the EHL and pull it distally.
- Most commonly, the laceration will be a clean cut, and so direct primary repair is possible.

SELECTED REFERENCES

1. Bastías GF et al: Technique tip: EDL-to-EHL double loop transfer for extensor hallucis longus reconstruction. Foot Ankle Surg. ePub, 2017
2. Habashy A et al: Peroneus quartus muscle. Am J Orthop (Belle Mead NJ). 46(6):E419-E422, 2017
3. Imre N et al: The peroneus brevis tendon at its insertion site on fifth metatarsal bone. Foot Ankle Surg. 22(1):41-5, 2016
4. Pellegrini MJ et al: Effectiveness of allograft reconstruction vs tenodesis for irreparable peroneus brevis tears: a cadaveric model. Foot Ankle Int. 37(8):803-8, 2016
5. Saragas NP et al: Peroneal tendon dislocation/subluxation - case series and review of the literature. Foot Ankle Surg. 22(2):125-30, 2016

(Left) *A 24-year-old female patient with persistent lateral ankle pain after an ankle sprain despite months of physical therapy is shown. MR shows a split tear of the peroneus brevis ➾.* **(Right)** *First of 4 sequential images in the same patient shows some discontinuity of the peroneus brevis ➾.*

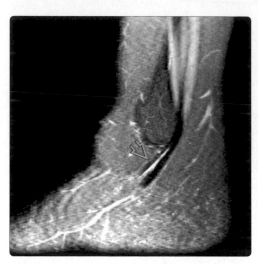
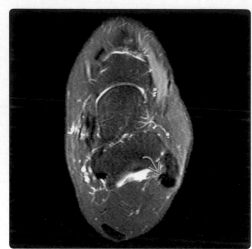

(Left) *Sequential image shows some discontinuity of the peroneus brevis ➾. Split tears can often be subtle and difficult to fully pick up on imaging. Correlation with physical examination is necessary.* **(Right)** *Sequential image shows some discontinuity of the peroneus brevis. Here, the abnormality is perhaps seen most clearly, as the tendon is flattened out ➾ with a fair amount of heterogeneity.*

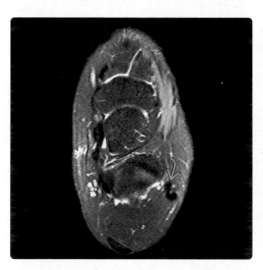
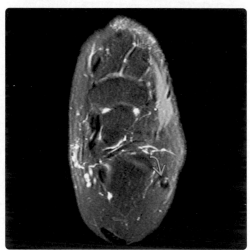

(Left) *Sequential image shows some discontinuity of the peroneus brevis. On this more distal image, the tendon can be seen to clearly split into 2 components, a more anterior part and a more posterior part ➾.* **(Right)** *A 74-year-old male patient 2 years status post total ankle arthroplasty who had persistent pain about the posterolateral hindfoot is shown. MR shows degenerative tear of the peroneus brevis ➾.*

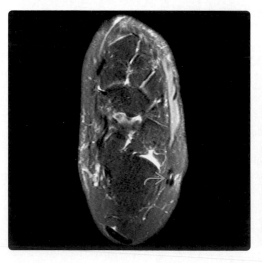
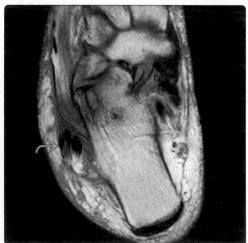

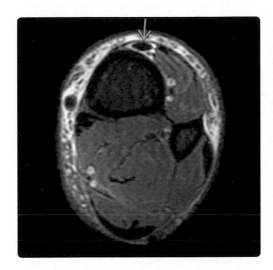

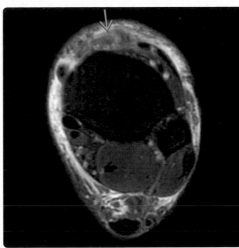

(Left) *First of 3 sequential axial images shows a 51-year-old male patient with anterior tibia tendon rupture. Here, we see the intact, more or less normal anterior tibial tendon* ➡. (Right) *The same 51-year-old male patient with anterior tibia tendon rupture is shown. Here, the tendon is not readily seen; a degenerative halo of tissue is seen where the tendon should be* ➡.

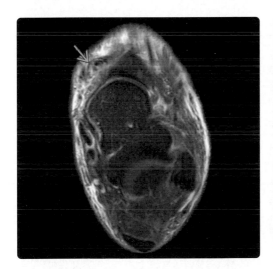

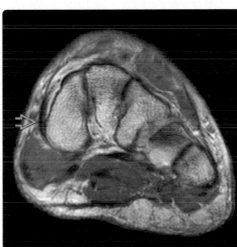

(Left) *The same 51-year-old male patient with anterior tibia tendon rupture is shown. Here, we see the residual distal tendon* ➡. *The rupture occurred in the distal tendon, although the insertion was not affected.* (Right) *The same 51-year-old male patient with anterior tibia tendon rupture is shown. In this coronal image, we see the intact anterior tibial tendon insertion* ➡.

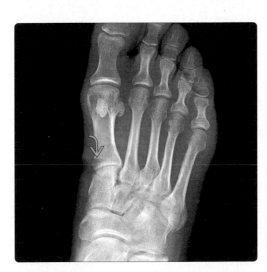

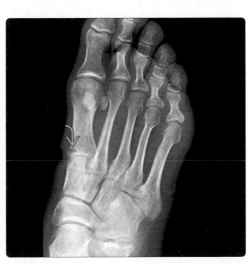

(Left) *A 45-year-old male patient who had a heavy blade fall on his foot causing the 1st metatarsal fracture* ➡ *as well as a laceration of the extensor hallucis longus tendon is shown.* (Right) *The oblique still shows the effect* ➡ *of the blade. The traumatic skin laceration was extended to repair the extensor hallucis longus tendon. The proximal tendon retracted requiring a 2nd incision over the anterior ankle; the extensor hallucis longus was identified there and passed distally with a suture passer.*

ANKLE INSTABILITY

- Ankle sprains are among the most common injuries seen by orthopaedic surgeons.
- A variety of pathologies can result from an ankle sprain mechanism. These individual pathologies should be actively sought, as the treatment is not the same for all of these different pathologies.
- The lateral ankle ligaments, as well as the syndesmotic ligaments, can be injured. Medial ankle injuries are less common, although sometimes all of the ankle ligaments can be injured to some degree.
  - The proximal fibula should be palpated so that a Maisonneuve injury is not missed.
- Fractures of the lateral process of the talus, anterior process of the calcaneus, or the base of the 5th metatarsal can occur. Even Lisfranc and other midfoot injuries can occur, and so all of these places should be palpated.
- Many, if not most, patients will completely recover without the need for any invasive treatment.

- If nonoperative treatment is unsuccessful, an MR may be warranted. The MR will typically show ligamentous injury; the chondral surfaces and the peroneal tendons should be closely assessed in these patients.
- When needed, surgery is often successful, although all pathology must be sought and addressed.

(Left) Note the fibular origin ⇨ of the calcaneofibular ligament (CFL) in this patient without ligamentous pathology. Just inferior to the CFL are the peroneal tendons, and just superior and medial is the posterior talofibular ligament. (Right) A thicker anterior talofibular ligament (ATFL) ⇨ is seen in this axial MR. Increased thickness can be related to a previous ankle sprain injury, whereas more overt instability can present with discontinuity in the ligament or its complete absence.

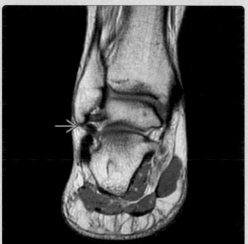
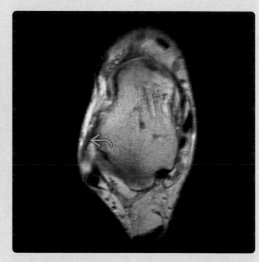

(Left) The CFL ⇨ is once again visualized. The coronal MR allows for the best view of the CFL. This patient did not have ligamentous ankle pathology. (Right) Another view of a normal ATFL ⇨ is shown. This ligament is completely normal with no thickening or other abnormality.

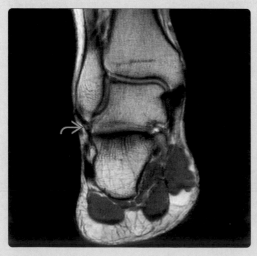
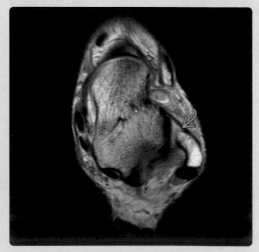

TERMINOLOGY

Ankle Sprains and Ankle Instability

- Ankle sprains are exceedingly common injuries. Virtually every person has sprained his or her ankle at some point. Many of these acute injuries will improve without any specific treatment or without a trip to the doctor. Ankle instability is essentially by its very definition a chronic condition, whereby the static and dynamic stabilizers no longer function to provide adequate stability for the ankle &/or subtalar joint.

ANATOMY/BIOMECHANICS

- The ligaments about the ankle are generally broken down into component groups that act together to provide certain components of stability about the ankle and hindfoot. The syndesmotic, or tibiofibular, ligaments provide stability to the syndesmosis, while the lateral ligament complex includes the anterior talofibular ligament (ATFL), calcaneofibular ligament (CFL), and lateral subtalar ligaments. The medial side of the ankle is stabilized by the deltoid ligaments in all its component parts.

Syndesmotic Ligaments

- The syndesmosis, or distal tibiofibular joint, is formed by the articulation of the incisura fibularis tibiae and the corresponding distal medial fibula. It is important to remember that the tibia and fibula come together to make a formal joint in this area.
- The ligaments stabilizing the tibiofibular syndesmosis include the anterior inferior tibiofibular ligament (AITFL), posterior inferior tibiofibular ligament, and interosseous ligament, in addition to the interosseous membrane and the transverse tibiofibular ligament.
- The primary motion of the fibula relative to the tibia is primarily rotation in the axial plane, although there is some medial translation with plantarflexion.

Lateral Ankle Ligament Complex

- This complex is made of the ATFL, CFL, and posterior talofibular ligament (PTFL).
- The ATFL and CFL are commonly injured, while the PTFL is rarely injured. The ATFL is a condensation of the lateral ankle joint capsule.
- The ATFL limits anterior translation of the talus, while the CFL limits inversion at both the ankle and subtalar joints, as it also crosses the subtalar joint.

Subtalar Ligament Complex

- The subtalar joint allows for inversion and eversion of the calcaneus relative to the talus.
- The lateral subtalar ligaments limit anterior and medial translation as well as inversion at the subtalar joint.
- There are 3 layers of lateral ligaments: Superficial (calcaneofibular and lateral talocalcaneal ligaments, lateral root of the inferior extensor retinaculum), intermediate (cervical ligament, intermediate root of the inferior extensor retinaculum), and deep (interosseous talocalcaneal ligament and the medial root of the inferior extensor retinaculum).

Deltoid Ligament

- Deltoid ligament is a large ligament with a deep and superficial component; it is confluent with other medial soft tissue structures and prevents eversion as well as anterior and posterior translation of the talus.

ACUTE LATERAL ANKLE LIGAMENT INJURIES

History

- Patients will typically describe an inversion ankle injury, although it is often difficult for the patient to remember the specifics of the injury.
- Patients will be variably limited in terms of their ability to ambulate, although some patients may be able to get around well.

Physical Examination

- Patients typically present with a swollen ankle; the swelling can be somewhat diffuse, extending to areas that may or may not be actually injured.
- Bruising tends to occur in the most dependent areas and can often often accumulate about the heel or even down the foot in between the toes.
- Palpation can be very helpful in terms of guiding the examiner as to what exactly is injured. Many structures can be injured with an inversion injury. The surgeon should steadfastly assess the following areas for tenderness to palpation: The proximal fibula (assess for Maisonneuve), distal fibula, 5th metatarsal (assess for Jones or other fracture), tarsometatarsal joints (assess for midfoot or Lisfranc injury), medial ankle (assess for deltoid injury), anterior syndesmosis, over the ATFL and CFL, peroneal tendons, anterior process of the calcaneus, and ankle joint line. An effort should also be made to palpate deep in the sinus tarsi to assess for a fracture of the lateral process of the talus, although palpation in this area is less specific and is often somewhat tender in those with an acute sprain.
- Range of motion should be assessed, especially in the hindfoot. Some patients, primarily but not exclusively adolescents, may be predisposed to ankle injuries due to a stiff hindfoot, most commonly from a tarsal coalition.

Imaging

- Ankle radiographs are appropriate to assess for any fracture; foot radiographs may be warranted in those patients whose physical exam is concerning for foot injury.
- In the acute setting, further imaging is seldom warranted unless there is concern for a specific injury that is not well visualized on plain radiography. An example would include a patient with pain concerning for a lateral process talus fracture. A CT scan would help to definitively assess whether a fracture was present, and, if so, its dimensions and extension.
- An MR is rarely needed in the acute ankle sprain, as it will rarely change the initial management. Most often, MRs obtained in this setting do not at all impact decision-making and are entirely extraneous, ultimately making for a poor use of resources.

Treatment

- Management of the acute ankle sprain is initially geared toward addressing the acute pain and swelling that accompany these injuries.

- A controlled ankle motion (CAM) boot can be very helpful for the patient in the initial few days to few weeks, as it simply protects the ankle and makes it easier for the patient to ambulate.
- Once the acute injury is not so painful, typically in 1-2 weeks, physical therapy is initiated. Physical therapy principally works on peroneal strengthening and balance utilizing a balance board. The return to full eversion strength typically heralds functional recovery.
- Physical therapy is remarkably successful in this setting with the overwhelming majority of patients getting completely better with no further need for treatment. If patients do not improve despite several months of physical therapy, then further and more aggressive treatment may be warranted.
- The proportion of patients with acute injury that will develop chronic issues is difficult to define. It is almost certainly overestimated by surgeons. Many patients in the acute phase may never seek formal treatment and are therefore not counted in the denominator of those injured.

CHRONIC ANKLE INSTABILITY

History

- It goes without saying, but it is important to establish the chief complaint. Some patients will have more pain than instability, while others will complain primarily of instability and less of pain.
- The patient's treatment up to the point of presentation must be understood. Not infrequently, the patient has had no formal treatment or at least insufficient treatment.
- It must be noted that some of this instability can come from the subtalar joint. Given the similarity of mechanism involved in injury to either joint, subtalar joint instability can often coexist with ankle instability or, less frequently, exist in isolation.

Physical Examination

- In the chronic setting, patients can present with variable degrees of swelling or may have no swelling at all.
- As in the acute setting, tenderness to palpation can be a good guide as to what may be injured or most symptomatic, although the relationship between the 2 is not as consistent as it is in the acute setting. The pain in the chronic setting can often be a bit more diffuse and difficult to pin down.
- Ankle and hindfoot range of motion should be assessed. As above, a stiff hindfoot can be a predisposing factor to injury.
- A cavovarus foot, or even a subtle cavovarus foot, can predispose to ankle instability. Surgeons should look for the "peek-a-boo" heel that can be seen in the subtle cavus foot, which is indicative of some hindfoot varus.
- Strength should be assessed, especially eversion strength. A lack of full strength generally or a lack of eversion strength can be indicative of incomplete rehabilitation efforts and may signal a need for further physical therapy prior to surgical intervention.

- The anterior drawer test is used to assess insufficiency of the ATFL. This test can be quite subjective; a surgeon must perform it many times to be able to attain the feel necessary to differentiate what are often subtle differences between degrees of anterior translation. Performing stress radiographs can lend more objectivity to this examination.
- While it is clinically difficult to differentiate between subtalar and ankle instability, one author noted a rotational component to subtalar instability. In this way, varus stress with internal rotation may cause medial shift of the calcaneus or increased lateral opening of the talocalcaneal joint.

Imaging

- Stress radiographs with an anterior drawer test (sagittal plane instability) and talar tilt (coronal plane instability) can help to objectively document instability.
- An MR is often warranted preoperatively, less to assess for ligamentous injury to the ankle than to assess the peroneal tendons for injury and any degree of intraarticular pathology that may need to be addressed. The subtalar ligaments can be also assessed on MR.
- If there is concern for a tarsal coalition, a CT scan may be warranted to document its presence and degree.

Treatment

- If the patient has not had any or has had insufficient rehabilitation, then a trial of physical therapy is warranted.
- Generally speaking, the 3 areas of concern with surgery are, obviously, the ligamentous insufficiency, but also the status of the ankle articular cartilage and peroneal tendons.
- Even if the preoperative MR shows no overt injury to the articular cartilage or the peroneal tendons, surgeons will often directly assess both at the time of surgery. Scar tissue &/or synovitis in the anterior or lateral ankle will often need to be debrided, and peroneal pathology can sometimes be incompletely visualized on an MR. A distal peroneus brevis muscle belly or peroneus quartus may need to be addressed.
- An ankle arthroscopy is performed with any intraarticular pathology addressed at that time. Surgeons will then often use a roughly transverse incision centered over the distal fibula that provides access to both the ATFL and CFL in addition to the peroneal tendons.
- As above, peroneal pathology can include a split tear, distal muscle belly, or peroneus quartus.
- While a host of nonanatomic ankle ligament reconstructions have been described, the Broström-Gould reconstruction is an anatomic reconstruction, is most commonly used today, and has an established track record of excellent clinical results. Some authors have used a slip of peroneus brevis to augment the reconstruction, although the need for this is unclear at best, and, given the prime role that a strong peroneus brevis plays in maintaining ankle stability, using the tendon in this fashion may not be the best idea.
- In the Broström-Gould reconstruction, the ATFL and CFL are incised off the fibula; any redundancy in the tissue may be incised to some degree. The ligaments are then repaired back to the fibula either through drill holes or with suture anchors. The Gould modification involves using the inferior extensor retinaculum, which is sutured to the fibular periosteum to back up the repair.

- In those patients with ligamentous laxity, it is often necessary to back up the repair to some degree given the patient's soft tissues are insufficient. Some surgeons will use allograft ligaments; another option is using a heavy suture to augment the ligament repair.

SYNDESMOSIS INSTABILITY

History

- Syndesmotic injury typically, although not necessarily, involves a different mechanism of injury than a typical lateral ankle sprain.
- The mechanism of injury will typically involve a forced external rotation mechanism of the ankle. In this setting, injury to the syndesmosis can be accompanied by injury to the deltoid ligament.
- The syndesmosis can be injured in part with the AITFL often injured to some degree in acute lateral ankle sprains.

Physical Examination

- In the acute phase, it can be difficult to differentiate syndesmotic injury from other lateral ankle injuries. However, patients will typically have distinct pain over the AITFL, indicating at least some involvement of the anterior syndesmosis. The posterior syndesmosis is deeper and more difficult to directly palpate.
- As previously mentioned, a thorough exam should be performed. Special tests have been described, including the squeeze test, although they are not very sensitive or specific.
- The proximal fibula should be palpated; tenderness to palpation in that area could be indicative of a Maisonneuve injury and may prompt more aggressive treatment.

Imaging

- Ankle radiographs should be assessed for any diastasis. If the patient has any proximal fibular tenderness, tib-fib films should be obtained to assess for a proximal fibular fracture, which may accompany syndesmotic injury.
- Conservative treatment is usually initiated prior to obtaining advanced imaging. In the athlete, early MR may be warranted to help guide treatment. Rarely, patients can completely tear the syndesmosis without fracture, which may warrant more aggressive early treatment.

Treatment

- Syndesmosis sprain is treated in much the same way as a lateral ankle sprain with a period of protection in a boot with the subsequent initiation of physical therapy.
- For reasons that are not entirely clear, syndesmosis sprains tend to be slow to fully recover, slower than lateral ankle sprains.
- In those patients with evidence of a tear of all the syndesmotic ligaments, surgical stabilization is warranted. The fibula is typically stabilized to the tibia with either screws or a suture device. Screws have traditionally been used with a protracted period of non-weight bearing to allow the ligaments to heal. Suture button devices may more easily allow for a more anatomic reduction as well as earlier weight bearing.

DELTOID INJURY

History

- The deltoid ligament can be injured in combination with any other ankle ligament injury. Isolated injury can also occur, typically with an eversion &/or external rotation mechanism. Further, the deltoid ligament can be injured with fracture of the ankle.
- Deltoid injury, much like syndesmotic injury, can be slow to improve. Some patients may be predisposed to a more protracted recovery, as those with pes planus put relatively more strain on the deltoid. In this setting, acute injuries are more likely to linger with full recovery taking months.

Physical Examination

- The deltoid ligament is a broad ligament with multiple component parts. Medial swelling is often seen with injury as well as tenderness to palpation over any of these component parts.
- External rotation stress can recreate pain or a sense of instability.
- In the flatfooted patient, it is necessary to rule out any pathology of the posterior tibial tendon based solely on exam. However, the ability to perform a single limb heel rise proves that the posterior tibial tendon is functional.

Imaging

- Ankle radiographs will often be normal acutely. Stress radiographs are rarely obtained without the presence of any fracture.
- If pain persists, an MR may be warranted to document the degree of injury and anatomically define what part of the deltoid is injured.

Treatment

- A thorough trial of conservative treatment is warranted to include a CAM boot, physical therapy, and potentially orthotics to correct pes planus.
- If pain persists despite appropriate nonoperative treatment, then surgical repair of the deltoid may be warranted. In this setting, the MR can be helpful to direct the surgeon to the area of pathology. Deltoid repair, reefing, or reconstruction can be performed depending on the pathology. Ligament augmentation has been used with some success to buttress repair or reconstruction.
- In those patients who do have a flatfoot, a discussion regarding possible flatfoot correction should be had with the patient. There is little guidance in the literature as to when this correction should be considered, and so, the surgeon can tailor the need for reconstruction to the individual patient.

SELECTED REFERENCES

1. Andersen MR et al: Randomized trial comparing suture button with single syndesmotic screw for syndesmosis injury. J Bone Joint Surg Am. 100(1):2-12, 2018
2. Coetzee JC et al: Functional results of open Broström ankle ligament repair augmented with a suture tape. Foot Ankle Int. 1071100717742363, 2018
3. Cho BK et al: The peroneal strength deficits in patients with chronic ankle instability compared to ankle sprain copers and normal individuals. Foot Ankle Surg. ePub, 2017
4. Cho BK et al: Minimal invasive suture-tape augmentation for chronic ankle instability. Foot Ankle Int. 36(11):1330-8, 2015
5. Huber T et al: Motion of the fibula relative to the tibia and its alterations with syndesmosis screws: a cadaver study. Foot Ankle Surg. 18(3):203-9, 2012

(Left) *Axial MR at the very distal tip of the fibula provides the best view of the often-injured ATFL* ⊡. *The ligament is intact on this image.* **(Right)** *This patient had many sprains over years. Note the significant attenuation of the ATFL* ⊡ *as well as the fracture fragment from the distal fibula* ⊡. *This patient had both injured the ligament itself and had an ankle sprain equivalent fracture. The patient ultimately needed ankle stabilization.*

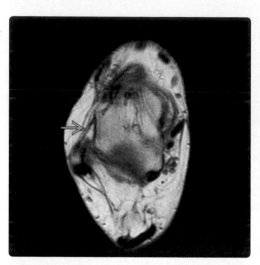
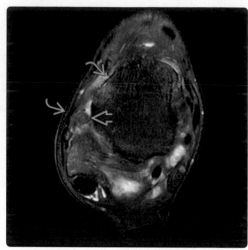

(Left) *This axial MR is perhaps most notable for what is not seen, i.e., there is no discernible ATFL* ⊡. *This patient was a college athlete who had had multiple sprains over years and was ligamentously lax. She ultimately required ligamentous stabilization.* **(Right)** *Note the attenuation of the CFL* ⊡ *seen on this MR in the same patient. This patient had both increased anterior translation as well as significant laxity on talar tilt testing.*

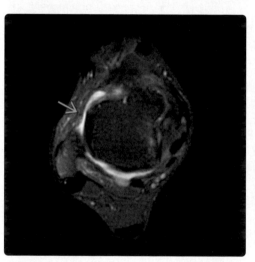
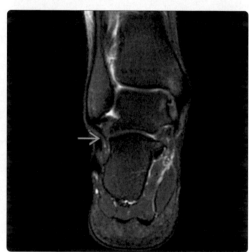

(Left) *Complete syndesmotic disruption in an American football player is shown. No clear attachment* ⊡ *is seen between anterior fibula and tibia, indicating disruption of AITFL. Further, note attenuation of the PITFL as it attaches to fibula* ⊡ *as well as fluid seen between PITFL and tibia* ⊡. *Fluid interspersed between PITFL and tibia can be a subtle indication of syndesmotic injury.* **(Right)** *The patient with complete syndesmotic disruption underwent syndesmosis ORIF with a suture button construct.*

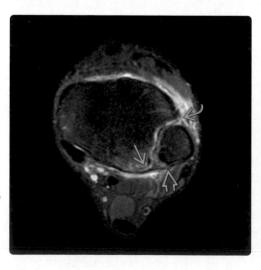
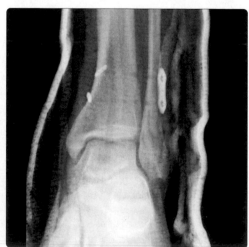

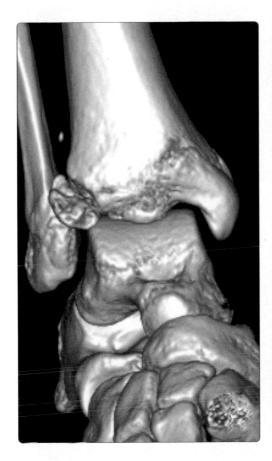

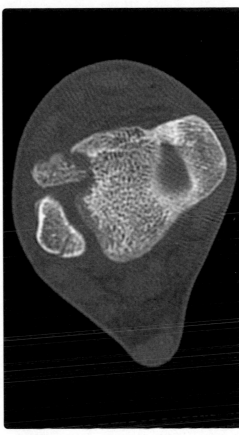

(Left) *3D reconstruction shows the fractured fragment. The AITFL remained attached to the fibula, while the ligament pulled a piece of bone off the tibia. The fractured fragment is externally rotated.* (Right) *A somewhat rare Chaput tubercle fracture is shown, which is essentially an AITFL injury in a skeletally immature 15-year-old male patient. The fractured fragment contained articular surface of both the plafond and syndesmosis.*

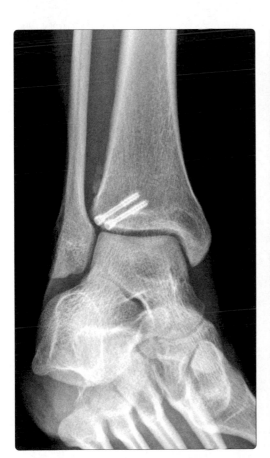

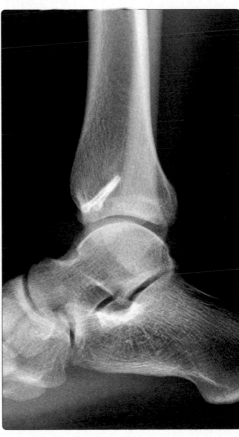

(Left) *Patient underwent ORIF of the fractured fragment with 2 headless, partially threaded screws. He was able to return to baseline activities upon full healing without any limitation.* (Right) *Lateral view of ankle status post ORIF is shown. Once again, the patient was able to return to baseline activity with full healing of the fracture.*

Core Knowledge in Orthopaedics: Foot and Ankle

KEY FACTS

- The natural history of osteochondral lesions of the talus appears to be fairly benign, especially as it relates to the risk of the development of arthritis.
  - Treatment is thus most appropriately based on the patient's symptoms, a very relevant fact given that many osteochondral lesions are incidental findings.
- There are a host of classifications for osteochondral lesions, although no 1 classification is used universally, as the classifications generally do not influence treatment nor do they predict prognosis.
- Nonoperative treatment is limited in terms of options; often activity modification is a central aspect. A boot or cast may be considered, and even a period of non-weight bearing in certain settings may be warranted.

- There are a variety of surgical treatment options; the size and location of the lesion will often steer the surgeon toward one treatment vs. another. Given the relatively mild morbidity associated with marrow stimulation, it is often used as the 1st-line treatment, while more invasive treatments are often reserved for the revision setting.

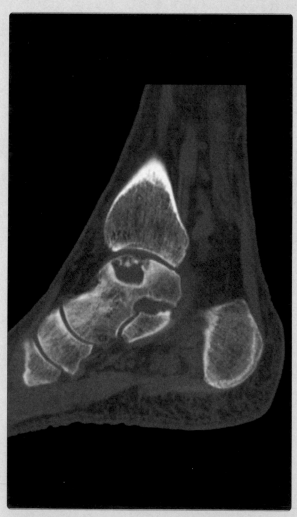

Sagittal CT shows a large cystic osteochondral lesion of the talus. In this setting, marrow stimulation is unlikely to be effective, and an osteochondral autograft would not be large enough; therefore, osteochondral allograft is most appropriate.

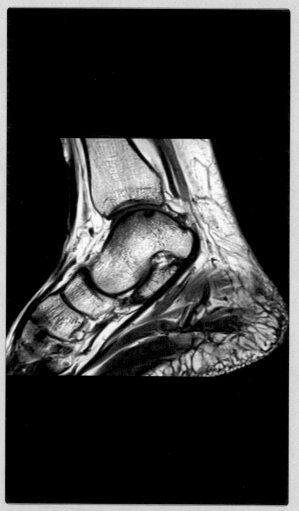

T1 MR shows the subchondral discontinuity in the posteromedial talus, which is the typical location for the traditional osteochondral lesion, as opposed to more lateral lesions, which are more often posttraumatic.

OVERVIEW

- Osteochondral lesions of the talus (OLT) represent a continuum of disease that is likely not 1 single pathology but a grouping of similar pathologies.
- The historical term for this grouping of pathologies, osteochondritis dissecans (OCD), emphasized a localized vascular deficiency within the talus as the principle pathology with the symptoms being secondary to loss of adequate chondral support &/or cyst formation within the talus. Traumatic chondral defects, on the other hand, are often related to shear.
- Traditionally, lateral defects were more likely to be traumatic in nature, while medial and posteromedial defects were more likely a true OCD.
- While treatment of these lesions has advanced considerably over the years, the underlying pathogenesis of the OCD (i.e., nontraumatic) lesions remains unclear.

NATURAL HISTORY

- Certainly, establishing the natural history of any pathology is critical to understanding if and when intervention is warranted.
- There is surprisingly little evidence that speaks to the natural history of OLTs.
- Some surgeons theorize that asymptomatic OLTs may lead to ankle osteoarthritis if left untreated. However, there is simply very little evidence to back up this statement. What little evidence that does exist suggests that the natural history of OLTs is relatively benign.
- Given this fact, treatment for OLTs should be based chiefly on symptoms referable to the lesion. Further, it appears that the asymptomatic OLT can be summarily ignored.

CLASSIFICATION

- There are no fewer than 4 classification schemes depending on various imaging modalities.

Plain Radiographs

- Berndt and Harty published their original description in 1959 on what they called transchondral fractures of the talus.
  - Stage I: Subchondral compression (fracture)
  - Stage II: Partial detachment of osteochondral fragment
  - Stage III: Completely detached fragment without displacement from fracture bed
  - Stage IV: Detached and displaced fragment
  - Stage V (added subsequently by Loomer et al in 1993): Radiolucent defect (i.e., subchondral cyst) present

CT (Ferkel and Sgaglione)

- This is an extension of Berndt and Harty on CT.
  - Stage I: Intact roof/cartilage with cystic lesion beneath
  - Stage IIa: Cystic lesion with communication to surface
  - Stage IIb: Open surface lesion with overlying fragment
  - Stage III: Nondisplaced fragment with lucency underneath
  - Stage IV: Displaced fragment

MR (Hepple et al)

- This staging system was devised to allow for earlier detection of lesions.
  - It is still largely based on Berndt and Harty.
    - Stage 1: Articular cartilage damage only
    - Stage 2a: Cartilage injury with underlying fracture and surrounding bony edema
    - Stage 2b: Stage 2a without surrounding bony edema
    - Stage 3: Detached but undisplaced fragment
    - Stage 4: Detached and displaced fragment
    - Stage 5: Subchondral cyst formation

How To Put All This Together

- As is readily apparent, there is a lot of overlap between these classifications. None of them consistently predicts treatment or prognosis, and so, based on what is typically desired from a classification scheme, none of these schemes are ideal. Practically speaking, radiographs are often used as a screening tool, while MR is typically the study of choice for identifying an OLT. CT can be useful in characterizing cyst and lesion morphology and size.

HISTORY AND PHYSICAL

History

- The history for a patient with a symptomatic osteochondral lesion can vary considerably.
- Not infrequently, patients will recall a history of trauma that they may or may not correlate with their symptoms.
- Most of the time, patients will have the insidious to relatively acute onset of pain in the ankle that is typically, at least initially, activity related.
- Patients sometimes will recall a similar episode in the past that resolved spontaneously.
- A history of an ankle fracture or repeated ankle sprains may be related to a more clear traumatic origin and therefore more chondral defects ± subchondral bone involvement.

Physical

- On inspection, an effusion of varying proportions may be the only outward sign of pathology.
- Based on the location of the lesion, patients may have some tenderness to palpation at the ankle joint line, although this finding is inconsistent at best.
- If a lesion has detached and become a loose body, then some limitation of motion may be noticeable relative to the contralateral side. For similar reasons, patients may rarely experience mechanical locking of the ankle.

TREATMENT

Nonoperative Treatment

- Recommendations for nonoperative treatment are largely lacking, as there is a dearth of evidence to provide much guidance.
- Generally, protection of the ankle in either a cast or a CAM walker boot is appropriate. Non-weight bearing can be considered, although the degree to which it provides benefit is questionable at best. Activity modification should be undertaken as well; it may often be the more attractive option than prolonged use of a boot or cast.

- As above, symptoms dictate treatment. Depending on symptom severity, it is often advisable to try nonoperative treatment for at least 1-3 months before moving to more aggressive treatment, as the symptoms can sometimes dissipate with time.
- Further, it is imperative to differentiate symptoms from an OLT from other symptoms. Given that OLTs can coexist with ankle instability, appropriate treatment should be instituted for the instability before aggressively treating the OLT.

Operative Treatment

- The treatment paradigms for OLTs are largely adapted from the treatment of osteochondral lesions and injury in other joints, most notably the knee.
- The different treatment options include marrow stimulation, osteochondral autograft, osteochondral allograft, and the various forms of autologous chondrocyte implantation (ACI).
- Marrow stimulation
  - The basic idea behind this treatment is the removal of injured or diseased cartilage and bone with the promotion of bleeding and clot formation in the resultant defect that will eventually allow for fibrocartilage fill of the defect.
  - The mechanism of marrow stimulation has varied over time. Abrasion arthroplasty was traditionally used, although microfracture is more commonly used today. Microfracture involves the perforation of the subchondral plate in several places within a lesion allowing for the egress of marrow elements.
  - It is understood that the fibrocartilage that fills these defects has inferior mechanical properties to the normal hyaline cartilage. However, the fibrocartilage can often be sufficient to take away a patient's symptoms referable to the defect.
  - Results from microfracture are generally good with success rates above 80-90% in terms of pain and functional outcome at early and midterm follow-up.
  - In an effort to improve the mechanical properties of repair tissue, a host of enhancements to microfracture have been proposed with varying results.
  - Platelet-rich plasma and bone marrow aspiration concentrate have been used in this setting with some success in terms of improving outcomes, although there is insufficient data to comment in a definitive way at this point.
  - Various forms of particulated cartilage have been used in an effort to provide allogeneic chondrocytes, which will hopefully increase the proportion of hyaline cartilage in repair tissue, although the results from these concoctions have been inconsistent.
- Osteochondral autograft
  - This treatment paradigm was developed to address some of the shortcomings of marrow stimulation.
  - The advantages of osteochondral autograft is principally the ability to get hyaline cartilage as opposed to fibrocartilage.

- There are potential downsides, however. Most notably, the graft must come from somewhere (most typically the lateral nonarticular trochlea) that is ostensibly normal, potentially introducing pathology into an otherwise normal joint. Also, an osteotomy is frequently necessary. Further, the graft is typically impacted into place, a trauma that can potentially cause the death of chondrocytes. Finally, if the graft fit is off, the ingress of synovial fluid can cause cyst formation underneath the graft.
- For all of these reasons, osteochondral autograft is probably best reserved for the revision setting in most cases.
- However, some authors have astutely noted that larger lesions tended to less well with microfracture, and so patients with larger lesions may be better served with a primary autograft.
- ACI
  - ACI was originally developed in the knee and subsequently used in the ankle.
  - It traditionally necessitated 2 surgeries. In the 1st surgery, native cartilage was harvested, which was subsequently grown in the lab. A 2nd surgery allowed for implantation of the autologous cartilage cells, which were historically placed under a periosteal sleeve.
  - Matrix ACI has been developed, allowing for the implantation of a matrix implanted with with autologous chondrocytes, thereby simplifying the implantation surgery significantly.
  - There is a limited amount of data on this treatment modality, although good results have been published in the revision setting.
  - Given the involved nature of this procedure, it is likely most appropriate in the revision setting.
- Osteochondral allograft
  - Large defects present a significant problem, especially when there is a cystic defect in the talus. Microfracture and osteochondral autograft will each have limited efficacy in this situation, as microfracture does not work well with large defects, and autograft is ultimately a limited resource.
  - ACI can be used with bone grafting, although maintaining the bone graft in position can be difficult.
  - In this setting, an osteochondral allograft can sometimes be the best, if not downright only, option.
  - Good results have been noted in this setting.
- Particulated cartilage allograft
  - Small pieces of juvenile or adult articular allograft can be implanted into the defect.
  - Evidence on the efficacy of particulated graft is pending.
- Postoperative care
  - When an osteotomy is necessary, postoperative care is usually dictated by the need for osteotomy healing.
  - In the setting of microfracture, weight bearing was historically restricted for 6 weeks so as to limit shear stress across the filling defect.
  - Recent evidence suggests 2 weeks of non-weight bearing are sufficient.

SELECTED REFERENCES

1. Adams SB et al: Prospective evaluation of structural allograft transplantation for osteochondral lesions of the talar shoulder. Foot Ankle Int. 39(1):28-34, 2018

2. Karnovsky SC et al: Comparison of juvenile allogenous articular cartilage and bone marrow aspirate concentrate versus microfracture with and without bone marrow aspirate concentrate in arthroscopic treatment of talar osteochondral lesions. Foot Ankle Int. 39(4):393-405, 2018

3. Dekker TJ et al: Efficacy of particulated juvenile cartilage allograft transplantation for osteochondral lesions of the talus. Foot Ankle Int. 39(3):278-283, 2017

4. Lanham NS et al: A comparison of outcomes of particulated juvenile articular cartilage and bone marrow aspirate concentrate for articular cartilage lesions of the talus. Foot Ankle Spec. 10(4):315-321, 2017

5. Guney A et al: Clinical outcomes of platelet rich plasma (PRP) as an adjunct to microfracture surgery in osteochondral lesions of the talus. Knee Surg Sports Traumatol Arthrosc. 23(8):2384-2389, 2015

6. Klammer G et al: Natural history of nonoperatively treated osteochondral lesions of the talus. Foot Ankle Int. 36(1):24-31, 2015

7. van Bergen CJ et al: Arthroscopic treatment of osteochondral defects of the talus: outcomes at eight to twenty years of follow-up. J Bone Joint Surg Am. 95(6):519-25, 2013

8. Donnenwerth MP et al: Outcome of arthroscopic debridement and microfracture as the primary treatment for osteochondral lesions of the talar dome. Arthroscopy. 28(12):1902-7, 2012

9. Lee DH et al: Comparison of early versus delayed weightbearing outcomes after microfracture for small to midsized osteochondral lesions of the talus. Am J Sports Med. 40(9):2023-8, 2012

10. Smyth NA et al: Establishing proof of concept: Platelet-rich plasma and bone marrow aspirate concentrate may improve cartilage repair following surgical treatment for osteochondral lesions of the talus. World J Orthop. 3(7):101-8, 2012

11. Lee KB et al: Arthroscopic microfracture for osteochondral lesions of the talus. Knee Surg Sports Traumatol Arthrosc. 18(2):247-53, 2010

12. Choi WJ et al: Osteochondral lesion of the talus: is there a critical defect size for poor outcome? Am J Sports Med. 37(10):1974-80, 2009

13. Lee KB et al: Second-look arthroscopic findings and clinical outcomes after microfracture for osteochondral lesions of the talus. Am J Sports Med. 37 Suppl 1:63S-70S, 2009

14. Chuckpaiwong B et al: Microfracture for osteochondral lesions of the ankle: outcome analysis and outcome predictors of 105 cases. Arthroscopy. 24(1):106-12, 2008

15. Ferkel RD et al: Arthroscopic treatment of chronic osteochondral lesions of the talus: long-term results. Am J Sports Med. 36(9):1750-62, 2008

16. Becher C et al: Results of microfracture in the treatment of articular cartilage defects of the talus. Foot Ankle Int. 26(8):583-9, 2005

17. Loomer R et al: Osteochondral lesions of the talus. Am J Sports Med. 21(1):13-9, 1993

18. McCullough CJ et al: Osteochondritis dissecans of the talus: the natural history. Clin Orthop Relat Res. 264-8, 1979

19. Berndt AL, Harty M. Transchondral fractures (osteochondritis dissecans) of the talus. J Bone Joint Surg Am. 1959;41-A:988-1020.

(Left) *A 44-year-old female patient with consistent medial ankle pain for several months refractory to nonoperative treatment is shown. A posteromedial osteochondral lesion is seen with a mild cystic component.* **(Right)** *Coronal image of the same patient is shown. There is mild reactive edema around the lesion, although it is not severe. This patient had tried to avoid surgery for some time, although her symptoms persisted.*

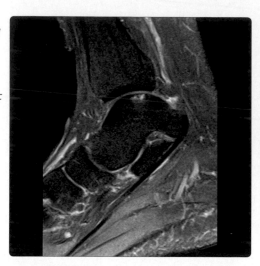 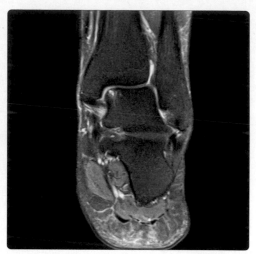

(Left) *Axial MR shows septations within the lesion in the cystic component of the lesion. These lesions can often have septa, especially when they have been present for some time.* **(Right)** *Closer look at the medial gutter with a cartilage lesion noted is shown. This area corresponded to the area of abnormality on the MR as well as the area where most of the patient's pain was centered.*

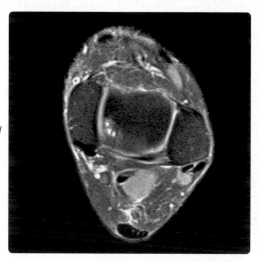 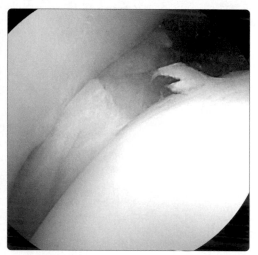

(Left) *The osteochondral lesion has been thoroughly debrided back to normal bone. Microfracture has been performed in the base of the lesion (not shown).* **(Right)** *The lesion has been filled with particulated cartilage allograft and overlaid with fibrin glue. Traditionally, this part of the procedure was not done, although it is performed currently in the hopes that more hyaline-like cartilage will form, as opposed to the fibrocartilage fill that typically occurs.*

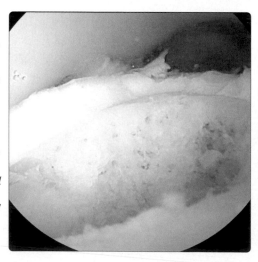 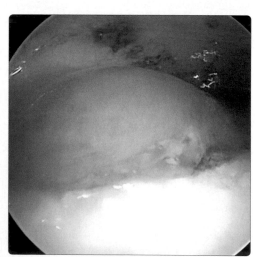

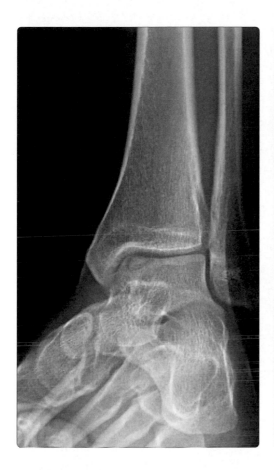

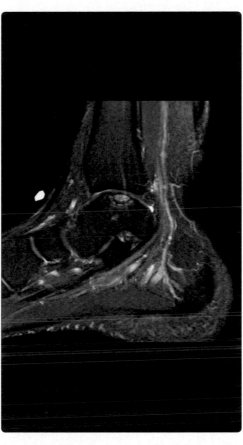

(Left) *A loose osteochondral lesion in a 23-year-old male patient is shown. This patient had had a previous ankle sprain and continued to have pain after the ankle sprain had been appropriately treated.* (Right) *The same lesion is shown. There is a clear delineation between the lesion and the rest of the talus with some reactive edema within the lesion itself and in the rim of bone around it.*

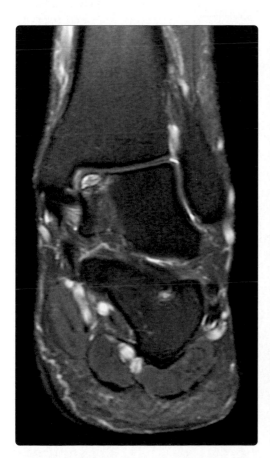

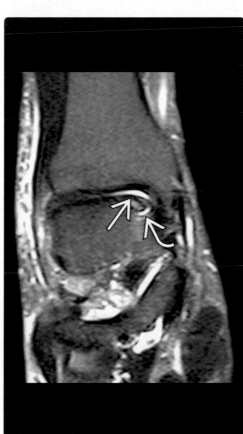

(Left) *The lesion is again seen; note the reactive edema inferior to the lesion. This reactive edema is quite extensive on this image and is thought to correlate to symptoms to some degree (i.e., more reactive edema = more symptomatic).* (Right) *MR shows an unstable image with fluid underneath the lesion ➦, although there is not a clear defect in the superior surface ➥. There is some reactive edema underneath the lesion. (From SI: Arthrography.)*

(Left) *A medial osteochondral lesion of the talus with a moderately large cystic component is shown. This patient presented with a long history of medial ankle pain refractory to conservative measures.* **(Right)** *Patient has undergone medial malleolar osteotomy with osteochondral autograft transplant from the ipsilateral knee. Given the large cystic nature of the lesion, it was felt that osteochondral autograft was more appropriate.*

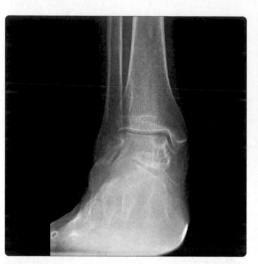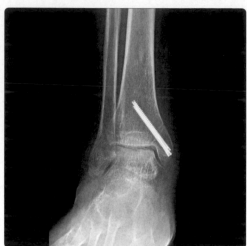

(Left) *A medial osteochondral lesion of the talus with a moderately large cystic component is shown.* **(Right)** *Patient has undergone medial malleolar osteotomy with osteochondral autograft transplant from the ipsilateral knee. The medial malleolar osteotomy was here fixed with 2 screws, although a plate can be utilized as well.*

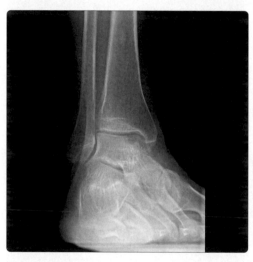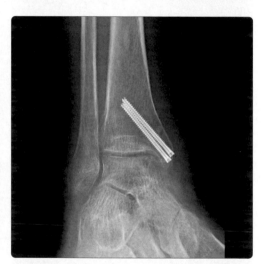

(Left) *A medial osteochondral lesion of the talus with a moderately large cystic component is shown. The anteroposterior extent of the lesion can be seen here.* **(Right)** *Patient has undergone medial malleolar osteotomy with osteochondral autograft transplant from the ipsilateral knee. The cystic lesion is no longer as readily apparent.*

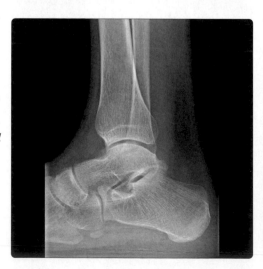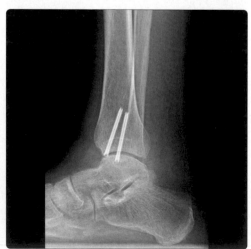

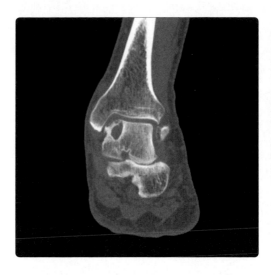
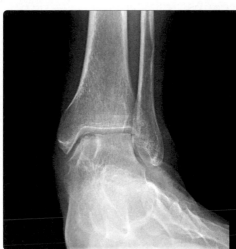

(**Left**) *Large medial osteochondral lesion of the talus with cyst involving much of the medial talus is shown. This patient was a manual laborer who had progressive ankle pain that left him unable to work.* (**Right**) *Large medial osteochondral lesion of the talus with cyst involving much of the medial talus is shown. The cyst involved much of the medial talus, although some of the medial wall was intact.*

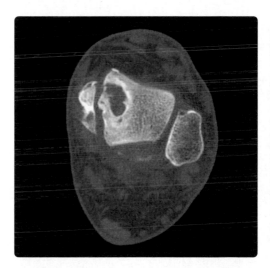
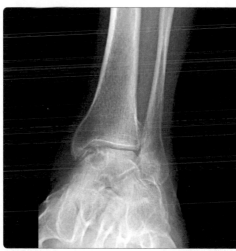

(**Left**) *Large medial osteochondral lesion of the talus with cyst involving much of the medial talus is shown. Given the size of this cyst, surgical treatment options are fairly limited.* (**Right**) *Large medial osteochondral lesion of the talus with cyst involving much of the medial talus is shown.*

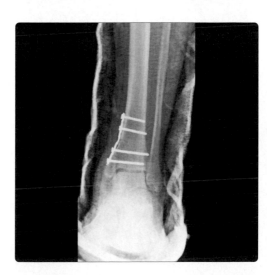
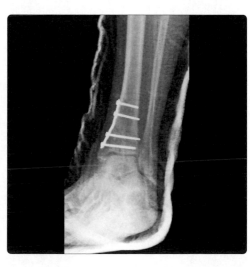

(**Left**) *Patient underwent medial malleolar osteotomy with osteochondral talar allograft. The osteotomy must be planned so as to allow adequate access to the talus.* (**Right**) *Patient underwent medial malleolar osteotomy with osteochondral talar allograft. The fill of the cyst can be seen to some degree on these postoperative images.*

KEY FACTS

- The treatment of ankle fractures is chiefly concerned with mitigating and minimizing the risk of posttraumatic arthritis.
- The relative stability of an ankle fracture will ultimately determine whether surgical intervention is warranted.
- Supination-external rotation ankle fractures are the most common rotational injuries.
- Syndesmotic stability must be assessed in all operative ankle fractures; sagittal plane instability is often a more sensitive indicator of the presence of a syndesmotic injury.
- While size has traditionally been the deciding factor as to whether a posterior malleolar fracture should undergo open reduction and internal fixation, the presence of syndesmotic instability and marginal impaction are also deciding factors.
- The presence of medical comorbidities, most notably osteoporosis and diabetes mellitus should influence surgical treatment options.

- More fixation may be warranted in poor bone or in those whose neuropathy may limit non-weight bearing.
- A1C > 7.5 has been linked with increased surgical complications.

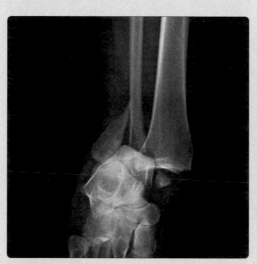
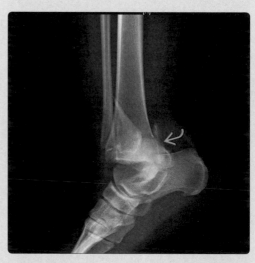

(Left) A displaced bimalleolar fracture in a 60-year-old female patient is shown. The patient was diabetic, although it was well controlled. There was also a posteromedial fracture of the tibia, which is not well visualized here. (Right) This fracture-dislocation also had a posteromedial distal tibia fracture ⊡ that can be seen here. In order to minimize the risk of posttraumatic arthrosis, all components of the fracture were fixed.

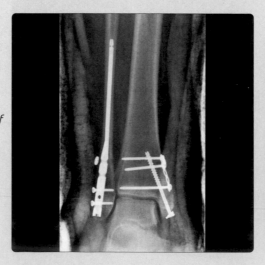
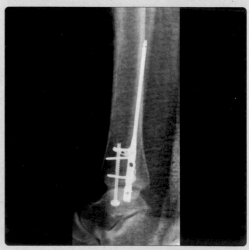

(Left) An intramedullary device was chosen for the fibula in this diabetic patient in an effort to minimize the surgical insult. Syndesmotic instability was noted, and a suture button device was placed. (Right) Lateral view shows anatomic restoration of the ankle. In this setting, an effort must be made to place the medial hardware in a way so as to minimize traffic.

OVERVIEW

- Ankle fractures encompass a broad range of pathology. Generally speaking, as surgeons, we differentiate low-energy rotational injuries (ankle fractures) from higher energy, axial-loading injuries (pilon or plafond fractures). The division between these 2 ranges of pathology can be somewhat gray, as there can obviously be overlap of the mechanisms with some rotation and some axial loading. These injuries more frequently involve the posterior plafond, and so we will talk about these injuries under the posterior pilon and include a discussion of these injuries with rotational ankle fractures. Also included with rotational injuries are coronal plane injuries that often tend to be low energy as well.
- Rotational ankle fractures, or malleolar fractures, are very common injuries with an incidence of almost 170 per 100,000 people in one 10-year incidence study.
- The principle concern with an ankle fracture is ultimately the risk of posttraumatic arthritis (PTA), and, therefore, the goal of treatment is to attempt to minimize the risk of PTA. The mechanisms of PTA are poorly understood. The risk of PTA is likely proportional to some degree to the initial cartilage injury. Any degree of malunion can also increase the risk of PTA in a joint as constrained as the ankle.
- Not all ankle fractures are treated operatively. Operative decision making, in a basic way, comes down to an assessment of stability. If the fracture is deemed to be unstable, then operative treatment is generally recommended. Generally speaking, trimalleolar, bimalleolar, and SER4 equivalent fractures are thought to be unstable and are therefore treated operatively in an effort to minimize the risk of malunion and PTA.

ANATOMY

Syndesmosis

- The syndesmosis is the articulation of the tibia and the fibula just proximal to the tibiotalar joint. It is a joint with articular cartilage and is stabilized by the syndesmotic ligaments [anterior-inferior tibiofibular ligament (AITFL), posterior inferior tibiofibular ligament (PITFL), and interosseous ligament].
- The incisura fibularis tibiae is the lateral cavity of the tibia with which the fibula articulates. This anatomic feature of the tibia can differ fairly significantly from the almost C shape in the axial plane to a much flatter shape.

Mortise

- The mortise is composed of the articulation between the tibia and fibula superiorly and the talus inferiorly.
- Much of the stability of the ankle mortise in stance comes from the bony conformity. A host of ligaments provide static restrictions to various ankle and hindfoot motions, while tendons can provide a dynamic component to this stability.
- The capsule of the ankle joint is confluent with ligamentous structures laterally, posteriorly, and medially, while extending a few centimeters proximal to the plafond anteriorly. The role of the ankle capsule in ankle function is currently unclear.

- The articular cartilage of the ankle is fundamentally different from that of the knee in ways that may relatively protect the ankle.
- The fibula extends distal to the tibia and should form a curve, whereby the distal fibula is confluent with the lateral process of the talus.

CLASSIFICATION

- There are different ways that ankle fractures can be classified, although Lauge-Hansen still greatly informs the fundamental concepts that dictate thought on ankle fractures.
- The Lauge-Hansen classification describes the position of the foot at the time of injury and then what force is exerted on the ankle to produce the given fracture, ultimately yielding 4 separate types of fracture: Supination-adduction (SAD), supination-external rotation (SER), pronation-abduction (PAB), and pronation-external rotation (PER).
- This system does not encompass all types of ankle fractures, although many fit into these categories. Generally speaking, it does not predict syndesmotic injury, although pronation injuries are thought to be higher risk for syndesmotic injury
- The simple Danis-Weber classification looks solely at the level of the fibula fracture and its relation to the ankle mortise. Those fractures below the plafond are Weber A, at the plafond Weber B, and above the plafond Weber C. Weber C fractures generally have a higher risk of syndesmotic injury.
- To be sure, neither of these classifications is perfect, as neither system directly guides treatment, nor do they clearly predict outcome.

GENERAL TREATMENT

Overview

- The central goal of treatment of an ankle fracture is the restoration of full function. Treatment should be tailored to maximize function and minimize the risk of PTA.
- Whether surgery is warranted or not will depend on injury and patient factors.
- If surgery is needed, then the general concepts of anatomic reduction with rigid fixation coupled with delayed weight bearing and early range of motion should generally be followed.
- More specifically with regards to surgery, length and rotation of the fibula must be restored, while intraarticular fractures must be anatomically reduced.
- Given the differences involved with different types of fractures, the discussion of treatment will be made for each individual type of fracture.

Supination-Adduction

- SAD fractures are coronal plane injuries that are essentially the same mechanism as an ankle sprain. With type 1 injuries, there is a Weber A fibula fracture, while type 2 fractures are characterized by impaction of the talus into the medial shoulder of the plafond, creating a characteristic vertical medial malleolus fracture.
- Marginal impaction can occur in the medial plafond; its presence should be actively sought and assessed with a CT scan if unclear on plain films.

- SAD 1 fractures are essentially ankle sprain-equivalent injuries and rarely require operative treatment. If operative treatment is necessary, a single longitudinal screw is usually sufficient.
- SAD 2 fractures will require operative treatment. A longitudinal anteromedial incision will allow access to the joint for disimpaction and anatomic reduction. Bone grafting is occasionally necessary. A medial buttress plate with subchondral lag screws provides optimal fixation.

Supination-External Rotation

- SER fractures occur through 4 stages.
  - SER 1 fractures: In original description, this injury consisted of tear of AITFL or fracture of Chaput (insertion of AITFL on tibia) or Wagstaffe tubercle (insertion of AITFL on fibula); practically, these injuries, unless they involve large fracture fragment, likely get grouped in with ankle sprains more than fractures; surgical treatment is only rarely necessary
  - SER 2 fractures: Each stage is progressive, and so this would involve an SER 1 and an oblique fracture (Weber B) of the distal fibula; typical fracture orientation runs from anterior inferior to posterior superior
  - SER 3 fractures: SER 2 with either PITFL tear or posterior malleolar fracture
  - SER 4 fractures: SER 3 with either deltoid ligament tear or medial malleolar fracture
- Generally speaking, SER 4 fractures are treated operatively. It can often be difficult to clearly diagnose SER 2 vs. SER 4 fractures on nonstress radiographs, especially when there is no medial fracture.
- External rotation stress radiographs can help to differentiate SER 2 from SER 4 fractures. Opening of the medial clear space generally signifies injury to the deltoid ligament, although there has been debate about what degree of opening is truly indicative of injury, and different surgeons have different thoughts. The longitudinal data that would allow for a better understanding of how best to treat these injuries is currently lacking.
- Some authors view opening of the medial clear space in a binary fashion, whereby a differentiation is made between those that nearly dislocate vs. those that widen a couple millimeters. Widening of a few millimeters is ultimately of unclear significance, especially given the inherent error in measurement, the lack of a consistently superior mode of measurement, and the inherent difficulty of standardizing how hard one should pull. Further, early results suggest that many of these equivocal injuries will stabilize under the mortise and attain stability over time, although, once again, more relevant long term data is lacking.

Pronation-Abduction

- Like SAD fractures, PAB fractures are strictly coronal plane injuries, although the injury starts on the medial side.
  - PAB 1 fractures: Transverse medial malleolar fracture
  - PAB 2 fractures: PAB 1 + disruption of the syndesmotic ligaments with possible posterior malleolar fracture
  - PAB 3 fractures: PAB 2 + Weber C comminuted fibula fracture
- These fractures will often need surgery, as they will be displaced; syndesmotic disruption is common with these injuries.

- Attaining appropriate length and rotation of the fibula can be challenging in these fibula fractures, especially with significant comminution.
- Talar dome fractures can occur from shear stresses associated with the fracture.

Pronation-External Rotation

- Like SER fractures, PER fractures occur through 4 stages.
  - PER 1 fractures: Transverse medial malleolar fracture
  - PER 2 fractures: PER 1 + AITFL tear
  - PER 3 fractures: PER 2 + spiral fibular fracture (Weber C), anterior superior to posterior inferior
  - PER 4 fractures: PER 3 + PITFL tear or posterior malleolar fracture
- As before, PER injuries are often associated with syndesmotic disruption.
- Operative treatment is the norm for these injuries.

Posterior Pilon Fractures

- Posterior pilon fractures can encompass any of the above if the injury has an axial component.
- You will often see some marginal impaction of the fracture with an impacted fragment anterior to the posterior malleolar fracture.
- They may necessitate a posterolateral approach to the ankle, utilizing the interval between the peroneal tendons laterally and the flexor hallucis longus medially. Care must be taken to protect the sural nerve given its proximity to the approach.
- While traditional thinking on posterior malleolar fractures focused on the size of the fractured fragment as the main feature influencing surgical decision making, surgeons now also take into account the presence of any marginal impaction and the effect of PITFL restoration on syndesmotic stability.
- Good results have been achieved with these injuries, although these injuries must be recognized and treated appropriately.

Syndesmosis Disruption

- Disruption of the syndesmosis often represents a diagnostic challenge. In the setting of an ankle fracture, the fibula is typically stabilized prior to assessing syndesmotic instability.
- The Cotton test is the most widely known test of syndesmotic instability, whereby the fibula is clamped, and any widening is sought in the coronal plane. A more sensitive measure of syndesmotic instability, however, may be seen in the sagittal plane where excess sagittal motion of the fibula relative to the tibia may indicate syndesmotic instability.
- Other authors have suggested using arthroscopic evaluation to assess for syndesmotic instability.
- An anatomic reduction of the syndesmosis is likely best achieved with an open reduction in order to directly place the fibula into the incisura. Further, some authors have noted that the quality of syndesmosis reduction correlates directly with outcome.

- Syndesmotic reduction can be maintained with either syndesmotic screws or suture button devices. Some evidence suggests that suture button devices may be more forgiving in terms of reduction and may allow for better results in terms of functional outcome, quality of life, and pain.

Perioperative and Postoperative Care

- Outpatient management of ankle fractures may be cheaper and associated with less medical morbidity postoperatively. A delay in timing between injury and surgery does not appear to adversely affect outcome.
- Pain management focuses on minimizing the use of opioid medications by providing multimodal analgesia.
- Deep vein thrombosis (DVT) prophylaxis appears unnecessary after ankle fracture given the low incidence of DVT and pulmonary embolism after ankle fracture. DVT prophylaxis should be considered in patients that are high risk.
- Weight-bearing recommendations after ankle open reduction and internal fixation (ORIF) surgery have historically been a source of significant variability, often based more on tradition than any objective criteria.
- Recent evidence has shown no difference in wound complications, infection, loss of reduction, or hardware failure with 2 weeks of non-weight bearing (NWB) as opposed to 6 weeks of NWB after ORIF of multiple types of ankle fractures.

OTHER CONSIDERATIONS

Diabetes Mellitus

- Although diabetes does not in and of itself portend any excess risk for ankle fracture patients, poorly controlled diabetes is another story.
- A displaced ankle fracture in a poorly controlled diabetic with neuropathy and arterial disease is a limb-threatening injury.
- Neuropathy, even without diabetes, significantly increases the risk of complications with surgery.
- A hemoglobin A1C > 7.5 has been found to increase the risk associated with surgery. Surgical management of ankle fractures in this setting should be circumspect.
- Surgical management of the diabetic should generally be cautious with attempts made to achieve greater fixation with longer periods of NWB.

Osteoporosis

- Ankle fractures are increasingly recognized as a source of morbidity in the elderly.
- These fractures have been associated with a lower 1-year morbidity than hip fractures, suggesting that these patients are healthier and more active than hip fracture patients and possibly indicating that more aggressive management of geriatric ankle fractures is appropriate.
- Delayed periods of NWB should be avoided in the elderly, where and if possible.
- Similar to diabetic fractures, attempts should be made to maximize fixation.

Use of Arthroscopy

- Many authors have noted the presence of articular cartilage injury with arthroscopy at the time of ankle fracture.

- Arthroscopy aids in the diagnosis of these defects, as well as potential treatment, although the effect of this treatment is currently unclear.
- Further, arthroscopy can aid in the visualization of fracture reduction, providing another data point in the assessment of articular congruence. Similarly, as above, syndesmotic instability can be visualized with the scope.
- Perhaps of greater significance, though, is the ability to wash away catabolic mediators that have been shown to be present after fracture and may promote cartilage degradation.

SELECTED REFERENCES

1. Andersen MR et al: Randomized trial comparing suture button with single syndesmotic screw for syndesmosis injury. J Bone Joint Surg Am. 100(1):2-12, 2018
2. Elsoe R et al: Population-based epidemiology of 9767 ankle fractures. Foot Ankle Surg. 24(1):34-39, 2018
3. Adams SB et al: Inflammatory microenvironment persists after bone healing in intra-articular ankle fractures. Foot Ankle Int. 38(5):479-484, 2017
4. Cancienne JM et al: Hemoglobin A1c as a predictor of postoperative infection following elective forefoot surgery. Foot Ankle Int. 38(8):832-837, 2017
5. Dehghan N et al: Early weightbearing and range ofmMotion versus non-weightbearing and immobilization after open reduction and internal fixation of unstable ankle fractures: a randomized controlled Trial. J Orthop Trauma. 30(7):345-52, 2016
6. Qin C et al: Safety and outcomes of inpatient compared with outpatient surgical procedures for ankle fractures. J Bone Joint Surg Am. 98(20):1699-1705, 2016
7. Hsu RY et al: Morbidity and mortality associated with geriatric ankle fractures: a medicare part A claims database analysis. J Bone Joint Surg Am. 97(21):1748-55, 2015
8. Swart E et al: How long should patients be kept non-weight bearing after ankle fracture fixation? A survey of OTA and AOFAS members. Injury. 46(6):1127-30, 2015
9. Warner SJ et al: The measurement and clinical importance of syndesmotic reduction after operative fixation of rotational ankle fractures. J Bone Joint Surg Am. 97(23):1935-44, 2015
10. Swart EF et al: Arthroscopic assessment of medial malleolar reduction. Arch Orthop Trauma Surg. 134(9):1287-92, 2014
11. Westermann RW et al: The effect of suture-button fixation on simulated syndesmotic malreduction: a cadaveric study. J Bone Joint Surg Am. 96(20):1732-8, 2014
12. Wukich DK et al: Neuropathy and poorly controlled diabetes increase the rate of surgical site infection after foot and ankle surgery. J Bone Joint Surg Am. 96(10):832-9, 2014
13. Franzone JM et al: Posterolateral approach for open reduction and internal fixation of a posterior malleolus fracture–hinging on an intact PITFL to disimpact the tibial plafond: a technical note. Foot Ankle Int. 34(8):1177-81, 2013
14. Sagi HC et al: The functional consequence of syndesmotic joint malreduction at a minimum 2-year follow-up. J Orthop Trauma. 26(7):439-43, 2012
15. Gardner MJ et al: Surgeon practices regarding operative treatment of posterior malleolus fractures. Foot Ankle Int. 32(4):385-93, 2011
16. Jameson SS et al: Venous thromboembolic events following foot and ankle surgery in the English National Health Service. J Bone Joint Surg Br. 93(4):490-7, 2011
17. Wukich DK et al: Outcomes of ankle fractures in patients with uncomplicated versus complicated diabetes. Foot Ankle Int. 32(2):120-30, 2011
18. Amorosa LF et al: A surgical approach to posterior pilon fractures. J Orthop Trauma. 24(3):188-93, 2010
19. Elgafy H et al: Computed tomography of normal distal tibiofibular syndesmosis. Skeletal Radiol. 39(6):559-64, 2010
20. Stufkens SA et al: Cartilage lesions and the development of osteoarthritis after internal fixation of ankle fractures: a prospective study. J Bone Joint Surg Am. 92(2):279-86, 2010
21. Candal-Couto JJ et al: Instability of the tibio-fibular syndesmosis: have we been pulling in the wrong direction? Injury. 35(8):814-8, 2004
22. Weber M: Trimalleolar fractures with impaction of the posteromedial tibial plafond: implications for talar stability. Foot Ankle Int. 25(10):716-27, 2004
23. Cole AA et al: Distinguishing ankle and knee articular cartilage. Foot Ankle Clin. 8(2):305-16, x, 2003

(Left) *A bimalleolar ankle fracture in an elderly patient is shown. This patient was lost to follow-up for almost 3 weeks after injury. Surgery was more challenging, as the fracture had begun healing to some degree.* **(Right)** *Open reduction and internal fixation of the same bimalleolar ankle fracture with 2 fibular plates is shown. Two fibular plates were used in order to maximize the amount of fixation both proximally and distally.*

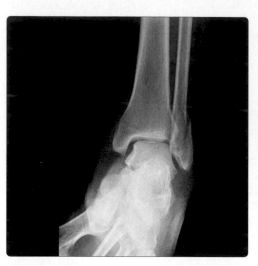 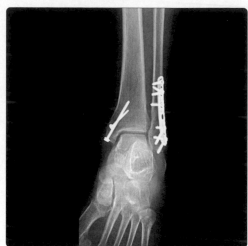

(Left) *A bimalleolar ankle fracture in an elderly patient is shown. Given that the patient was older with possibly compromised bone quality, an effort should be made to maximize fixation so as to decrease the risk of loss of fixation.* **(Right)** *Open reduction and internal fixation of a bimalleolar ankle fracture with 2 fibular plates is shown. The medial malleolar fracture extended somewhat superior and anterior, necessitating screws in different planes medially.*

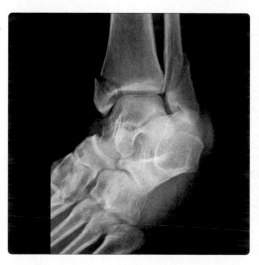 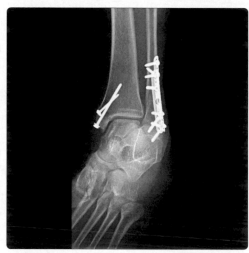

(Left) *The fractures are not well visualized on this lateral image. Delayed presentation can lead to relative osteopenia, which can be another reason to try to maximize fixation.* **(Right)** *Open reduction and internal fixation of a bimalleolar ankle fracture with 2 fibular plates is shown. The 2 plates are seen most clearly here with 4 screws on each side of the fracture. The medial screws proximal and distal are seen more readily here as well.*

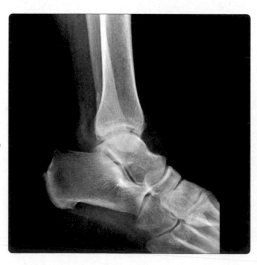 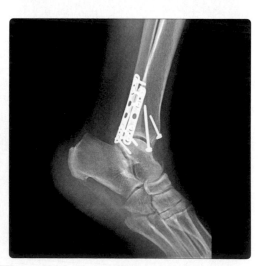

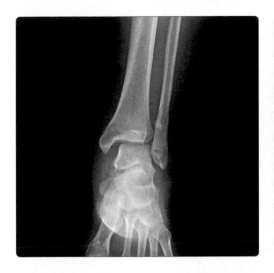

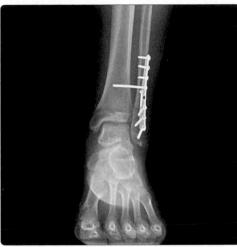

(Left) *Supination-external rotation (SER) 4-equivalent fracture with syndesmotic injury is shown. Medial clear space widening with syndesmotic widening is seen here.* (Right) *Open reduction and internal fixation of an SER 4-equivalent fracture with syndesmotic screw and posterolateral fibular plating is shown. A posterolateral plate has the advantage of allowing stronger bicortical distal fixation. A syndesmotic screw is used here.*

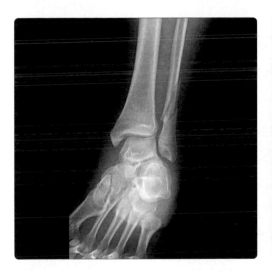

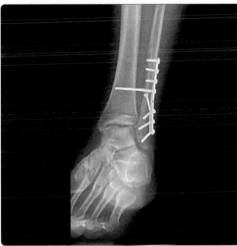

(Left) *SER 4-equivalent fracture with syndesmotic injury is shown. The fibula fracture is seen more easily here as an oblique Weber C-type fracture.* (Right) *Open reduction and internal fixation of an SER 4-equivalent fracture with syndesmotic screw and posterolateral fibular plating is shown. The syndesmotic screw can be removed or left, although it will typically either loosen or break if not removed.*

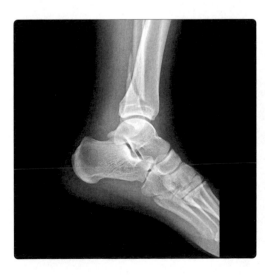

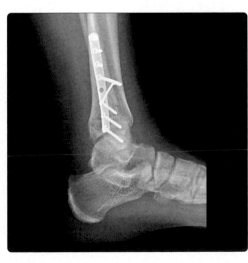

(Left) *SER 4-equivalent fracture with syndesmotic injury is shown. The fracture is perhaps seen most fully on this lateral image.* (Right) *Open reduction and internal fixation of an SER 4-equivalent fracture with syndesmotic screw and posterolateral fibular plating is shown. The posterior to anterior distal fibular screws can be seen better.*

Core Knowledge in Orthopaedics: Foot and Ankle

(Left) *Trimalleolar ankle fracture in a 24-year-old female patient is shown. The posterior malleolus can be difficult to see on this AP view, although the cortical fracture line ⇗ is often visible.* **(Right)** *Trimalleolar ankle fracture in a 24-year-old female patient is shown. Note the size of the posterior malleolar fracture and the marginal impaction ⇒ anterior to the posterior malleolar fracture.*

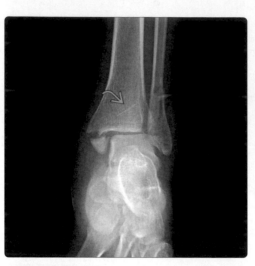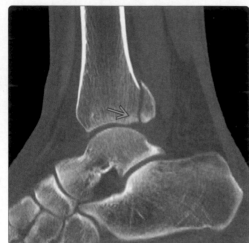

(Left) *Trimalleolar ankle fracture in a 24-year-old female patient is shown. Once again, the posterior malleolus fracture can be seen primarily in terms of the cortical fracture line ⇒.* **(Right)** *Open reduction and internal fixation of trimalleolar ankle fracture in the same 24-year-old female patient is shown. A posterolateral approach was used for the posterior malleolus and the fibula.*

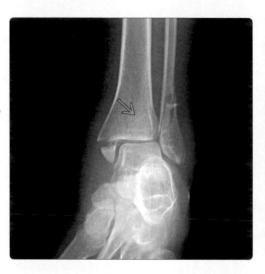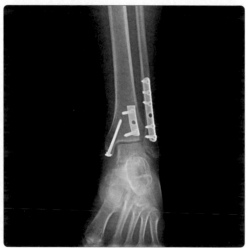

(Left) *Trimalleolar ankle fracture in a 24-year-old female patient is shown. The posterior malleolus can be seen in conjunction with the fibular fracture.* **(Right)** *Open reduction and internal fixation of trimalleolar ankle fracture in the same 24-year-old female patient is shown. The anatomic reduction of the mortise is seen here. Visualizing anterior to the posterior malleolus is often difficult.*

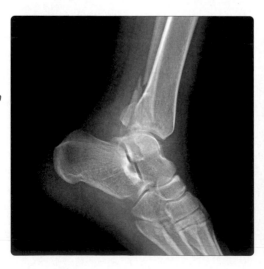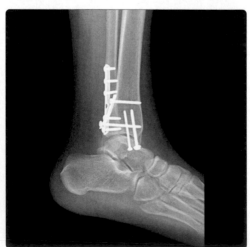

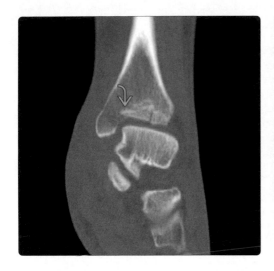

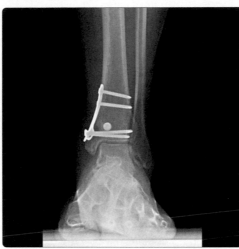

(Left) *Supination adduction fracture in a 33-year-old female patient is shown. Note the impaction of the medial plafond ➡. This patient was snowboarding and sustained a forced dorsiflexion injury.* (Right) *Open reduction and internal fixation of a supination adduction fracture in a 33-year-old female patient is shown. The medial plafond was disimpacted, and bone graft was placed in the resultant defect.*

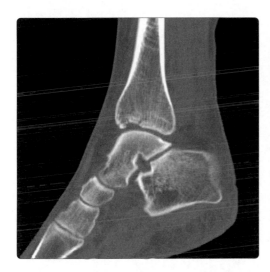

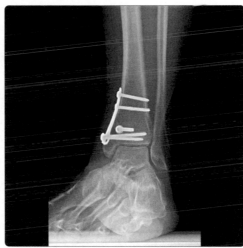

(Left) *Supination adduction fracture in a 33-year-old female patient is shown. Note the impaction of the anteromedial plafond. Arthroscopy can sometimes be an aid in these injuries to allow for better articular evaluation.* (Right) *Open reduction and internal fixation of a supination adduction fracture in a 33-year-old female patient is shown. In many ways, these injuries are like upside down tibial plateau fractures, as the principles are often the same. The anatomic articular reduction is seen here.*

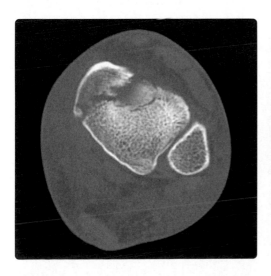

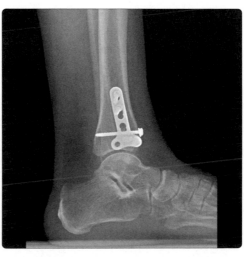

(Left) *Supination adduction fracture in a 33-year-old female patient is shown. Note the impaction of the anteromedial plafond.* (Right) *Open reduction and internal fixation of a supination adduction fracture in a 33-year-old female patient is shown. Fixation options vary; in this case, a distal radius plate was used and placed upside down.*

Tibial Pilon Fractures

KEY FACTS

- The tibial pilon fracture is a rare, yet devastating injury.
  - Despite the best treatment, patients sustaining high-energy pilon fractures generally do not return to their previous state of general health or function.
  - After recovery from pilon fractures, many patients continue to have debilitating pain and ankle stiffness.
- Pilon fractures can occur from both low- and high-energy mechanisms.
- The pilon fracture usually has an anterolateral (Chaput) fragment and a posterolateral (Volkmann) fragment.
  - Fragments usually remain attached to the distal fibula segment by the anterior and posterior tibiofibular ligaments.
- Initial management of pilon fractures depends as much on the soft tissue as the bony injury.
  - Understanding the soft tissue injury accompanying pilon fractures is of utmost importance for providing optimal treatment while minimizing complications.

- Indications for closed reduction and cast treatment of pilon fractures are limited.
  - Pilon fractures treated with a cast have led to poorer outcomes than those managed operatively.
- Surgical timing and type of fixation utilized is largely dictated by the condition of the soft tissues.
  - Surgical options include the following: Bridging external fixation, external fixation with limited internal fixation, nonspanning external fixation ± limited internal fixation, and staged open reduction and internal fixation.
- Complications following surgical management of pilon fractures, particularly wound breakdown, were historically common.
  - Wound complications can be minimized with appropriate treatment strategies and soft tissue handling.
- Other common complications seen following treatment of tibial pilon fractures are arthrofibrosis and posttraumatic arthritis.

Pilon fracture map.

Pilon comminution pattern.

(Left) *Primary fracture lines of 40 OTA-type 43C3 fractures are shown. Fracture lines were mapped from axial CT cuts 3 mm above the plafond after an external fixator had been applied. Appreciate the consistent Y pattern creating 3 main articular fragments.* (Right) *Impaction most commonly occurs at the dome between the 3 main fracture fragments. Anterolateral comminution is commonly encountered with high-energy fractures. Collectively, these 2 maps aid the surgeon in predicting necessary surgical tactics and approaches.*

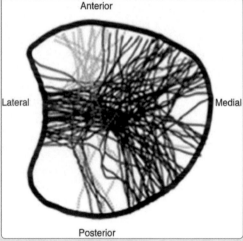

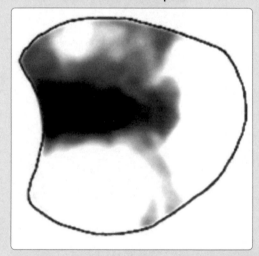

(Left) *Arbeitsgemeinschaft für Osteosynthesefragen/OTA pilon fracture classification system is shown.* (Right) *Axial CT shows fracture lines ➡ dividing the plafond into 3 major fragments: Anterolateral, posterior, and medial. There are also multiple small, comminuted fragments. Sclerosis ➡ is due to impacted bone fragments/trabeculae. The small flake of bone medially ➡ is consistent with flexor retinaculum avulsion. (From DI: MSK Non-Trauma.)*

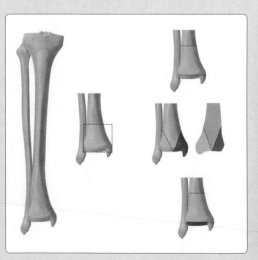

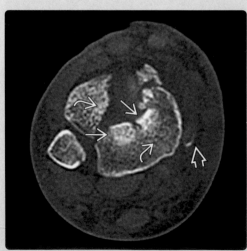

TERMINOLOGY

Definitions

- Pilon is a French term used to describe a fracture of the distal tibia usually characterized by high-energy traits, including dissociation of the articular surface from the tibia shaft.
  o Destot coined the term pilon, as he thought that the distal tibial metaphysis resembled a pharmacist's pestle.
- Plafond is also a French term, described by Bonin, referring to the distal tibial articular surface as the roof (ceiling) of the ankle joint.

ANATOMY

Normal Anatomy

- At the level of the ankle, the distal tibia is intimately associated with the fibula through strong ligamentous attachments.
  o The attachments are as follows:
    - Anterior inferior tibiofibular ligament
    - Posterior inferior tibiofibular ligament
    - Interosseous ligament
    - Inferior transverse ligament
- The articular surface of the distal tibia is concave in both the coronal as well as the sagittal plane.
- The talus has the opposite geometry of the tibial plafond and therefore serves as a perfect template for assessing articular reduction of the distal tibia.
- The concave tibial plafond provides ~ 40% more posterior than anterior coverage.

Fracture Anatomy

- The pilon fracture usually has an anterolateral (Chaput) fragment and a posterolateral (Volkmann) fragment, which usually remain attached to the distal fibula segment by the anterior and posterior tibiofibular ligaments.
- In the vast majority of pilon fractures, the fracture lines propagate from the fibular incisura laterally in the shape of a Y to exit anterior and posterior to the medial malleolus.
- Comminution, which frequently occurs with high-energy pilon fractures, is most typically located in the anterolateral and central regions of the plafond.

Surrounding Soft Tissue Anatomy

- There simply is not a lot of soft tissue around the distal tibia, as compared to more proximal parts of the leg.
  o There is no muscle tissue to "cushion" or protect the bone if skin is injured.
- The tendons of the anterior compartment, the dorsalis pedis artery, and the superficial and deep peroneal nerves can be encountered with anterior exposures at the level of the ankle joint.
- The tendinous and neurovascular structures are covered proximally by the investing fascia of the anterior compartment and distally by the extensor retinaculum.
- The superficial peroneal and saphenous nerves are superficial to the fascia.
  o The superficial peroneal nerve pierces the fascia of the lateral compartment ~ 12 cm proximal to the ankle joint en route to provide sensation to a majority of the dorsum of the foot.

- Anterolateral exposures for pilon fractures risk injury to the superficial peroneal nerve.
- The dorsalis pedis and deep peroneal nerve are at risk with an anterior exposure.
  o They run together in the pericapsular fat between the extensory digitorum and extensor hallucis longus tendons.

UNDERSTANDING INJURY

Context and Mechanism

- The tibial pilon fracture is a rare yet devastating injury.
- Despite the best treatment, patients sustaining high-energy pilon fractures generally do not return to their previous state of general health or function.
  o After recovery from pilon fractures, many patients continue to have debilitating pain and ankle stiffness (Babis et al 1997, Sands et al 1998, Pollak et al 2003).
- Fortunately, pilon fractures compose a minority of tibia or lower extremity fractures, occurring in ~ 7% and 1% of all cases, respectively.
- Pilon fractures can occur from both low- and high-energy mechanisms.
  o Low-energy fractures typically occur due to rotational forces imparted to the distal tibia.
  o High-energy fractures are generally due to axial force that drives the talus into the tibial plafond, causing an "implosion" of the articular surface.
- In the most severe plafond fracture patterns, the articular segment is fractured into numerous pieces with certain segments driven proximally into the metaphysis, creating marked joint incongruity and associated metaphyseal defects.
- An associated fibula fracture is often present in pilon fractures.
- The most common fracture pattern occurs with the ankle in dorsiflexion (i.e., the foot on the brake pedal during a motor vehicle accident).
  o When the ankle is dorsiflexed at the time of injury, pilon fracture patterns involve the anterior articular surface of the tibial plafond.
- Central articular (implosion) injury is the result of an axial load on the foot in neutral position.
- A severely traumatized soft tissue envelope accompanies the higher energy pilon fractures.
  o Although many pilon fractures are open injuries, closed fractures have significant soft tissue compromise as well.
- Initial management of pilon fractures depends as much on the soft tissue as the bony injury.
  o Understanding the soft tissue injury accompanying pilon fractures is of utmost importance for providing optimal treatment while minimizing complications.

Classification

- Classification systems have been developed to stratify both severity of fracture pattern and soft tissue injury.
- Although the Arbeitsgemeinschaft für Osteosynthesefragen (AO)/Orthopaedic Trauma Association (OTA) classification system is the most widely accepted fracture classification system, the Ruedi-Allgower system is the classic fracture scheme often known and used for this injury throughout the world.

- Ruedi-Allgower type 1 fractures are minimally displaced cleavage fractures, in contrast to type 2 injuries, which are displaced. Type 3 injuries portend the worst prognosis as a consequence of articular comminution and metaphyseal impaction.
- Moderate interobserver reliability makes the AO/OTA system reliable for classifying pilon fractures (Swiontkowski et al 1997).
  - The distal tibia is designated as #43 (4 = tibia, 3 = distal segment).
  - The fractures are divided into types and further into groups then subgroups.
- 43C patterns are high-energy injuries with a compromised soft tissue envelope.
  - Irreversible damage to the articular cartilage, and at times the soft tissues, occurs at the time of injury.
- Soft tissue injury has been standardized using the method of Tscherne for closed fractures and the Gustilo-Anderson classification for open injuries.
  - The Tscherne scheme has 4 grades of increasing severity for soft tissue injury in closed fractures.
    - Tscherne grades 0 and 1 have negligible soft tissue injury and superficial abrasions/contusion, respectively.
    - Type 2 Tscherne injury describes advanced muscle contusion and deep, potentially contaminated abrasions.
    - Pilon fractures with extensive crush, degloving, or vascular injury are considered type 3.
  - The most widely accepted open fracture classification is credited to Gustilo and Anderson.
    - Gustilo type 1 open fractures are generally clean with a < 1-cm skin laceration.
    - Type 2 open fractures have more extensive soft tissue injury with minimal to moderate crushing, typically with a laceration > 1 cm.
    - Open pilon fracture with extensive soft tissue injury and a severe crush component are graded as type 3.
      - Type 3A open fractures have adequate soft tissue coverage over the fracture.
      - Type 3B are usually contaminated with extensive periosteal stripping and bone exposure necessitating flap coverage.
      - Open fractures with vascular injury requiring repair along with extensive soft tissue compromise are considered type 3C.

Evaluation

- In view of the fact that most pilon fractures usually occur as the result of violent trauma (i.e., motor vehicle accident), associated bodily injuries must be considered in the work-up of these patients.
- Examination should document the presence of both closed and open soft tissue injury as well as location and extent of lacerations, abrasions, and contamination.
- A systemic motor and sensory examination is warranted in addition to documentation of distal pulses.
- Leg compartment syndrome should be diagnosed based on clinical examination and confirmed if necessary with compartment pressures.

- Radiographs are critical for characterization of the bony injury and joint position and must include an ankle anteroposterior, mortise, and lateral view.
  - Traction views may be valuable for further characterization of the pilon fracture.
- Computed tomography (CT) examination is best delayed until restoration of length in shortened fractures because ligamentotaxis helps to better approximate fragments closer to their native position, making interpretation easier.
- Initial splinting in the emergency room decreases further soft tissue trauma, and fracture dislocations should be reduced with adequate anesthesia to restore joint alignment.
- Open wounds are covered with moist gauze, and antibiotic and tetanus protocols are employed.

Historical Discussion

- Ruedi and Allgower revolutionized the management of pilon fractures after reporting their operative strategy in 1969.
- The series reported by Ruedi and Allgower described superior outcomes after formal open reduction and internal fixation (ORIF) in their patient population with few major complications.
- The operative principles described by the AO group for operating pilon fractures serves as a working paradigm for ORIF of these injuries.
  - Principle 1: Length and rotation is restored by ORIF of the fibula.
  - Principle 2: Anatomical reconstruction of the articular surface of the tibial plafond is performed after the acute phase of the injury.
  - Principle 3: Metaphyseal bone defects are bone grafted to buttress the articular surface.
  - Principle 4: Buttressing of the tibial metaphysis is then required while connecting the articular block to the diaphysis.
- These principles (perhaps with #3 optional), restoration of articular surface, realign joint surface to shaft, then bridge metaphyseal comminution with fixation, can be applied to any periarticular fracture.
- The results of the classic study from the Swiss AO group could not, however, be reproduced by all surgeons.
  - Reports describing ORIF of tibial pilon fractures revealed a concerning complication rate with higher energy pilon fractures, including wound problems, deep infection, nonunion, and malunion (McFerran et al 1992, Teeny and Wiss 1993).
- Recognition of a different category of higher energy pilon injuries emerged, which was quite different than those treated by Ruedi and Allgower, who treated lower energy injuries primarily in healthy skiers: So-called "boot top injuries."
- New research was undertaken to determine the best way to manage higher energy fractures of the tibial plafond in response to the higher rates of infection.
- External fixation alone became popular for managing complex pilon fractures associated with both closed and open compromised soft tissue envelopes.
  - The rate of deep infection decreased with external fixation, however, at a cost.

- o The quality of reduction with external fixation alone was suboptimal, leading to poor outcomes secondary to joint arthrosis.
- Initial external fixator constructs spanned the ankle joint until fracture union, resulting in unacceptable ankle stiffness.
- Small wire epiphyseal-diaphyseal ring fixators were then employed to treat pilon fractures to allow for early ankle motion in an effort to minimize long-term ankle stiffness.
- Limited ORIF to improve articular reductions without formal operative exposures was then employed to supplement external fixation strategies.
- Unsatisfied with the limitations of external fixation strategies, including compromised articular reduction, pin tract complications, and patient dissatisfaction, new strategies to allow for ORIF were investigated.
- Protocols developed to enhance soft tissue recovery prior to definitive operative fracture fixation, including greater waiting time for such recovery, became the mainstay.
- A common modern algorithm is to apply a spanning external fixator to maintain length urgently following injury.
  - o Once the swelling has peaked and regressed 1-3 weeks after injury, open reduction of the tibia (and fibula) can be performed with removal of the temporary external fixator.
- Some surgeons have found that immediate (within a few hours of injury) open reduction, prior to significant swelling, can be performed safely.
  - o There may be some benefits to this technique with possibly less swelling and stiffness.
  - o This is still an emerging technique, and the risk of opening a pilon fracture during the initial stages of swelling could be devastating.

MANAGEMENT OF PILON FRACTURES

Nonoperative Treatment

- Indications for closed reduction and cast treatment of pilon fractures are limited.
  - o This is especially appropriate for nondisplaced injuries, but late displacement is possible.
- No articular displacement should be accepted unless the patient is not an appropriate surgical candidate.
  - o Patients with medical infirmity precluding operative intervention may be candidates for conservative fracture management.
- Pilon fractures treated with a cast have led to poorer outcomes than those managed operatively.
  - o After closed reduction, maintaining lower limb alignment is very difficult in a cast, particularly due to a propensity for the fracture to fall into varus.
- The ability to impart a closed reduction relies on the principle of ligamentotaxis.
  - o Impacted joint segments, found in most plafond fractures, do not have capsular attachments and will not reduce with closed reduction techniques.
- Prolonged immobilization of the ankle joint after fracture can lead to "cast disease."
  - o Cast immobilization until fracture union promotes ankle stiffness, dystrophic changes, muscle atrophy, and disuse osteopenia.

- o Cartilage nutrition is promoted by early ankle joint motion after articular injury, and arthrosis is hastened with cast treatment for pilon fractures.
- Furthermore, monitoring/managing the traumatized soft tissue envelope associated with high-energy pilon fractures cannot be efficiently performed if cast treatment is utilized.

Bridging External Fixation

- An ankle-spanning external fixator can be used for both temporary as well as definitive management of distal intraarticular tibia fractures.
  - o Definitive ORIF is not advisable through a compromised soft tissue envelope.
- Spanning external fixation as a temporary strategy can serve as so-called "traveling traction."
- The fixator can be applied so that the soft tissues and fracture fragments are held out to appropriate length, allowing for recovery of the traumatized tissue envelope.
- Many different frame configurations have been used to effect stability.
  - o A delta frame may be the most popular, and this configuration forms a triangle with a calcaneus transfixion pin attached medially and laterally to 2 pins placed in the tibia, proximal to the zone of injury.
  - o A medially based external fixator can also be used, typically employing half-pins placed in the tibia, talar neck, and calcaneus.
- External fixator application should be placed in such a way to allow for easy management of soft tissues, including access for flap procedures.
- Although fracture union can be achieved with external fixation, malunion rates are higher than with ORIF.

Bridging External Fixation With Limited Internal Fixation

- The most important limitation of external fixation alone as definitive management for pilon fractures is incomplete articular reduction, which portends a worse clinical outcome.
- Limited open approaches to impart an improved reduction of the distal tibia joint surface can be used in conjunction with external fixation.
  - o The rationale of this approach is based on minimizing iatrogenic periarticular soft tissue injury.
- Strategic screws are used in an attempt to restore joint incongruity of the tibial plafond.
  - o In the absence of comminution or displacement at the joint surface, lag screw techniques are utilized to impart compression and stability across joint fragments.
- External fixation decreases the incidence of wound dehiscence (compared to plate fixation) while imparting length, alignment, and rotation.
- Some degree of major and minor pin site problems and septic arthritis is inevitable with the use of external fixation.
- The incidence of malunion may be increased with external fixation, as stability is not as reliably imparted.
- Most concerning is the compromise of the articular reduction in the name of "minimally invasive" or "biologic" surgery.
- Early joint motion, a basic goal of definitive internal fixation, is not possible with spanning frames ± limited internal fixation.

Nonspanning External Fixation ± Limited Internal Fixation

- Joint immobilization has detrimental articular effects, at least in adults with intraarticular fractures.
- Nonbridging external fixators have been used for the management of high-energy pilon fractures to promote the possibility of early motion and weight bearing.
- Frame constructs consist of thin wire fixation into the epiphyseal or articular block with attachment to the diaphyseal segment via rods that are connected to either thin wires (Ilizarov frame) or larger half-pins (hybrid designs).
- The distal fixation consists of tensioned wires connected to a ring.
- "Olive" wires can be placed strategically in the distal segment to assist in compression of articular fragments if open reduction is not performed.
  - The olive part of the wire impinges against the cortex of an articular fragment, which is then pulled toward an adjacent joint segment, imparting an indirect reduction.
- If limited ORIF is used, direct articular reduction can be performed with screw fixation and then a nonspanning external fixation can be placed to align the articular segment with the tibial shaft.
- Standard position of wires after limited open techniques consists of a posterolateral to anteromedial technique (transfibular) as well as a posteromedial to anterolateral placement.
- Encouraging clinical outcomes have been realized with nonspanning fixators by experienced surgeons using Ilizarov techniques.
- However, pin site problems, septic arthritis, patient dissatisfaction with external frames, sacrifices in articular reduction, and high-maintenance follow-up care are inherent challenges.

Staged Open Reduction and Internal Fixation

- The concept is to initially restore length with an external fixator (but not formal incisions), allowing the soft tissues to swell and then return close to normal.
  - If length is not maintained, the tissue will contract, making it impossible to close the wounds without tension when ORIF is eventually performed.
- Although it is possible to reduce and fix the fibula through a posterolateral incision at the initial surgery, along with external fixation, it may be preferable to delay any open incisions until the final plan is made.
- Respect for the soft tissue envelope is paramount if considering ORIF.
  - This includes the following:
    - Conservative timing for definitive incisions
    - External fixation for recovery phase from soft tissue trauma
    - Carefully chosen incisions developing periosteocutaneous flaps
    - Preservation of blood supply to major fracture fragments
    - Gentle soft tissue handling during case
    - Meticulous skin closure technique
- Numerous reports detail the serious complications encountered after untimely ORIF of high-energy tibial plafond fractures.

- These complications include the following:
  - Skin necrosis
  - Wound dehiscence
  - Deep infection
  - Nonunion
  - Malunion
  - Amputation
- During the period of temporary external fixation, the surgeon can get to know the patient and his or her injury.
- Understanding the patient's resources for assistance, job status, personality, recreational preferences, and comorbidities can play a role in decision-making.
- Staged reconstruction also allows the surgeon to develop a relationship with the patient and begin the process of education of what is sure to be a difficult period for the patient.
- Education should cover everything from smoking cessation to injury perspective; it uses the patient's "negative circumstance" for an extraordinary opportunity, often beginning a process of healthy personal discipline: Working on compliant preoperative care and postoperative rehabilitation.
- This period of time affords the surgeon the opportunity to study the injury pattern, obtaining appropriate studies and formulating a surgical tactic.
  - An anteroposterior, mortise, and lateral ankle radiograph in a nonsplinted ankle is obtained 1st in the emergency setting.
  - It is optimal to wait on CT until after the 1st stage of surgery (restoration of length with an external fixator).
- Early intraoperative consultation with a microvascular surgeon is particularly important in the management of open Gustilo type 3B pilon fractures.
  - The goal for this patient may be a bit different; avoiding amputation and getting skin coverage is just as important as obtaining an anatomic reduction.
- Mature clinical judgment is required to determine when the definitive reconstruction should be performed.
  - This stage is enhanced and expedited by strict limb elevation and mechanical pneumatic compression.
  - Clinical signs of a maturing soft tissue envelope include return of the skin wrinkle sign and reepithelization of fracture blisters.
- Traditional teaching is that it is necessary to have at least a 7-cm skin bridge between incisions.
  - However, about the ankle, it is safe to have only a 5-cm bridge, if careful soft tissue handling is performed.
- Based on the CT scan, a final surgical plan is made.
  - This is often performed 1-3 weeks following injury but may need to be delayed even longer if the tissues are not ready.
- There are different surgical approaches commonly used.
- The posterolateral approach uses a long incision, often threatening the superficial peroneal nerve.
  - It is possible to access the fibula and tibia through the same incision, although it may not be as "friendly" to the soft tissues.
- Alternately, the fibula can be approached through a separate posterolateral incision and the tibia through anterior approaches (anterior or anteromedial).

- Anterior or anteromedial approaches to the tibia give good access to the anterior joint, but it is difficult to manipulate the posterolateral fragment.
- For partial articular fractures, where the posterolateral tibial fragment is still connected to the shaft, this is not a problem.
- For complete articular fractures, where the posterolateral fragment is displaced from the shaft, anterior approaches alone may not effect a good reduction.
  - For these patients, the fibula and the posterolateral tibia can be reduced through a posterolateral approach.
  - An anterior approach can be performed at the same setting or a week later, depending on soft tissues, to restore the anterior tibia.
  - The need for a separate posterior approach to the tibia is debated.

Posterolateral Approach

- This approach can be used for the fibula as well as to reduce the posterolateral tibia.
- The patient is preferably prone.
- The incision runs along the peroneal tendons
  - It is generally a long incision.
- The sural nerve is medial (midline) to the incision.
- After incising the fascia over the peroneal tendons, the tendons can be retracted medially to access the fibula.
  - Simple fracture patterns can be directly reduced.
  - Extensive comminution will require bridging.
    - Either way, a plate holds the fibula out to length.
- The peroneal tendons are retracted laterally, over the fibula, if the tibia is to be accessed.
  - The fascia over the flexor hallucis longus (FHL) is incised, and that muscle belly is retracted medially, to expose the posterior tibia.
- The posterior tibial periosteum is thick and may require incising.
- The extraarticular fracture lines of the posterolateral fragment are keyed in to the tibial shaft.
- A plate with short screws can be placed posteriorly to hold this fragment, but it is essential not to place screws into other fragments at this time.
  - Such screws would block the ability to reduce fragments from the anterior approach.
- For closure, the peroneal fascia (superior peroneal retinaculum) is repaired distally but can be left open proximally.
  - The FHL fascia is not repaired.

Anterior Approaches to Tibia

- Preoperative CT scanning assists the surgeon in defining the number and size of fracture fragments, orientation, and sites of articular impaction.
- Preoperative planning includes determining approaches, reduction of fragments, and provisional and definitive fixation.
- Smaller plates and screws may be needed to stabilize articular fragments, while a precontoured periarticular plate will bridge the metaphyseal comminution.
  - Several studies have shown that the anterolateral precontoured plates may not achieve sufficient fixation in the medial articular fragment(s).

- Many of the precontoured implants offer locking options, but at least 1 study has not shown any benefit to locked screws overall.
  - Certain cases may benefit from locked fixation.
- The most direct operative exposure reduces the need for excessive periosteal stripping, which would further denude the fracture segments of their critical blood supply.
- Only full-thickness flaps should be raised, and delicate soft tissue handling is performed.
- Self-retaining retractors should be used sparingly, if at all, for pilon fracture surgery.
- Although the classic operative exposure is an anteromedial approach, medial to the tibialis anterior tendon, current thinking is that the surgeon should be prepared for whatever interval gets the surgeon to the fracture plane with the least dissection.
  - A direct anterior approach passes between the anterior tibialis and the extensor hallucis longus.
    - This approach accesses the entire anterior tibia well.
  - An anterolateral approach is performed lateral to the extensor digitorum longus and requires a bit more dissection to get the to the medial fragment.
    - This approach has the greatest potential to injure the superficial peroneal nerve and may be the least "friendly" to soft tissues.
- A femoral distractor can be used to aid visualization of the articular surface.
  - The distractor is placed medially and can utilize the pins from the temporary bridging external fixator, if that was placed medially.
- A head light also is very helpful.
- Fracture reduction should proceed in a stepwise manner, typically building from the posterior to anterior
  - The lateral fragments will typically be out to length due to their attachments to the fibula through the tibiofibular ligaments (assuming that the fibula length and rotation have been restored).
  - Impacted articular fragments must be brought into their appropriate position, and some bone void filler should be packed behind the associated metaphyseal defect.
  - Provisional K-wires and bone reduction forceps should maintain the reduction before definitive fixation is placed.
- The articular reduction needs to be critically assessed with visual inspection in addition to intraoperative fluoroscopy.
  - It is imperative to have a large fluoroscopy field of view, which allows for analysis of ankle alignment as well as articular reduction.
- The talar articular surface can be used as a template for judging the accuracy of the tibial plafond after the traction from the femoral distractor is let down.
- Strategic lag screws are placed to rigidly fix and, if appropriate, compress the articular fragments.
- The typical periarticular plates are anterolateral and medial.
  - Either can be used.
  - Some surgeons use both plates for each case, but it is possible to make a "dead bone sandwich" with anterior tibial avascular necrosis.
    - In general, single bridging plate is adequate.
  - The plate can be slid under the soft tissues with small stab incisions for proximal screw placement.

- This keeps main incision and dissection limited to articular surface.
- After capsular repair, the investing distal fascia and extensor retinaculum should be reapproximated.
- Subcutaneous sutures can be carefully placed to minimize tension on the skin layer.
- Skin is closed using a meticulous Allgower-Donati technique to maximize blood flow to the wound edges.
  - Vertical mattress sutures can be appropriate as well.

Postoperative Care

- A splint is generally applied for 2 weeks; such immobilization aids in wound healing.
- From week 2 onward, a removable cast boot can be used to prevent equinus contracture along with active range of motion exercises for ankle and foot.
- Weight bearing begins once there is metaphyseal healing, usually 7-10 weeks after surgery.
- Pool therapy is a helpful adjunct for patients during the phase of increasing weight bearing.

Special Considerations in Open Fractures

- An open fracture is typically the result of high-energy trauma, implying significant bone and soft tissue injury.
- The open wound is usually medial, where the soft tissue is thinnest.
- Prompt surgical debridement and irrigation is the mainstay of early operative management.
- Bridging external fixation is appropriate management at the 1st debridement to allow for soft tissue recovery and wound management.
- As an adjunct to surgical strategies, antibiotic and tetanus protocols should be administered in all open plafond fractures.
- Early wound coverage is important.
  - In some cases, direct closure may be possible.
  - In many cases, free tissue transfer (muscle free flap) will be required.
  - Ideally, the wound should be closed within a week, and certainly within 2 weeks, to decrease chance for deep infection.
- Although with modern surgical techniques, limb salvage is typically the best option for open pilon fractures, amputation should be considered in the mangled extremity in nonambulators and in the multiply injured elderly patient with comorbidities.
- Elective bone grafting procedures to fill bone voids from open fracture management should be planned at 6-12 weeks.
- Primary ankle fusion can be a useful tool in the worst cases.
  - Usually, the ankle can be narrowed to facilitate closure, and there may be less need for dissection of soft tissue off bone.

OUTCOMES

- Many studies have shown relatively worse outcomes when compared to other fractures or other diseases.
- Some studies suggest an anatomic reduction of the articular surface as well as restoration of limb alignment may correlate with a better outcome.

- Studies comparing external fixation with ORIF have mixed results.
  - In general, external fixation is associated with more infections (pin tract, not necessarily deep infection).
  - ORIF is associated with higher chance of subsequent surgery for hardware removal.
  - Outcomes are sometimes better with ORIF but not in all studies.
- In one study, restoration of fibular length correlated with outcome.
- Outcomes probably depend on a combination of factors: Patient, injury, and surgeon.

COMPLICATIONS

Wound Problems and Infection

- Historically, an alarmingly high percentage of pilon fracture surgeries have developed wound complications, reported in the range of 12-40%.
- Wound complications after pilon fracture management often are a precursor to the development of deep infection.
- Partial- and full-thickness skin necrosis, wound dehiscence, superficial infection, and deep infection are all reported complications of pilon fracture management.
- Application of the principles previously described should help to decrease such problems to a manageable incidence somewhere below 5% in closed fractures.
- Early soft tissue coverage, ideally within 7 days, will minimize such complications in open injuries.

Arthrofibrosis

- Ankle function rarely returns to normal, even with superior operative strategies.
- Periarticular scar formation limits the final range of motion in high-energy pilon patterns.
- Temporary bridging external fixation, which immobilizes the ankle joint, may contribute to ankle arthrofibrosis.
- Early motion protocols after treatment with nonspanning external fixation or ORIF improves ankle range of motion at union.
- However, in the typical case with initial external fixation and then short-term postoperative splinting (after definitive ORIF), motion exercises do not begin until more than a month after injury.

Arthritis

- Quality of articular reduction positively correlates with clinical outcome.
- Nonanatomical reductions with articular step-offs and gaps predispose the ankle joint to pain as well as early arthrosis.
- However, a perfect-looking joint on x-ray does not equate to a perfect or even good outcome, and an imperfect reduction does not always guarantee bad results.
- In cases of anatomical joint reductions after high-energy pilon fractures, degenerative joint disease may still occur.
- At the time of plafond fracture, an unpredictable percentage of the cartilaginous surface is irreversibly damaged.
  - Impacted articular segments are often devascularized at the time of injury, occasionally resulting in osteonecrosis of the joint segment and cartilage loss.

- Injudicious periosteal or capsular stripping during ORIF can also devascularize segments of articular surface, leading to iatrogenic-induced focal osteonecrosis and resultant joint arthrosis.
- Particular emphasis should be given by the surgeon to preserve the blood supply to the major fragments, particularly the vulnerable anterolateral fragment and its soft tissue hinge that receives blood supply from the anterolateral sleeve of tissue corresponding with anterior syndesmotic attachments.
- This anterior fragment, often associated with the greatest degree of comminution, is vulnerable to avascular necrosis and, thus, susceptible to collapse with premature loading.
- An ankle orthosis, such as a double upright brace, functionally prevents ankle motion and may decrease arthritis symptoms.
- The Intrepid Dynamic Exoskeletal Orthosis (IDEO) is a custom AFO with energy-storing ability and may give the patient with a stiff ankle some push-off energy.
  - It may be very helpful for the active young patient trying to regain more athletic activity, but availability of the brace is limited.
- Ankle fusion is the gold standard salvage procedure for the treatment of posttraumatic ankle arthrosis.
  - A properly performed ankle arthrodesis can restore the mechanical alignment of the hindfoot and achieve solid union across the tibiotalar interface.

SELECTED REFERENCES

1. Pollak AN et al: Outcomes after treatment of high-energy tibial plafond fractures. J Bone Joint Surg Am. 85-A(10):1893-900, 2003
2. Watson JT et al: Pilon fractures. Treatment protocol based on severity of soft tissue injury. Clin Orthop Relat Res. 78-90, 2000
3. Anglen JO: Early outcome of hybrid external fixation for fracture of the distal tibia. J Orthop Trauma. 13(2):92-7, 1999
4. Patterson MJ et al: Two-staged delayed open reduction and internal fixation of severe pilon fractures. J Orthop Trauma. 13(2):85-91, 1999
5. Pugh KJ et al: Tibial pilon fractures: a comparison of treatment methods. J Trauma. 47(5):937-41, 1999
6. Sirkin M et al: A staged protocol for soft tissue management in the treatment of complex pilon fractures. J Orthop Trauma. 13(2):78-84, 1999
7. Sands A et al: Clinical and functional outcomes of internal fixation of displaced pilon fractures. Clin Orthop Relat Res. 131-7, 1998
8. Babiş GC et al: Results of surgical treatment of tibial plafond fractures. Clin Orthop Relat Res. 99-105, 1997
9. Swiontkowski MF et al: Interobserver variation in the AO/OTA fracture classification system for pilon fractures: is there a problem? J Orthop Trauma. 11(7):467-70, 1997
10. McDonald MG et al: Ilizarov treatment of pilon fractures. Clin Orthop Relat Res. 232-8, 1996
11. Tornetta P 3rd et al: Axial computed tomography of pilon fractures. Clin Orthop Relat Res. (323):273-6, 1996
12. Helfet DL et al: Intraarticular "pilon" fracture of the tibia. Clin Orthop Relat Res. 221-8, 1994
13. Bone L et al: External fixation of severely comminuted and open tibial pilon fractures. Clin Orthop Relat Res. 101-7, 1993
14. Teeny SM et al: Open reduction and internal fixation of tibial plafond fractures. Variables contributing to poor results and complications. Clin Orthop Relat Res. 108-17, 1993
15. Tornetta P 3rd et al: Pilon fractures: treatment with combined internal and external fixation. J Orthop Trauma. 7(6):489-96, 1993
16. McFerran MA et al: Complications encountered in the treatment of pilon fractures. J Orthop Trauma. 6(2):195-200, 1992
17. Bourne RB et al: Intra-articular fractures of the distal tibia: the pilon fracture. J Trauma. 23(7):591-6, 1983

(Left) *Soft tissue injury associated with a pilon fracture at 72 hours is shown. Skin incisions are not advisable at this time due to wound healing and infection risk. Blood-filled blisters represent injury of the dermoepidermal junction.* **(Right)** *Initial management goals are achieving length and skeletal alignment. A common strategy includes restoring the lateral column with internal fixation of the fibula through a posterolateral approach. Medial stability can be achieved with a spanning external fixator.*

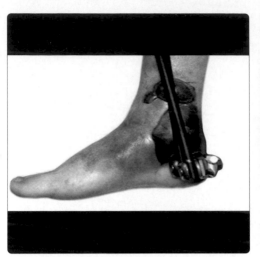

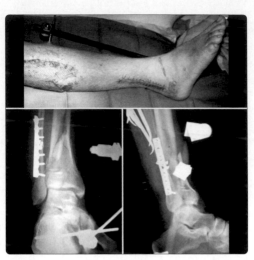

(Left) *A nonspanning (hybrid) external fixator is shown. Typically, tensioned thin wires attached to a ring are placed in the articular segment. Proximal to the fracture, conventional Shantz pins can be placed in the tibial shaft. The fracture is then spanned with bars from the proximal Shantz pins to the distal ring.* **(Right)** *External fixator placement at the 1st debridement allows access for early flap coverage when necessary. Better outcomes and lower complication rates are associated with flap coverage within 72 hours.*

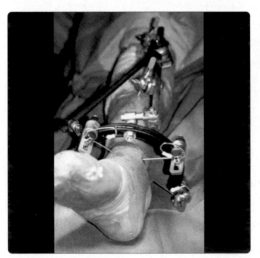

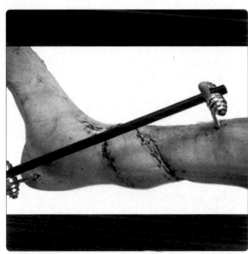

(Left) *Open pilon fracture management consists of meticulous debridement, irrigation, and, sometimes, antibiotic beads. A vacuum-assisted closure dressing is useful between presentation and flap coverage.* **(Right)** *A femoral distractor is useful during definitive reconstruction. A proximal Shantz pin is placed in the medial tibia cephalad to the zone of injury, and a distal pin is typically placed in the talar body. Distraction allows for maintenance of longitudinal alignment while the articular surface is reconstructed.*

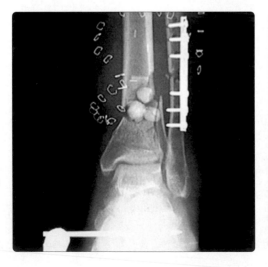

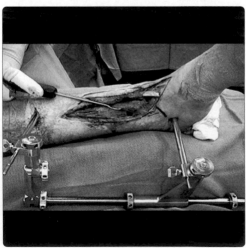

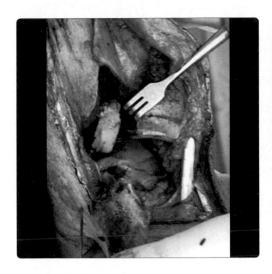

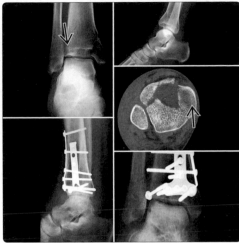

(Left) Distractor allows for superior joint visualization during plafond reduction. Talus serves as a template for determining position of comminuted articular segments. (Right) Note definitive reconstruction of 43B pilon fracture. Anterior approach was utilized to anatomically reduce anterior impaction injury ➡. Anterior & medial buttress plate fixation is necessary, in addition to lag screw fixation of joint surface. Bone void filler was used to fill metaphyseal defect left after disimpaction of articular segment.

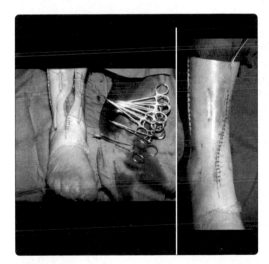

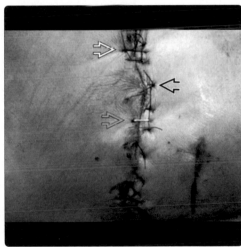

(Left) The Allgower-Donati technique is the recommend closure, as it maximizes blood flow to the wound edges. (Right) Allgower-Donati technique ➡ compared with simple suturing ➡ and skin stapling ➡ is shown. Note that with the other techniques, the skin edges are not perfectly opposed, and significant blanching of the skin is evident.

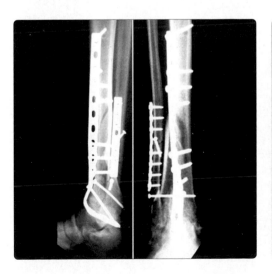

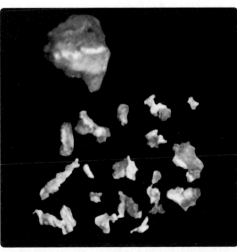

(Left) Ankle arthrodesis is both a primary as well as a later reconstruction option for pilon fractures. While extremely rare, consideration for primary fusion surgery should be contemplated when extensive comminution of the articular surface precludes stable reduction and anatomical restoration of the joint surface. However, more commonly, arthrodesis is indicated for posttraumatic ankle degenerative joint disease. (Right) Fusion was chosen as a primary treatment option in this severely comminuted pilon fracture.

KEY FACTS

- Calcaneus fractures account for ~ 2% of all fractures.
- The calcaneus is the most frequently fractured tarsal (hindfoot) bone.
  - It represents 60% of all tarsal fractures.
  - Minor avulsion fractures off anterior process are common and usually benign.
- Most intraarticular calcaneus fractures are the result of an axial load applied directly to the heel.
- A high-energy calcaneus fracture is often a life-altering event for the affected individual.
- The socioeconomic burden of calcaneus fractures is significant.
  - 90% of these fractures occur in working individuals between 20-40 years of age.
- The mechanism of injury (axial loading) often results in concomitant injuries to the lower extremities and the spine.
- Always evaluate patients for signs and symptoms of compartment syndrome.

- Radiographic examination should include a lateral of the foot and ankle, a mortise view of the ankle, dorsoplantar and oblique x-rays of the foot, and an axial (Harris) view.
- Definitive management of intraarticular calcaneus fractures consists of either operative or nonoperative treatment.
- The historical aversion to operative treatment of the calcaneus was related to severe complications, including compartment syndrome, nerve injury, wound-healing problems and infection, malunion, subtalar arthritis, and nerve injury.
- Treating orthopedists have been guilty of focusing too much attention on the articular reduction of the posterior facet.
- Attention to all aspects of the injury, both osseous and soft tissue, will yield the best results.

(Left) The history of calcaneus fractures demonstrates an oscillation between nonoperative treatment and surgical intervention. Advances, such as antibiotic therapy, the discovery of the CT scan, and improved surgical techniques, have led to improved outcomes for surgical treatment in the past 2 decades. (Right) Two characteristic fracture lines, ⇒ and ➡, of intraarticular calcaneus fractures as described by Carr et al are shown.

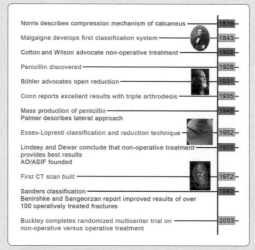

Norris describes compression mechanism of calcaneus	1839
Malgaigne develops first classification system	1843
Cotton and Wilson advocate non-operative treatment	1908
Penicillin discovered	1928
Böhler advocates open reduction	1931
Conn reports excellent results with triple arthrodesis	1935
Mass production of penicillin / Palmer describes lateral approach	1948
Essex-Lopresti classification and reduction technique	1952
Lindsey and Dewar conclude that non-operative treatment provides best results / AO/ASIF founded	1958
First CT scan built	1972
Sanders classification / Benirshke and Sangeorzan report improved results of over 100 operatively treated fractures	1993
Buckley completes randomized multicenter trial on non-operative versus operative treatment	2003

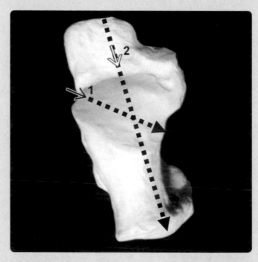

(Left) CT scan demonstrates the characteristic fracture lines, ⇒ and ➡. (Right) Harris axial x-ray of the calcaneus demonstrating a characteristic fracture line ⇒ is shown.

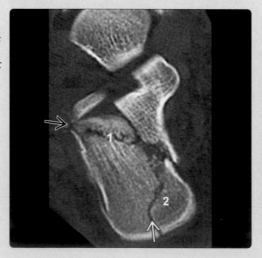

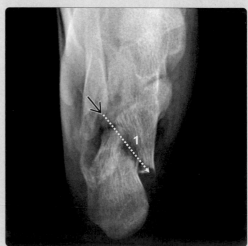

HISTORICAL PERSPECTIVE

- Surgical treatment of the calcaneus was discouraged through most of the early 20th century.
  - The treatment of acute fractures was all but abandoned.
  - Focus of treatment was on late reconstruction of healed malunions.
- In 1916, Cotton and Henderson concluded that, "The man who breaks his heel bone is done."
- In 1926, Conn wrote, "Calcaneus fractures are serious and disabling injuries in which the end results continue to be incredibly bad."
- Böhler advocated open reduction of calcaneus fractures as early as 1931.
  - However, due to the limitations of poor diagnostic tools and the lack of appropriate implants to achieve stable fixation, the complication rate (i.e., wound problems, infection, and loss of reduction) was high.
- Throughout North America, primary triple or isolated subtalar arthrodesis was popularized during the 1930s and 1940s.
  - The results of those treatments continued to be poor.
  - In 1942, Bankart concluded, "the results of crush fractures of the os calcis are rotten."
- In 1958, Lindsey and Dewar studied the long-term outcome of calcaneus fractures and concluded that nonoperative treatment provided the best outcome.
  - Throughout the 1960s and 1970s, nonoperative treatment continued to be the treatment of choice.
- Treatment options for calcaneus fractures remain controversial.
  - However, advances in radiographic imaging, surgical technique, and a better understanding of the pathoanatomy of calcaneus fractures have led to improved results with surgical treatment of these challenging fractures over the past 20 years.

MECHANISM OF INJURY

- Most intraarticular calcaneus fractures are the result of an axial load applied directly to the heel.
  - High-energy intraarticular calcaneus fractures are usually the result of a fall from height or a motor vehicle accident.
  - The actual fracture pattern is influenced by the position of the foot and the subtalar joint, the force of the impact, and the quality of the patient's bone.
- Extraarticular fractures are more frequently the result of a twisting or an avulsive force.
  - Isolated fractures of the anterior process of the calcaneus may be the result of forced inversion of the plantar flexed foot, resulting in an avulsive force created by the insertion of the bifurcate ligament.
    - Alternatively, forced dorsiflexion and eversion may compress the anterior process between the cuboid and the talus.
  - Avulsion fractures of the tuberosity may be caused by a sudden forceful contraction of the gastrocnemius-soleus muscle complex.
    - They may occur in patients with a previously tight heel cord (e.g., diabetics).

- In intraarticular fractures, the energy imparted to the calcaneus during axial loading results in 2 characteristic primary fracture lines.
  - The 1st fracture line usually starts at the crucial angle of Gissane.
    - The lateral process of the talus acts as a wedge, dividing the calcaneus into an anterior and a posterior 1/2.
  - The anteromedial fragment, also called the constant fragment, usually maintains its relationship with the talus, tethered by the strong interosseous and medial ligaments.
  - The posterolateral fragment usually displaces laterally and into varus alignment.
  - Secondary fracture lines travel in the sagittal plane along the length of the bone in an anterior and a posterior direction.
    - These fracture lines can travel into the calcaneocuboid joint, split the anterior facet, or exit the body of the calcaneus medially or laterally.
- In higher energy fractures, additional secondary fracture lines develop, resulting in higher degrees of comminution.

INITIAL EVALUATION AND MANAGEMENT

- Initial evaluation of all patients with calcaneus fractures involves a thorough physical examination.
- The mechanism of injury (axial loading) often results in concomitant injuries to the lower extremities and the spine.
  - Lumbar spine fracture
  - Tibia fracture (pilon, plateau)
  - Ankle fracture
  - Additional foot fracture
  - Acetabular fracture
- Lumbar spine fractures are most commonly associated, especially in cases of bilateral calcaneus fractures.
  - Some would argue for routine lumbar spine radiographs in any patient with a calcaneus fracture from a fall.
- The injured foot is placed into a bulky dressing or a foam boot and is elevated.
- The neurovascular status of the fractured extremity should be carefully tested and documented.
  - Numbness or a subjective decrease in sensation may be an early warning sign of impending compartment syndrome.
- Evaluation for compartment syndrome is essential on initial evaluation.
  - Carefully monitor for developing or impending compartment syndrome with serial examinations.
  - Compartment syndrome of the foot may present as excruciating pain, an alteration in sensation, or pain with passive motion of the toes.
  - Many patients with calcaneus fractures will have pain with passive toe motion, because the origin of the flexor digitorum brevis is on the calcaneus.
  - It is also common to see plantar nerve paresthesias with high-energy injuries, so the entire clinical picture must be taken into account when evaluating for compartment syndrome.
- A patient with suspected compartment syndrome should undergo invasive measurement of the compartments of the foot.

- Absolute compartment pressure > 30 mm Hg or a 40-mm Hg difference between the measured pressure and the patient's diastolic pressure is an indication for foot fasciotomies.
- The energy imparted to the foot in calcaneus fractures is shared equally by the bone and soft tissues.
  - Therefore, evaluation and close monitoring of the soft tissues is important.
  - Patients will often present with fracture blisters, which result when there is cleavage at the dermal-epidermal junction.
    - Blisters should be covered with sterile dressings and allowed to drain on their own.
- If the patient is to undergo surgical treatment, the operation is delayed until the blisters have reepithelialized, and skin wrinkles are visible over the lateral aspect of the hindfoot.
  - Sequential compression devices for the foot may be of some use in helping to control edema in the preoperative phase.
- An exception to delayed treatment is in cases where the soft tissue may be threatened by a displaced fracture.
  - Tuberosity avulsion fractures may result in pressure over the skin of the posterior heel.
  - The surgeon should consider urgent reduction to prevent additional soft tissue injury, which may quickly lead to full-thickness skin necrosis.
- Severe injuries may result in open fractures.
  - Open calcaneus fractures are rare and account for < 10% of all calcaneus fractures.
  - The traumatic wound tends to be on the medial side, caused by the sharp spike of the medial wall created by the primary fracture line.
  - The tuberosity is dislocated laterally.
- Open fractures should be treated with urgent debridement.
  - The medial wound is debrided.
  - Closed or minimally invasive techniques to realign the calcaneus can be performed at the time of debridement.
    - Given the severe soft tissue injury, extensile approaches should be avoided until the soft tissues have recovered.
  - Typically, wires are used to hold the tuberosity in a relatively reduced position until time of definitive treatment.
- Occasionally, higher energy injuries will result in fractures with open wounds laterally.
  - Care must be taken in the debridement of these wounds, as the lateral exposure may be later utilized for stabilization of the fracture.
- Inspection and palpation of the peroneal tendons should also be performed on initial examination.
  - Often, the initial examination is difficult due to swelling and patient discomfort.
  - The examination is repeated under anesthesia.
  - Dislocated tendons usually reduce to their anatomical location with adequate reduction of the fracture.

Radiographic Evaluation

- Initial radiographic examination of the injured foot should include:
  - Lateral of foot and ankle
  - Mortise view of ankle
  - Dorsoplantar and oblique x-rays of foot
- In addition, an axial (Harris) view is obtained.
  - The Harris view is obtained with the foot in maximal dorsiflexion, and the x-ray beam angled 45° cephalad.
- A lateral and axial view of the contralateral foot should be obtained for comparison.
- All patients with calcaneus fractures should undergo axial computed tomography (CT) scan of the foot.
  - Coronal images can be obtained by flexing up the knee and resting the foot plantigrade on the CT table.
  - Alternately, coronal and sagittal reconstructions can be created with appropriate software.

CLASSIFICATION

- Several systems have been developed for classification of calcaneus fractures.
- Calcaneus fractures can be divided into 2 broad categories: Intraarticular and extraarticular.
  - 30% of calcaneus fractures are extraarticular.
    - Anterior process fractures represent the majority of extraarticular injuries.
      - They account for 10-15% of all calcaneus fractures.
      - They are more common in women.
  - Intraarticular fractures comprise 70% of all calcaneus fractures.
- In 1952, Essex-Lopresti classified intraarticular calcaneus fractures into 2 broad types: Tongue type and joint depression.
  - The Essex-Lopresti classification was primarily descriptive but also helps to distinguish those fractures that could be approached through percutaneous techniques (Essex-Lopresti maneuver).
- In 1993, Sanders classified calcaneus fractures based on the number and location of articular (posterior facet) fracture fragments as seen on CT scan.
  - The Sanders classification is unique in that it is prognostic as well as descriptive.
  - One of the limitations of the Sanders classification is that it is based purely on the posterior facet and does not address injuries to the remainder of the calcaneus.
- More recently, the Foot and Ankle Study Group of the Arbeitsgemeinschaft für Osteosynthesefragen has developed the Integral Classification of Injuries to the bones, joints, and ligaments.
  - This system provides a precise descriptive classification for injuries to the foot, including calcaneus fractures.
  - In this fracture classification scheme, the foot is divided into 3 zones:
    - Hindfoot
    - Midfoot
    - Forefoot
  - A numeric system is used to describe the location of the fracture.
    - 81.2 is number used to designate calcaneus
  - The fracture is then determined to be:
    - A (extraarticular)
    - B (intraarticular)
    - C (fracture-dislocation)

- Additional subgroups are included for direction of dislocation, number of joints involved, and soft tissue injury.
- Although this system provides a comprehensive classification scheme, its reproducibility and usefulness remain to be seen.

OPERATIVE VS. NONOPERATIVE TREATMENT

- Definitive management of intraarticular calcaneus fractures consists of either operative or nonoperative treatment.
- Several factors determine which method of treatment is used, including patient factors, type of fracture, and surgeon experience.
- A number of patient-related factors can affect the outcome of intraarticular calcaneus fractures and, therefore, will impact the decision to pursue operative or nonoperative treatment.
  - Patients with drug and alcohol addiction, organic brain disease, or other forms of mental incapacitation, and who are unable to cooperate with the postoperative rehabilitation plan, are probably better treated nonoperatively.
- Patient factors that may result in an inability to heal surgical wounds are also considered to be relative contraindications for operative treatment.
  - Smoking or other regular nicotine use impairs wound healing.
  - Patients with diabetes mellitus or peripheral vascular disease carry a higher risk of complications with surgery.
- The specific nature of the fracture also influences this decision.
  - Minimally displaced fractures can be treated without surgery.
  - There is some evidence that dramatically displaced fractures (particularly those with a negative Böhler angle) may have a poor outcome regardless of the treatment.
- Occasionally, the fracture type may supersede other factors in determining operative vs. nonoperative approach.
  - For example, an Essex-Lopresti tongue-type fracture that can be reduced and stabilized through percutaneous methods may be treated operatively with a low risk of complications, even in a smoker with diabetes mellitus.
- Finally, surgeon experience plays an important role in the operative treatment of calcaneus fractures.
  - The learning curve for surgical repair of the calcaneus is well documented.
  - Complications and poor results may occur more frequently if complex fractures are managed by inexperienced surgeons.
- In 2002, Buckley et al reported the results of a prospective randomized study of operative vs. nonoperative treatment of calcaneus fractures at 2 years' follow-up.
  - 309 patients with 371 calcaneus fractures were randomized to receive a standardized operative or nonoperative treatment conducted at 4 trauma centers.
  - Based on 36-Item Short-Form Health Survey and visual analog scores, there was no difference in outcome based on treatment groups.

- However, when the treatment groups were stratified, operative treatment was shown to be superior in women and patients who were not on workers' compensation.
  - Within the nonworkers' compensation group, the following groups had better results with operative treatment:
    - Younger patients
    - Patients with injury Böhler angle of 0-14°
    - Patients with lighter workload
  - This study is helpful in identifying patients who may have an improved outcome with operative treatment.
- However, the decision for operative or nonoperative treatment must be made on an individual basis.
  - Although Buckley contends that nonoperative treatment may provide better outcomes at 2 years in certain cases, the surgeon should also consider the long-term effects of a malaligned calcaneus on the remainder of the joints in the foot and ankle.
    - Later foot reconstruction is easier and safer with a well-aligned foot.

TREATMENT OF EXTRAARTICULAR CALCANEUS FRACTURES

- Extraarticular calcaneus fractures are often missed on initial evaluation and often result in a painful foot and delayed diagnosis.
- The most common extraarticular calcaneus fracture is the anterior process fracture.
- Depending on the extent and symptoms of the fracture, treatment consists of nonoperative treatment with functional rehabilitation, open reduction and internal fixation (ORIF), or excision of symptomatic fracture fragments.
- Extraarticular fractures of the calcaneal tuberosity often are minimally displaced and can be treated nonoperatively in the majority of cases.
- Displaced fractures, however, may threaten the thin posterior soft tissue envelope and lead to full-thickness necrosis.
  - Fractures with soft tissue compromise must be reduced emergently to prevent potentially devastating wound complications and infection.

TREATMENT OF INTRAARTICULAR CALCANEUS FRACTURES

- The outcome of a calcaneus fracture is affected by:
  - Surrounding soft tissue
  - Height and shape of bone
  - Articular surface alignment
- The impact of injury, as well as soft tissue handling during surgery, can lead to scarring and stiffness of adjacent tissues.
- Loss of height is universal with displaced intraarticular calcaneus fractures.
  - This loss of height alters the position of the talus and adversely affects both ankle and subtalar mechanics.
    - The worst outcomes are often seen with calcaneal malunions with loss of height.
- Articular incongruity can lead to posttraumatic arthritis of the subtalar or calcaneocuboid joints.

Nonoperative Treatment

- Patients treated nonoperatively are splinted in a neutral position.
- After initial discomfort improves and soft tissue swelling diminishes, patients are treated with early range of motion of the ankle, subtalar joint, and intrinsic muscles of the foot.
- Dorsiflexion splints are useful in preventing plantar flexion contracture.
- Weight bearing is delayed until radiographic fracture consolidation is evident.
  - This typically occurs ~ 2 months after the injury.

Operative Treatment

- Operative treatment can be done through an extensile lateral approach, which gives good access to most parts of the bone (except for the medial sustentaculum).
  - However, soft tissue scarring and subtalar stiffness is common.
  - Wound-healing problems, including deep infection, can occur as well.
- Percutaneous and minimally invasive techniques have been described and are most appropriate for tongue-type fractures.
  - There is less chance of wound-healing problems and often better subtalar motion.
  - Reduction of more complex fractures may be incomplete.
- More recently, sinus tarsi approaches with access to the posterior facet and tuberosity have gained popularity.
  - Less soft tissue dissection may lead to better wound healing and possibly better motion.
- Multiple studies have shown sinus tarsi approaches, and other less invasive approaches, have lower rates of wound-healing problems and may offer faster healing and return to activity.
  - However, it is not clear if these less invasive approaches also result in less good reductions.
    - And it is not clear if they lead to better or worse outcomes.
- Outcomes of calcaneus fractures are hard to study.
  - Surgery for these injuries is challenging, and different surgeons will have varying abilities to effect a good reduction.
    - This is one of the many reasons why it has been so difficult to prove what treatment options are best.
- Outcomes of surgery will tend to improve as surgeon experience improves.

Open Treatment

- Surgical approaches for open treatment include medial, lateral, or combined approaches.
- The medial approach allows for the direct visualization of the medial wall and direct reduction of the tuberosity fragment.
  - This approach does not allow for direct visualization of the subtalar joint.
    - Subtalar reduction is performed indirectly using manipulation through the primary fracture line with the aid of fluoroscopy.
  - Furthermore, this approach does not allow for decompression of the lateral wall.

- The major risk of the medial approach is damage to the neurovascular structures.
  - The main nerve at risk from this approach is the medial calcaneal sensory branch.
    - It is reported to be injured in up to 20% of cases.
  - As the medial soft tissues are often severely compromised by the extreme shear forces produced by the fracture displacement, the risk of wound complications is high with this approach.
- The extensile lateral approach is the most commonly utilized approach for ORIF of the calcaneus.
  - The approach utilizes a lateral flap based on the lateral calcaneal artery.
  - An L-shaped incision (on the left foot, it is more like a J than an L) is made over the lateral calcaneus, and a full-thickness flap containing the skin, peroneal tendons, sural nerve, and periosteum is elevated sharply off the lateral calcaneal wall.
  - The lateral approach allows for direct visualization of the entire subtalar joint from the anterior process of the calcaneus to the tuberosity.
- The major risks for the extensile lateral approach are wound complications related to healing of the lateral calcaneal flap.
  - However, if performed carefully, the complication rate is low.
  - Benirschke and Kramer reported a 1.8% infection rate in closed fractures and a 7.7% infection rate in open fractures in 379 cases with an extensile lateral approach.
- The fragments are stabilized with strategically placed lag screws and bridging plates.
  - Several different plates are available from different manufacturers, but the reduction is more important than the plate.
- Locking plates have recently been introduced and may provide better fixation for the highly comminuted fracture.
  - Locking plates are probably not necessary for most calcaneus injuries.
- The use of bone graft is controversial.
  - Once reduction is achieved, there is consistently a void below the critical angle bone.
    - Depression of the posterior facet crushes the loose cancellous bone normally found in this location at the time of injury.
  - Cancellous autograft or allograft can be packed into the defect prior to plate application.
  - In theory, the graft provides better support and makes a better construct, although no studies have shown an advantage to grafting.
- Recently, calcium phosphate cements have been developed to provide better buttressing than cancellous graft.
- Better constructs raise the possibility of earlier weight bearing.
  - It is unclear whether the use of locked plates or calcium cements will allow earlier weight bearing.

Percutaneous/Minimally Invasive Technique

- Minimally invasive or percutaneous techniques allow for an alternative approach to calcaneus fractures.

- These techniques are particularly useful in patients who have contraindications or significant risk factors that preclude open approaches.
- The technique was originally described by Essex-Lopresti and is best indicated for fractures that fall into the tongue-type variety of the Essex-Lopresti classification scheme.
- Fractures treated by this method must be approached early (< 2 weeks).
  - Organized hematoma can interfere with fracture reduction beyond this time frame.
- The potential advantages of this technique include decreased wound complications, improved early postoperative motion, and decreased stiffness.
  - Tornetta (1998) reported 87% good or excellent results utilizing this technique.
- Tongue-type fractures can be reduced well with this technique.
- Percutaneous reduction techniques usually do not achieve an anatomic reduction for joint depression fractures.
- The decrease in wound complications and postoperative scarring may actually lead to better outcomes.
- It is hoped that a comparative study will define the exact role of percutaneous surgery in the future.

Sinus Tarsi Approach

- A relatively small incision is made parallel to the peroneal tendons, along the sinus tarsi.
- This approach provides good visualization of the posterior facet and allows direct manipulation of those fragments.
- The tuberosity can be reduced with half-pins through small incisions, and a bridging plate can hold the reduction of the tuberosity to the posterior facet.
- This approach potentially can minimize wound-healing problems while also achieving a good reduction.
- As with all surgical approaches, surgeon experience is essential for a good result

External Fixation

- External fixation is rarely used to treat fractures of the calcaneus.
- However, external fixation may play a role, particularly in the definitive treatment of some open calcaneus fractures or in patients with a severely compromised soft tissue envelope.
  - Two recent series (Ebraheim et al, 2000 and Emara and Allam, 2005) reported good results with external fixation, particularly in cases of soft tissue injury.
- A pin through the tuberosity holds the bone out to length.
- Other pins may be placed in the tibia and midfoot.
- When holding the reduction of an open calcaneus fracture temporarily while awaiting definitive surgery, a transfixion pin through the calcaneus should not be used, because the pin site will compromise definitive exposure.
  - The displaced tuberosity should be maintained with axial K wires ± a bridging external fixator (tibia to midfoot, no pins in calcaneus).

Primary Arthrodesis

- In cases of severe comminution, the surgeon may consider primary subtalar arthrodesis for the treatment of calcaneus fractures.

- Although no randomized, controlled studies exist to date, subtalar fusion is a treatment option often proposed for patients with Sanders type 4 fractures.
- When performing subtalar fusion, the shape and alignment of the calcaneus must be restored prior to proceeding with fusion.
- One study suggested a faster return to work for comminuted fractures treated with early fusion.

BLAST INJURIES

- The changing nature of military conflict has seen more frequent blast injuries, occurring from explosive devices.
- Severe open fractures of the calcaneus with extensive soft tissue disruption are the result.
- Initial treatment requires debridement and soft tissue coverage.
  - If soft tissues can heal without deep infection, reconstruction can be considered.
- If deep bone infection is established, amputation at a higher level (usually transtibial) is probably the best solution.

COMPLICATIONS

- The historical aversion to operative treatment of the calcaneus was related to the severe complications that are often encountered with these complex fractures.
- Complications of calcaneus fracture treatment include:
  - Compartment syndrome
  - Nerve injury
  - Wound-healing problems and infection
  - Malunion
  - Subtalar arthritis
  - Nerve injury
- The sequelae of compartment syndrome in the foot can be debilitating in patients with calcaneus fractures.
  - Complications include clawing of the lesser toes, chronic pain, and atrophy.
- Nerve injury can occur during surgical approach or may be the result of the injury.
  - The sural nerve is at risk for injury during the extensile lateral approach.
    - Injury to this nerve may result in loss of sensation or the development of a painful neuroma near the proximal or distal end of the incision.
  - In open fractures or high-energy calcaneus fracture-dislocations, the posterior tibial nerve may be at risk.
    - The posterior tibial nerve may also become entrapped medially.
- Wound-healing problems and infection are the result of a multifactorial process, including the subcutaneous nature of the calcaneus, the injury imparted to the soft tissues, and patient factors.
  - Improper soft tissue handling and surgical technique can result in additional injury to the tissues at the time of surgery.
- Risk factors for wound healing include:
  - Smoking
  - High body mass index
  - Single-layered closure
  - Peripheral vascular disease

o Diabetes mellitus

o Open fractures

- These patient factors have been shown to have an additive effect.
  - o With multiple risk factors, the rate of complications approaches 100%.
- Mild cellulitis can be treated with antibiotics.
  - o Wound drainage or severe cellulitis warrants a return to the operating room.
- Wound-healing problems tend to occur at the apex of the extensile lateral approach.
  - o Chronic osteomyelitis may require hardware removal.
  - o Soft tissue defects are best treated with a free flap.
    - The rare case of unresolved osteomyelitis with soft tissue loss may be best treated by amputation.
- Malunion of the calcaneus may be the result of operative or nonoperative treatment.
  - o The most common deformities are heel widening, varus of the hindfoot, and loss of heel height with subsequent Achilles tendon contracture.
  - o Every effort should be made during surgery to restore the normal anatomy of the hindfoot to avoid these complications.
  - o Malunion resulting in a wide heel and subfibular impingement may also result in pain and irritation of the peroneal tendons and sural nerve.
- Subtalar arthritis may result despite anatomical reduction of the calcaneus.
  - o The development of posttraumatic arthritis is dependent on a number of factors, including initial injury and quality of reduction.
  - o Risk factors for subsequent subtalar fusion include:
    - Low Böhler angle (< 0°)
    - Comminution
    - Workers' compensation status
    - Nonoperative treatment

LATE RECONSTRUCTION

- Pain following a calcaneal fracture can arise from:
  - o Plantar fat pad atrophy
  - o Subtalar or calcaneocuboid arthritis
  - o Prominent hardware
  - o Peroneal tendon problems
  - o There also may be nerve damage from original injury or, rarely, sural neuromas from surgical approach.
- If the previous treatment restored the overall shape and height of the calcaneus, posttraumatic arthritis can be treated with in situ arthrodesis.
- But if the calcaneus is shortened, subsequent surgery is more complex.
  - o Loss of calcaneal height will allow the talus to drop down and become less plantar flexed.
  - o It is very common to see anterior tibiotalar impingement from the loss of talar plantar flexion.
- In these cases of calcaneal malunion, reconstruction is performed with subtalar distraction arthrodesis.
  - o A structural block of bone is inserted into the posterior facet to "jack up" the talus and restore more normal anatomy.

o Because this increases the height of the heel acutely, it is common to see wound-healing problems following surgery.

- Even with successful subtalar fusion, varying degrees of discomfort and disability will remain.
  - o Calcaneus fractures often include injury to the plantar fat pad, the calcaneocuboid joint, and other surrounding soft tissues.
- Treating orthopedists have been guilty of focusing too much attention on the posterior facet.
  - o Attention to all aspects of the injury, both osseous and soft tissue, will yield the best results.

SELECTED REFERENCES

1. Carr JB: Surgical treatment of intra-articular calcaneal fractures: a review of small incision approaches. J Orthop Trauma. 19(2):109-17, 2005
2. Emara KM et al: Management of calcaneal fracture using the Ilizarov technique. Clin Orthop Relat Res. 439:215-20, 2005
3. Aldridge JM 3rd et al: Open calcaneal fractures: results of operative treatment. J Orthop Trauma. 18(1):7-11, 2004
4. Benirschke SK et al: Wound healing complications in closed and open calcaneal fractures. J Orthop Trauma. 18(1):1-6, 2004
5. Zwipp H et al: Integral classification of injuries (ICI) to the bones, joints, and ligaments--application to injuries of the foot. Injury. 35 Suppl 2:SB3-9, 2004
6. Csizy M et al: Displaced intra-articular calcaneal fractures: variables predicting late subtalar fusion. J Orthop Trauma. 17(2):106-12, 2003
7. Barei DP et al: Fractures of the calcaneus. Orthop Clin North Am. 33(1):263-85, x, 2002
8. Buckley R et al: Operative compared with nonoperative treatment of displaced intra-articular calcaneal fractures: a prospective, randomized, controlled multicenter trial. J Bone Joint Surg Am. 84-A(10):1733-44, 2002
9. Abidi NA et al: Wound-healing risk factors after open reduction and internal fixation of calcaneal fractures. Foot Ankle Int. 19(12):856-61, 1998
10. Miric A et al: Pathoanatomy of intra-articular fractures of the calcaneus. J Bone Joint Surg Am. 80(2):207-12, 1998
11. Tornetta P 3rd: The Essex-Lopresti reduction for calcaneal fractures revisited. J Orthop Trauma. 12(7):469-73, 1998
12. Sanders R et al: Operative treatment in 120 displaced intraarticular calcaneal fractures. Results using a prognostic computed tomography scan classification. Clin Orthop Relat Res. 87-95, 1993
13. ESSEX-LOPRESTI P: The mechanism, reduction technique, and results in fractures of the os calcis. Br J Surg. 39(157):395-419, 1952

Compartment Syndrome of Foot

Compartment syndrome of foot should be suspected in all patients with calcaneus fractures

Most sensitive sign of compartment syndrome in foot is severe pain with passive motion of toes; altered neurologic examination (diminished sensation) is also early sign of compartment syndrome

Surgeon should not be deterred by presence of pulses; if compartment syndrome is suspected, compartment pressures of foot should be measured using catheterization or portable pressure monitor

Indications for Fasciotomies

Absolute compartment pressure > 30 mm Hg

Difference of < 40 mm Hg between compartment pressure and patient's diastolic blood pressure

Measuring Compartment Pressures in Foot

There are at least 9 compartments in foot, and compartment pressures are measured in 4 different locations

Needle of pressure monitor is first inserted 4 cm inferior to medial malleolus, which allows for measurement of medial compartment in hindfoot; needle is then advanced through medial intermuscular septum into deep calcaneal compartment, and pressure is measured

Next, needle is inserted near medial arch of foot in order to measure superficial compartment

Needle is then inserted just inferior to base of 5th metatarsal to measure lateral compartment pressure

Finally, needle is inserted in between 1st and 2nd metatarsals distally on dorsum of foot in order to measure interosseous compartment; needle is then advanced deeper to measure adductor compartment in forefoot

Additional interosseous compartment measurements can be made by inserting needle between other metatarsals

Surgical Procedure: Fasciotomies of Foot

If compartment releases are indicated, 3 incisions should be utilized

2 incisions are made over dorsum of foot, centered over 2nd and 4rth rays; skin is divided, and interosseous compartments are released on both sides of metatarsal through each incision

Additional medial incision is also made; through this medial incision, fascia overlying abductor hallucis muscle is released; muscle is then retracted superiorly, and dense fascia of medial intermuscular septum is divided in order to release deep calcaneal compartment; care is taken in release of this layer, as lateral and medial plantar nerves lie just below intermuscular septum

Operative vs. Nonoperative Treatment of Calcaneus Fractures

Factors Associated With Improved Outcome in Operated Patients

Female gender

Nonworkers' compensation status

Factors Associated With Improved Outcome in Nonworkers' Compensation Group

Younger age (age < 29 years)

Low injury Bohler angle (0-14°)

Light workload occupation

Comminuted fracture

Anatomical reduction (< 2-mm step-off)

Buckley et al. (2002).

(Left) *The primary fracture line usually begins at the crucial angle of Gissane ➡. The angle is subtended by a line drawn along the anterior process and the posterior facet ➡.* **(Right)** *Compartment pressures in the foot are measured in 4 different locations.*

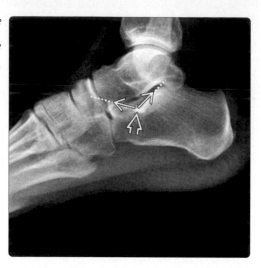

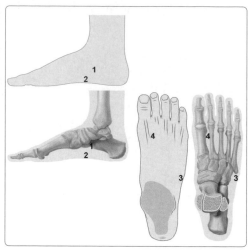

(Left) *Three incision approaches to compartment release of the foot are shown.* **(Right)** *Displaced tuberosity fracture tenting the skin over the posterior heel is shown. Urgent percutaneous reduction and fixation was performed to prevent skin necrosis.*

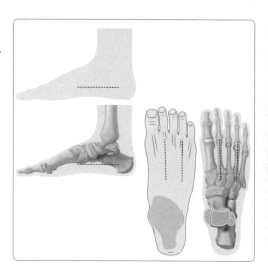

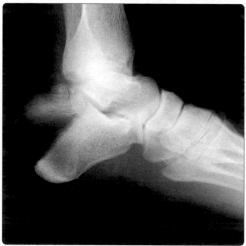

(Left) *The percutaneous reduction and fixation described by Essex-Lopresti is shown. Initially, a Steinmann pin is inserted into the tongue fragment. The fragment is then reduced using the Steinmann pin.* **(Right)** *Provisional K-wire fixation holds the fragment reduced.*

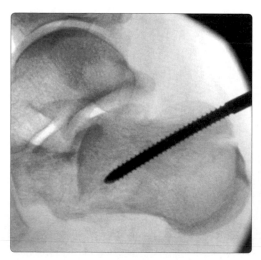

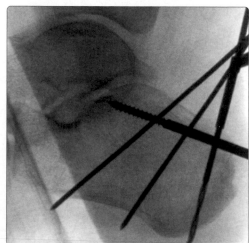

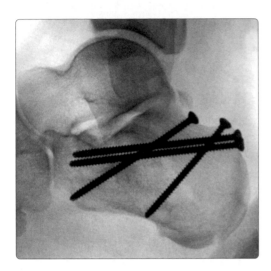

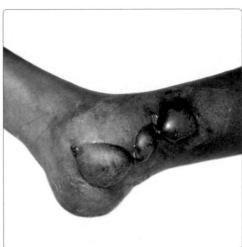

(Left) *Essex-Lopresti technique is shown. Definitive fixation is carried out with percutaneous screws.* (Right) *Fracture blisters around a calcaneus fracture following a motorcycle accident is shown.*

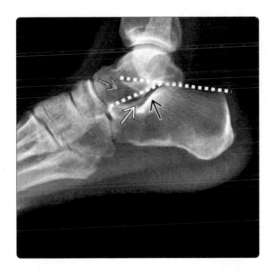

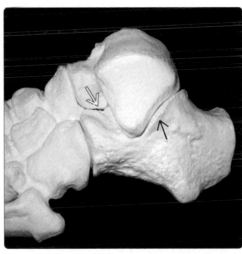

(Left) *Lateral view allows for the assessment of the posterior ⊟ and middle facet ➡ positions as well as an assessment of calcaneal height (Böhler angle ⊟). The Böhler angle is formed by drawing 2 lines. The 1st is drawn from the highest point on the anterior process to the highest point on the posterior facet. The 2nd line is tangential to the superior edge of the tuberosity. The normal value of the Böhler angle is 20-40°.* (Right) *Middle ➡ and posterior facets ⊟ visualized on a model are shown.*

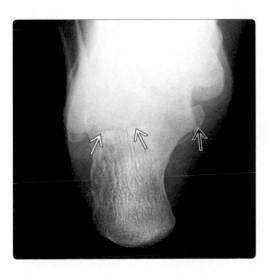

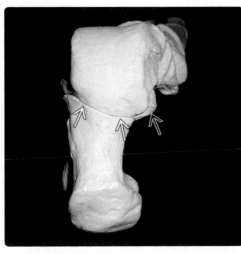

(Left) *Axial view of a normal heel demonstrating the subtalar joint ➡ and the sustentaculum ⊟ is shown. This view is useful for determining displacement of the tuberosity, varus angulation, fibular abutment, and displacement of the lateral wall.* (Right) *Subtalar joint ➡ and sustentaculum ⊟ visualized on a foot model is shown.*

(Left) *Lateral view of a calcaneus fracture shows a flattened Böhler angle ⇨ and a displaced posterior facet ⇨.* **(Right)** *Axial view of a calcaneus fracture shows lateral wall blowout ⇨ with subfibular impingement ⇨ and varus heel alignment ⇨.*

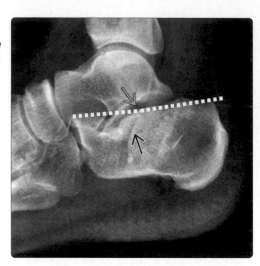

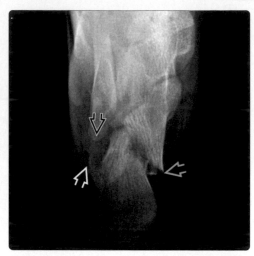

(Left) *CT scan of the calcaneus is useful for preoperative planning. Axial CT scan provides information on the extent of lateral wall blowout ⇨, the calcaneocuboid joint ⇨, and the sustentaculum.* **(Right)** *Coronal CT scan allows for the assessment of heel width, subfibular impingement, and the subtalar joint. The coronal CT scan is also the basis for the Sanders classification. Types 2 and 3 fractures are subclassified based on the location of the fracture lines (A-C).*

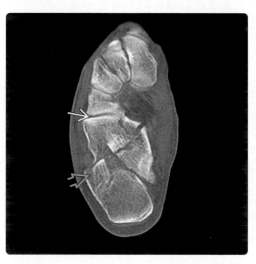

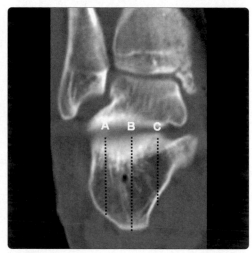

(Left) *Sagittal CT provides information about the anterior process ⇨ and the subtalar joint ⇨ and is useful in distinguishing joint depression from tongue-type fractures.* **(Right)** *The Sanders classification is based on the fracture pattern through the posterior facet on the coronal CT. Type 1 fractures are nondisplaced. Type 2 fractures have 2 parts. Type 3 fractures have 3 parts. Type 4 fractures are highly comminuted. The prognosis for calcaneus fractures worsens as the comminution of the posterior facet worsens.*

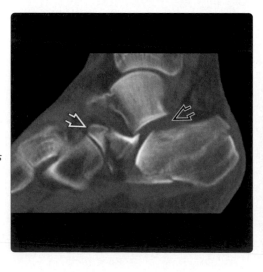

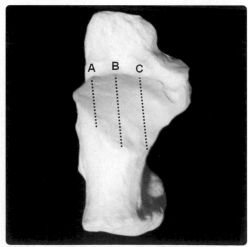

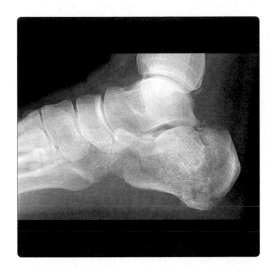

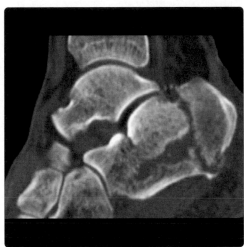

(Left) *In 1952, Essex-Lopresti described 2 distinct fracture patterns. In the tongue-type fracture, the tuberosity is continuous with the articular surface.* (Right) *A tongue-type fracture is shown. Essex-Lopresti based his classification on plain radiographs. However, the classification is aided by sagittal CT images.*

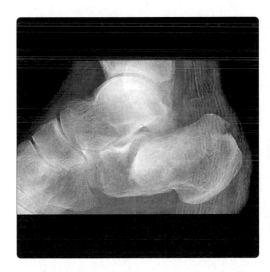

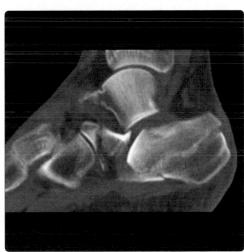

(Left) *A joint depression-type fracture is shown. In the joint depression fracture, the tuberosity fragment is separated from the articular fragment by an additional fracture line.* (Right) *A joint depression-type fracture is shown. This classification system is useful in determining treatment but does not provide prognostic information.*

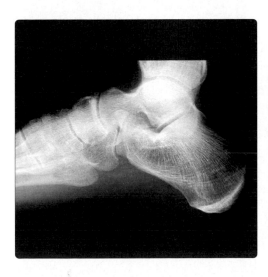

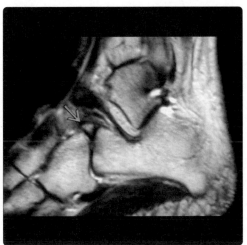

(Left) *Lateral foot x-ray of a patient with an anterior process fracture of the calcaneus is shown. The patient's fracture was not diagnosed at the time of injury, and he went on to develop a painful nonunion of the fracture.* (Right) *Selected MR scan of the missed anterior process fracture ⇒ is shown. The patient was treated with simple excision of the fragment.*

KEY FACTS

- The talus is the 2nd most commonly fractured tarsal bone (after the calcaneus).
- The blood supply of the talus can be tenuous, as there are limited spaces at which vessels can enter the bone, given its morphology and participation in multiple joints.
  - The blood supply of the talar body is retrograde through the talar neck.
- Although there is great concern for osteonecrosis after talar neck and body fracture, posttraumatic arthritis is a more common outcome.
  - Posttraumatic arthritis is likely related to the initial severity of the injury but also the quality of the ultimate reduction, and every effort should be made for as anatomica reduction as possible.
- For the rare posteromedial talar body fracture, it is important to understand that medial malleolar osteotomy is not helpful and does not improve visualization, as the fracture line is typically posterior to the medial malleolus.

- Lateral process talus fractures are increasingly common and should be considered in the setting of an acute ankle sprain.
- While nonunion is rare after talar neck fracture, malunion, especially varus malunion, is not. Compression of a comminuted medial talar neck should be avoided in an effort to minimize the risk of this complication.

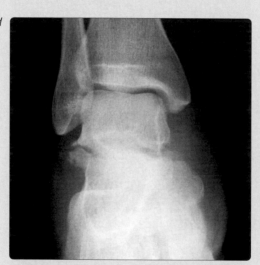

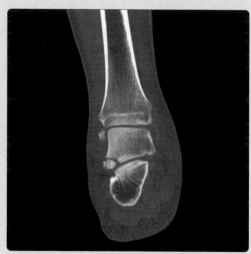

(Left) *A male patient in his mid 20s was skateboarding when he sustained an injury to his right ankle. Once he was able to get radiographs, a large lateral process talus fracture was seen.* **(Right)** *CT scan of the same patient shows a large displaced fragment. In this young patient, the concern for posttraumatic arthrosis is high, and the decision was made to perform open reduction internal fixation.*

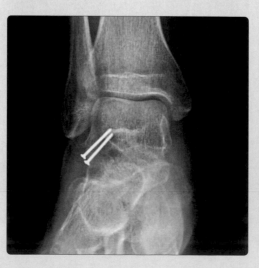

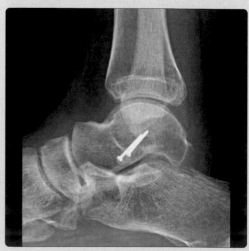

(Left) *The bony fragment was reduced though an Ollier-type lateral incision. Two 2.0-mm noncannulated screws were used with lag by technique, provided excellent compression for this anatomic reduction.* **(Right)** *Lateral view shows the relative anterior to posterior position of the screws. Given the nature of the injury, bicortical fixation is not possible, and some surgeons will consider headless screws if more traditional screws do not provide adequate fixation. These headed screws compressed the fracture well.*

Talus Fractures

BACKGROUND

- Talus fractures fall into a difficult middle ground of injuries that are infrequent enough that they are difficult to study but frequent enough and often severe enough that they cause significant functional morbidity for a number of people that is not insignificant.
  - Injuries are typically high energy, such as a fall from a height or a motor vehicle accident. As with any high-energy injury, initial evaluation consists of a thorough clinical examination with a search for other injuries.
  - As the talus is mostly covered with articular surface, any significant fracture displacement requires a joint subluxation or dislocation. In other words, most displaced talar fractures are also dislocations.
  - All dislocations should be reduced emergently to prevent further soft tissue injury. Historically, these injuries, especially talar neck fractures, were treated emergently, as this was thought to decrease the risk for osteonecrosis (ON), although more recent data suggests that this is likely untrue.
  - Radiographic examination consists of anteroposterior, lateral, and mortise images of the ankle and anteroposterior, lateral, and oblique views of the foot. Canale views are beneficial and can increase the ability to visualize the talar neck.
  - Computed tomography (CT) scanning of talus fractures is crucial; it aids in understanding the extent of injury as well as being critical for surgical planning. Imaging studies should be carefully reviewed for the presence of other fractures of the foot or ankle.

ANATOMY

Introduction

- "Talus" comes from taxillus, Latin, which means dice. The Romans used the heel bone of the horse to make dice. The Greeks used the 2nd cervical vertebrae of sheep to make dice, and astragalus is vertebra in Greek.
- 2/3 of the talus is covered by articular cartilage. There are no tendon or muscular attachments to the talus, but many muscles cross the talus, all of which also influence the subtalar and other hindfoot joints.
- It is a weight-bearing bone that transfers all the weight from the foot to the tibia and fibula. For descriptive purposes, it is divided into the body, neck, and head.

Talar Body

- The body includes the talar dome and posterior facet, which make up the ankle and subtalar joints, respectively. The superior portion of the body is articular. It is shaped like a pulley in the coronal plane with the trochlear portion lying offset more medially. In the axial plane, the superior surface is shaped like a trapezoid with the anterior portion wider than the posterior.
- The lateral talus becomes somewhat triangular and articulates with the fibula. The perimeter of the lateral articular portion is called the lateral process. It serves as the site of attachment for the lateral talocalcaneal ligament as well as the anterior and posterior talofibular ligaments. The undersurface of the lateral process makes up the lateral portion of the posterior facet of the subtalar joint, so that most lateral process fractures are intraarticular.

- The medial portion of the talus has a large articular surface for the medial malleolus. In the anterior nonarticular area, there are vascular foramina. The posterior body serves as insertion for the deep deltoid ligament.
- The posterior process of the talus is made up of posteromedial and posterolateral tubercles, between which lies a groove for the flexor hallucis longus tendon.

Talar Head

- The head primarily articulates with the navicular anteriorly. Inferiorly in the head are the anterior and middle subtalar facets, which are sometimes fused into a single facet. These joint surfaces make a socket in which the talar head rotates (or, more accurately, the socket rotates around the talar head). There are attachments for the spring ligament, deltoid ligament, and sustentaculum tali.

Talar Neck

- The neck lies between the body and head and has multiple ligamentous attachments. It is oriented 15-20° medial to the talar body and lies directly over the sinus tarsi and tarsal canal. This region has numerous capsular attachments and vascular foramina.

VASCULAR ANATOMY

- The vascular supply of the talus has been of special interest due to association of ON with talus injuries.
  - Since 2/3 of the talus is covered by articular cartilage, and there are no muscular attachments, the blood supply is limited. There are contributions from the capsular and ligamentous attachments to the tibia, calcaneus, and navicular.

Extraosseous Arterial Supply

- Branches of the posterior tibial, dorsalis pedis, and peroneal arteries contribute to the talus; however, there are multiple variants on the branches. There is a delicate network of anastomoses between the arteries, which envelops all the nonarticular areas of the talus.
- The posterior tibial artery gives off the artery to the tarsal canal and a vascular plexus for the posterior process. The deltoid branch of the artery to the tarsal canal supplies the medial talar body.
- The dorsalis pedis leads to the anterior lateral malleolar artery and branches over the superior surface of the neck to supply the head. The anterior lateral malleolar artery anastomoses with the peroneal artery supply to form the artery of the tarsal sinus.
- The peroneal artery sends branches to the posterior process to anastomose with the posterior tibial vessels. In addition, it contributes to the artery of the tarsal sinus via the perforating peroneal artery.
- The arteries of the tarsal canal and sinus anastomose, forming the artery of the tarsal sling. This supplies the inferior neck and lateral body. The arteries of the tarsal canal and sinus, along with the medial periosteal vessels, are the most essential supply to the talus.

Intraosseous Blood Supply

- The head receives its blood supply from the dorsalis pedis superiorly and artery of the tarsal sling inferiorly.
- The talar body blood supply enters the bone in 5 places.

- These vessels enter in those areas without articular cartilage:
  - Anastomosis between posterior tibial and peroneal branches at posterior process
  - Superior surface of talar neck
  - Inferior surface of talar neck
  - Anterolateral surface of talar body
  - Medial surface of talar body (from deltoid ligament)
- The artery of the tarsal canal supplies the lateral 2/3 of the talar body, while the deltoid branch supplies the medial 1/3. There are also multiple intraosseous vascular anastomoses between the supplying arteries.

TALAR BODY FRACTURES

Background

- These are typically, but not necessarily, high-energy injuries. Inokuchi et al defined the difference between talar neck and body fractures based on the inferior articular surface of the talus. If the major fracture line exits at or posterior to the lateral process, it is considered a body fracture. Thus, talar body fractures are intraarticular ankle and subtalar joint injuries. Fractures that exit anterior to the lateral process are neck fractures.

Evaluation

- As these are often high-energy injuries, a full secondary survey should be performed. Radiographs typically do not demonstrate the full extent of articular injury and comminution; therefore, CT imaging is required. The full degree of articular and cartilage injury often cannot be fully appreciated until the time of surgery.

Treatment

- Nonoperative treatment is reserved for those fractures that are completely nondisplaced. Even then, many surgeons will still opt for internal fixation to allow for early range of motion exercises.
- Emergent surgical treatment is necessary in all open injuries and in all dislocations that cannot be reduced, with irrigation and debridement of open wounds, and reduction of dislocations. Definitive reduction and fixation can wait.
- For the definitive surgery, anatomic reduction with stable fixation is the goal. Fragment specific fixation is often used.
- Surgical approach is dictated by the area of injury.
  - A medial approach through the interval between the tibialis anterior and the tibialis posterior is often required. This approach can be extended proximally to incorporate a medial malleolar osteotomy for greater visualization of the medial talar dome. The medial malleolus is predrilled for lag screws prior to the osteotomy.
  - An anterolateral Ollier-type approach can be used for lateral visualization.
- After provisional fixation, the reduction should be critically assessed. Once anatomic reduction is confirmed, final fixation is placed. It is occasionally necessary to countersink screw heads into the articular cartilage. The type of fixation used is much less important than the quality of reduction. Bone grafting is occasionally required to support articular segments that have been disimpacted.

- Postoperatively, the patient is splinted for 2 weeks, then a CAM boot is applied. With stable fixation, range of motion is begun at 2 weeks after surgery. All patients should remain non-weight bearing for 6-8 weeks depending on the injury.

Outcomes

- Outcomes are often dictated by the severity of the initial injury, quality of joint reduction, and degree of articular injury.
- Posttraumatic arthrosis, malunion, and ON are more common in severe crush injuries and are associated with the severity of the initial injury.
- Sneppen et al reviewed 21 patients with talar body fractures. Eighteen of these fractures were treated nonoperatively, and 3 underwent open reduction and internal fixation (ORIF). In this series, 60% of the patients had malunion. The subtalar and ankle joints were found to have very high rates of posttraumatic arthritis. 95% of patients had moderate to severe complaints.
- Vallier et al reviewed clinical, radiographic, and functional outcomes after operative treatment of talar body fractures. ON was observed in 10 of 26 patients, 5 advanced to collapse, while the other 5 showed signs of revascularization. Higher rates of ON were observed in open fractures and those with associated talar neck fractures. Posttraumatic arthritis was reported in 65% of tibiotalar joints and 35% of subtalar joints. Twenty of 30 patients returned to prior level of employment. Eight patients did not return to work. Worse outcomes were found with fractures with open injuries and associated talar neck fractures.
- Lindvall et al found no difference in union rates, ON, posttraumatic arthritis, or American Orthopaedic Foot and Ankle Society outcome scores between fractures of the talar neck and body. Posttraumatic arthritis was a more common finding than ON.

POSTEROMEDIAL TALAR BODY FRACTURES

- Fractures of the posteromedial aspect of the talus represent a rare variant of talar body fractures. The radiographic findings are subtle and can be missed without a thorough review of the radiographs. In several case series, > 50% were missed initially.
- Results of nonoperative treatment for this injury are poor with arthrodesis rates as high as 83%. Like all talar body fractures, they involve both the tibiotalar and the subtalar joints. CT evaluation greatly improves understanding of the extent of injury.
- Due to unacceptably high rates of posttraumatic arthritis with conservative treatment, displaced fractures should be treated with ORIF or excision of the fragment if it is small.
- The fracture cannot be adequately visualized with a medial malleolar osteotomy, as the majority of the injury is further posterior than can be visualized with this surgical approach.

- One option is to position the patient prone and approach the posteromedial aspect of the talus through the interval between the Achilles tendon and the flexor hallucis longus. The authors prefer an approach with the patient supine, utilizing the interval between the posterior tibialis and flexor digitorum longus. Visualization of the relationship of the tendons to the fracture, especially on the axial images, can be greatly beneficial in terms of preoperative planning.
- There is a limited area of extraarticular surface on the posterior talus, and fixation can be problematic. Headless screws can be helpful.
- Postoperative care consists of non-weight bearing for 6 weeks with initiation of ankle and subtalar range of motion exercises at 2 weeks. There is a lack of long-term data on these rare injuries.

TALAR NECK FRACTURES

Background

- Fractures of the neck of the talus account for 50% of all talus fractures.
- While neck fractures are not intraarticular, they disrupt the normal relationships between the articular facets of the subtalar joint. The fracture line often divides the posterior facet from the anterior and middle facets. For this reason, it is essentially an intraarticular injury, and anatomic reconstruction is critical. An in vitro study showed that displacement of the talar neck by 2 mm greatly increases contact pressures in the posterior facet.
- Injury begins with forced dorsiflexion, which causes impaction of the neck on the anterior distal tibial crest. As the forces progress, the posterior capsular structures, deltoid tear, and talar body can dislocate posteriorly.
- Most talar neck fractures occur as a result of a motor vehicle accident or a fall. Historically, talar neck fractures were seen with early airplane crashes, thus the name "aviator's astragalus."

Evaluation

- Patients typically present with swelling and gross deformity. Skin and soft tissues should be carefully assessed, as major displacement can compromise tissue perfusion and lead to necrosis.
- All obvious dislocations should be reduced emergently. Radiographic evaluation should include anteroposterior, lateral, and oblique images of the foot and 3 views of the ankle. Canale views can increase the ability to visualize the talar neck.
- CT evaluation is required in all talus fractures so that a full understanding of fracture morphology can allow for optimal treatment.

Classification

- The most widely used classification is the Hawkins classification. Higher rates of ON are seen as the Hawkins group number increases, providing prognostic value.

- Type 1 fractures are nondisplaced. These are uncommon injuries. If any displacement is present, even 1 mm, it is defined as displaced. If after CT review the fracture is truly nondisplaced, and there is no fracture debris present in the subtalar joint, then the injury can be treated with non-weight bearing for 8 weeks. Fractures treated conservatively need to be monitored closely for any late displacement, which would require operative reduction and fixation.
- Type 2 fractures of the talar neck demonstrate some subluxation or dislocation of the subtalar joint. The neck of the talus is typically malaligned in varus and has rotational deformity.
- Type 3 fractures have dislocation of the talar body at both the ankle and the subtalar joints. This usually requires disruption of most or all soft tissue from the talar body. Closed reduction of the dislocation (to get the talar body back under the tibia) should be attempted. Failure with closed reduction requires emergent open reduction. It is helpful to use a distractor between the tibia and calcaneus to create room for the talar body. In many cases, the body dislocates posteromedially and can compress the neurovascular bundle. Associated medial malleolus fracture is not uncommon and can be used to facilitate reduction. The talar head is still well aligned with the navicular in group 3 fractures. This implies that some soft tissue remains attached to the talar neck, so that at least 1 fragment will have a viable blood supply.
- Type 4 fractures have all the characteristics of group 3 with dislocation of the talar head at the talonavicular joint. There may not be any soft tissue attachments left on any fragment of the talus. The series reported by Canale and Kelly, who 1st reported this injury, found that only 3 of 71 fractures were group 4, and all had unsatisfactory results.

Treatment

- Operative approach should be by 2 incisions in most fractures. Medial and lateral approaches as previously mentioned are often most appropriate to facilitate anatomic reduction. Medial malleolar osteotomy may be necessary. Stripping of any remaining soft tissue should be avoided to preserve the remaining blood supply to the talus.
- Fractures are typically more comminuted medially, as the neck commonly displaces into varus. Comminution is evaluated through the medial incision. Fixation can be inserted from distal to proximal. Screws can be countersunk into the head of the talus.
- For a simple neck fracture, 2 lag screws are adequate, although care should be taken not to compress the comminuted medial talar neck, which can lead to a varus malunion and possible "acquired clubfoot." Lag screws may be inserted from the posterior process back into the neck, but the area for screw insertion is more limited. In an in vitro study, posterior to anterior screw placement had better mechanical strength when compared with standard anterior to posterior screws.

- Minifragment plating has also been used successfully in treating talar neck fractures, particularly in injuries with higher levels of comminution. There is a lateral nonarticular shelf where the neck meets the body that can be used for plating if necessary. In general, it is best not to be dogmatic about fixation schema, as flexibility is often required for each individual injury to figure out what makes the most sense. Postoperative treatment is not different than for other talus fractures.

Outcomes of Talar Neck Fractures

- Traditionally, talar neck fractures have been associated with high complication rates. There are many contributing factors, including the odd shape of the bony anatomy, relatively poor vascularity, high energy of the injury, comminution, and associated fractures and soft tissue injuries. Most surgeons rarely treat these injuries, so inexperience can also contribute to poor outcomes.
- Higher rates of ON are seen with increasing displacement. Hawkins found no ON in group 1 patients, but it was present in 42% of group 2 and 91% of group 3 patients. Subsequent studies have generally shown lower rates of ON but with the same trend.
- Historically, surgical delay was believed to lead to higher rates of ON. However, recent literature has shown no difference in complication rates with delayed treatment. The key is to reduce dislocations emergently but wait until soft tissues are appropriate for definitive reduction.
- Vallier et al reviewed 102 fractures in 100 patients. Each fracture was treated with ORIF. Functional outcomes were not great but were especially poor in high-energy injuries. Fracture comminution was associated with a poorer result. Of the 45 patients who completed outcome questionnaires, 32 returned to work, 6 with job modifications. Timing of ORIF had no bearing on the risk ON, which was associated with open fractures and increased comminution, suggesting that ON was more related to the force imparted at the time of injury than to timing of ORIF.
- In a subsequent study, the risk of ON was related to the amount of initial fracture displacement. ON did not occur in those fractures in which there was no dislocation.
- Posttraumatic arthritis appears to be a much greater concern after talar neck fracture than ON, as it is more common and more likely to be symptomatic. A recent metaanalysis noted that the rate of posttraumatic arthritis approached 80% with longer term follow-up.

LATERAL PROCESS FRACTURE

Background

- Fracture of the lateral process occurs in < 1% of all ankle injuries. These injuries are thought to occur from a combination of dorsiflexion and eversion, as happens in snowboarders. It is possible for them to occur with other ankle motions, though, including dorsiflexion and inversion.
- These injuries can often be mistaken for ankle sprains, given the similarity in terms of where the patient is tender and possibly similar mechanisms. Careful palpation can help to differentiate the 2, although any unclear diagnosis should be made explicitly clear with CT scan.

Evaluation

- On examination, the patient will have swelling and tenderness to palpation over the lateral side of the foot just distal to the tip of the fibula. The anterior talofibular ligament inserts on to the lateral process; therefore, these patients may present with symptoms of instability.
- Late presentation often consists of lateral-sided ankle pain made worse with uneven walking surfaces and prolonged standing. Decreased subtalar range of motion can be seen clinically in fractures presenting late for treatment.
- Fractures often are not readily apparent on plain radiographs. In cases with a high index of suspicion for this injury and negative plain radiographs, a CT scan should also be obtained. CT improves fracture understanding and can allow for identification of any fracture debris in the subtalar joint.
- Hawkins classified these injuries into 3 groups.
  - Type 1 is an extraarticular avulsion fracture.
  - Type 2 is a large fragment with a single fracture line that traverses both the superior (ankle) and inferior (subtalar) articular surfaces.
  - A type 3 fracture is comminuted and involves both articulations.

Treatment

- Acute fractures that are nondisplaced or small in size can be treated with a boot non-weight bearing for 6 weeks. Some surgeons will consider ORIF of larger nondisplaced fragments so as to allow for early ankle and hindfoot range of motion.
- Displaced fractures, fractures of larger size, and fractures with debris present in the subtalar joint require operative treatment to restore congruity to the talofibular and subtalar articular surfaces.
- Subtalar joint debridement should be performed in all cases with intraarticular debris identified on CT scans. It is imperative to restore congruity to the posterior subtalar facet. If the fracture is comminuted and not amenable to internal fixation, then the fragment should be excised to minimize the risk of subtalar arthrosis.
- Small fragments that present late can be treated by simple excision if symptomatic. Excision of up to a 1-cm³ fragment has not been shown to lead to ankle or subtalar instability on radiographic stress examination. Larger fragments should be treated by ORIF after all fibrous and calcified material is removed from the fracture plane.
- Lateral process fractures identified and treated early have better results than those with delay in diagnosis. The principle concern with these injuries is the potential development of arthrosis in both the hindfoot and the ankle. There are few longer term studies of these injuries, which show a wide range of subsequent arthrosis (15-45%).

OSTEONECROSIS

- ON is a unique complication of talus fractures. Talar neck or body fractures, or dislocations without fracture, can all lead to this potentially devastating complication.
- As above, it is directly related to the displacement at the time of injury and disruption of the tenuous vascular supply to the talar body.

- It is not always easy to recognize, and the timing of its presence is not always consistent, although, if present, some evidence will be seen by 2-3 months after injury.
- Radiographs should be obtained 6-8 weeks after injury or surgery to assess for the presence or absence of a **Hawkins sign**, a relative osteopenia of the subchondral portion of talar dome indicating that the vascularity is retained (the body is developing disuse osteopenia), and development of ON is unlikely. A negative Hawkins sign does not confirm that ON will occur; serial radiographic assessment should be performed.
- Hawkins' classic paper reported risk of ON by fracture type. More recent data links risk to increased initial fracture displacement, comminution, and open fractures, all indicators of the amount of energy involved in the original injury.
- ON can lead to collapse of the talar dome with painful ankle and subtalar arthritis. However, many patients with ON never develop clinical symptoms, and the talus revascularizes on its own. Both Hawkins and Canale found that even prolonged non-weight bearing does not prevent collapse. Additionally, it may take up to 36 months for revascularization to occur, and non-weight bearing for this duration is impractical, if not downright impossible.
- Vallier et al found that 37% of their patients with ON after a talar neck fracture demonstrated revascularization without limitations in weight bearing or bracing. Fracture healing should be assessed to determine weight-bearing status. If union has been achieved, weight bearing should be advanced even if concern exists for ON. Continued non-weight bearing is recommended if union has not been achieved.
- Core decompression and bone grafting have been performed for ON of the talus, mainly in atraumatic ON, although there are currently no long-term data. The results of these procedures in the traumatic population are largely unknown.
- Once the talar dome collapses, or for those with persistent pain after decompression, combined ankle and subtalar arthrodesis can be performed. Nonunion rates are higher than normal, as the talus is at least partially, if not completely, nonviable. A host of techniques have been described in an effort to increase union rates, perhaps most notably a Blair fusion (fusion of the viable talar neck to the anterior tibia). For the rare young and active patient, transtibial amputation may be considered.

NONUNION AND MALUNION

- Nonunion is a rare complication of talus fractures. Reported rates vary from 0-12%. Nonunion is more common in open fractures and fractures with extensive comminution. Traditional nonunion techniques are applicable, including bone graft, rigid fixation, and prolonged non-weight bearing.
- Malunion is probably more common than is reported. It is difficult to assess rotational and varus angulation on plain radiographs. Varus malunion of a talar neck fracture is most common. Malalignment in the talar neck by as little as 2 mm alters joint contact characteristics in the subtalar joint.

- Varus malalignment can be corrected by osteotomy of the talar neck and bone grafting, although this procedure is technically difficult. Arthrodesis is another salvage option, appropriate once posttraumatic arthritis develops. In cases with varus malunion, the medial column of the foot is shortened. At the time of arthrodesis, the medial column needs to be lengthened by bone grafting to obtain prior length, or the lateral column needs to be shortened.
- The determination of which joints to fuse is made by assessing the status of the tibiotalar, subtalar, and talonavicular joints. Whenever possible, joints are left mobile.
- Dorsal malalignment can cause anterior impingement of the ankle. If identified early, impingement can be treated by removing the prominence off the talar neck with an osteotome to create more room for the anterior tibial plafond.
- Ankle arthroplasty is an option in patients who have tibiotalar arthritis from anterior impingement and concomitant subtalar arthritis. However, arthroplasty should not be performed in cases of unresolved ON, as the likelihood of failure is significant. Tibiotalocalcaneal fusion may be the more appropriate option in this setting.

SELECTED REFERENCES

1. DeFontes KW 3rd et al: Tibiotalocalcaneal arthrodesis with bulk talar allograft for treatment of talar osteonecrosis. Foot Ankle Int. 39(4):506-514, 2018
2. Hernigou P et al: Stem cell therapy in early post traumatic talus osteonecrosis. Int Orthop. ePub, 2018
3. Annappa R et al: Functional and radiological outcomes of operative management of displaced talar neck fractures. Foot (Edinb). 25(3):127-30, 2015
4. Dodd A et al: Outcomes of talar neck fractures: a systematic review and meta-analysis. J Orthop Trauma. 29(5):210-5, 2015
5. Vallier HA et al: A new look at the Hawkins classification for talar neck fractures: which features of injury and treatment are predictive of osteonecrosis? J Bone Joint Surg Am. 96(3):192-7, 2014
6. Capelle JH et al: Fixation strength of anteriorly inserted headless screws for talar neck fractures. Foot Ankle Int. 34(7):1012-6, 2013
7. Attiah M et al: Comminuted talar neck fractures: a mechanical comparison of fixation techniques. J Orthop Trauma. 21(1):47-51, 2007
8. Langer P et al: In vitro evaluation of the effect lateral process talar excision on ankle and subtalar joint stability. Foot Ankle Int. 28(1):78-83, 2007
9. von Knoch F et al: Fracture of the lateral process of the talus in snowboarders. J Bone Joint Surg Br. 89(6):772-7, 2007
10. Charlson MD et al: Comparison of plate and screw fixation and screw fixation alone in a comminuted talar neck fracture model. Foot Ankle Int. 27(5):340-3, 2006
11. Valderrabano V et al: Snowboarder's talus fracture: treatment outcome of 20 cases after 3.5 years. Am J Sports Med. 33(6):871-80, 2005
12. Lindvall E et al: Open reduction and stable fixation of isolated, displaced talar neck and body fractures. J Bone Joint Surg Am. 86-A(10):2229-34, 2004
13. Vallier HA et al. Talar neck fractures: results and outcomes. J Bone Joint Surg Am. 2004;86:1616-24
14. Swanson TV et al: Fractures of the talar neck. A mechanical study of fixation. J Bone Joint Surg Am. 74(4):544-51, 1992

Hawkins Classification as Modified by Canale and Kelly

Type	Characteristics	Risk of Osteonecrosis (%)
I	Nondisplaced	0
II	Displaced with subtalar dislocation	42
III	Displaced with subtalar and ankle dislocation	91
IV	Displaced type 3 with talonavicular dislocation	100

Sneppen Classification of Talar Body Fractures

Type	Fracture
I	Transchondral dome fracture
II	Shear fracture
III	Posterior tubercle fracture
IV	Lateral process fracture
V	Crush fracture

Hawkins Classification of Lateral Process Talus Fractures

Type	Fracture	Percentage	Management
I	Simple	42	Open reduction and internal fixation (ORIF) if displaced &/or large
II	Comminuted	34	Can consider ORIF vs. removal of fragments
III	Chip	24	Treatment is typically conservative

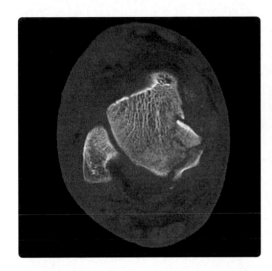

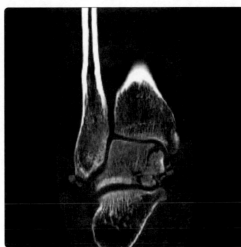

(**Left**) *A 39-year-old male patient fell down some stairs, injuring his right ankle. He presented 10 days out with an inability to bear weight and swelling of his ankle. Ankle and hindfoot motion was painful. A comminuted posteromedial talar body fracture is seen here.* (**Right**) *The fracture in another plane is shown. The significance of the fracture is much more readily apparent on this image with its extension, including much of the medial 1/2 of the talar body.*

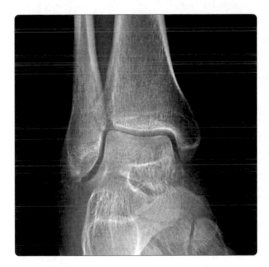

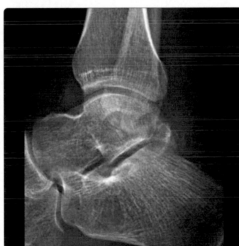

(**Left**) *Mortise radiograph of the same ankle is shown. Radiographs can often be underwhelming, especially given the severity of the injury on the CT scan. In the right traumatic setting, the medial ankle should be scrutinized on x-ray.* (**Right**) *This lateral radiograph is not very revealing either, although there is some abnormality more posteriorly. A high index of suspicion should lead a physician to getting a CT scan to better evaluate the injury.*

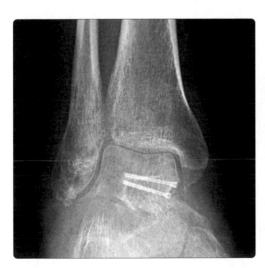

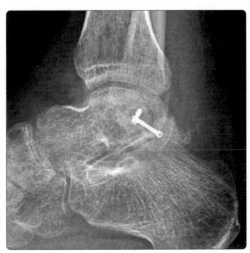

(**Left**) *A posteromedial approach was undertaken through the flexor digitorum longus subsheath. The major fracture fragments were reduced and fixed with buried headless screws. Some of the comminuted fragments were excised.* (**Right**) *Fixation was placed in 2 planes to optimize reduction and maximize compression. Headless screws are often helpful to maximize the footprint on the articular fragments while allowing excellent compression.*

(Left) *The talus is generally split into thirds in order to talk about the relative contributions to blood flow in each region. The relative contributions differ somewhat depending on the region of the talus.* **(Right)** *In the medial 1/3 of the talus, branches that run within and around the deltoid ligament supply much of the blood flow, accounting for the reason why the deltoid ligament should never be sectioned. If more proximal access is necessary, a medial malleolar osteotomy is performed.*

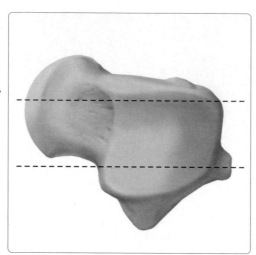
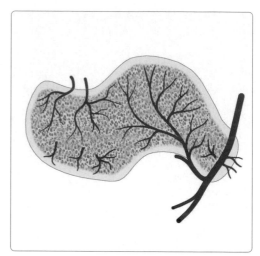

(Left) *In the middle 1/3 of the talus, blood flow from the artery to the tarsal canal predominates with some dorsal and posterior branches supplementing.* **(Right)** *In the lateral 1/3 of the talus, the artery of the sinus tarsi, a branch from the peroneal artery provides much of the blood flow. An anastomotic sling is formed between the sinus tarsi and the tarsal canal arteries.*

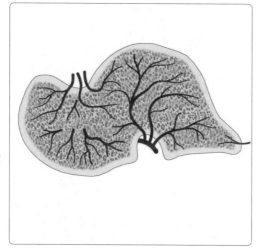
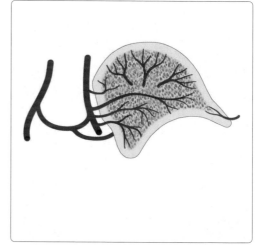

(Left) *Lateral radiograph shows a nondisplaced fracture (Hawkins type I) extending vertically through talar neck. Slight separation and offset of the fracture dorsally make this case easier to detect than many fractures of this type. (From DI: MSK Non-Trauma.)* **(Right)** *Lateral radiograph shows a Hawkins type III fracture. Body of talus is rotated 90° relative to tibia and calcaneus, indicating complete dislocation of both ankle and posterior subtalar joints. The talonavicular joint remains intact. (From DI: MSK Non-Trauma.)*

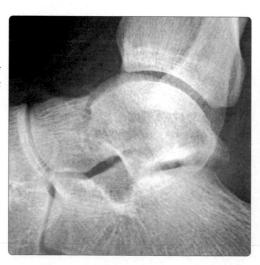
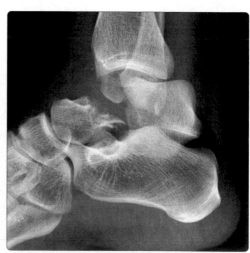

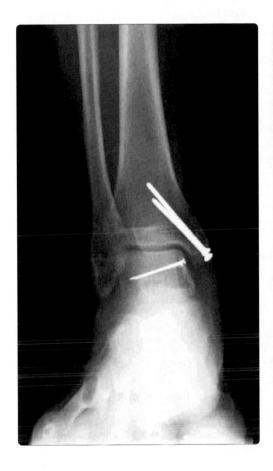

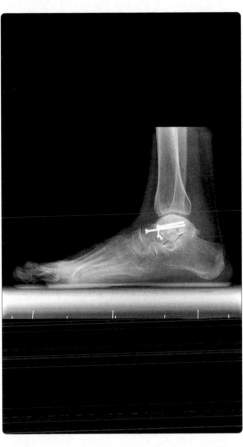

(Left) *A medial malleolar osteotomy may be necessary to fully access talar body fractures, as in this case. The osteotomy should be predrilled to ensure anatomic placement.* **(Right)** *Fragment specific fixation is often used in talar neck fractures. Retrograde lag screws along the neck can be used, although medial lag fixation should be avoided if there is comminution in the medial neck. The lateral shelf of the neck-body junction can be used for plate fixation.*

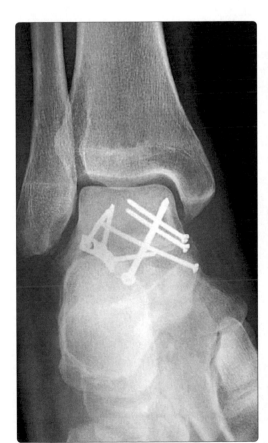

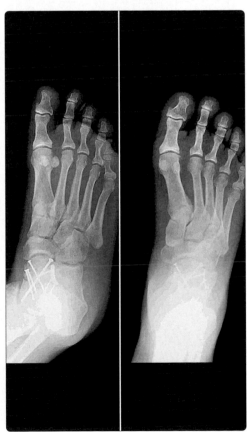

(Left) *Plate fixation at the lateral neck-body junction can be seen here, along with several fragment-specific lag screws of various sizes. As with many injuries, a flexible approach to what hardware to use is most appropriate, as 1 size does not often fit all.* **(Right)** *These foot films from the same patient show the combination of lag fixation with a combination of some degree of fixed angle construct in the plate. Mixing and matching what fits best and provides the most thorough fixation is an appropriate approach.*

KEY FACTS

NAVICULAR FRACTURES

- Three types of navicular fractures generally occur: Avulsion fractures, high-energy fractures with other associated injuries, and stress fractures.
- Avulsion fractures can generally be treated nonoperatively, except in those cases in which the fragment is large enough to warrant open reduction and internal fixation. These injuries are by far the least severe of the 3.
- High-energy injuries will require a plan that takes into account all associated injuries, understanding that many of the joints in the hindfoot and midfoot work in tandem, such that injury to one will directly affect the other. Some joints may need to be temporarily spanned in order to provide sufficient stability for the injury to heal. As a result, stiffness is often a concern after these injuries.
- Many stress fractures can be managed nonoperatively, although some will require surgery. Vigilance is required either way, as it can be difficult to get long-term nonunions to heal.

CUBOID FRACTURES

- There are rarer injuries still, and they will rarely occur in isolation.
- Injury will not infrequently lead to insufficiency of the lateral column of the foot, such that treatment will often require some distraction to regain that length.

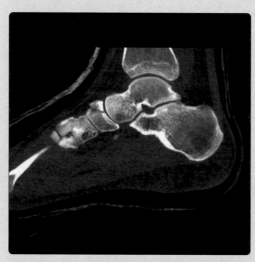
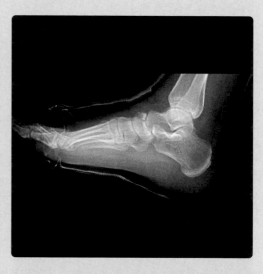

(Left) *A 23-year-old male patient with a large dorsal avulsion fracture fragment from the navicular is shown. He had simply tripped and sustained a trivial injury. This fragment is much larger than the typical avulsion fracture.* **(Right)** *Dorsal avulsion fracture off the navicular is shown. The radiograph shows the fragment to be somewhat large as well. A thorough discussion was had with the patient, and operative treatment was elected, given the large size of the fragment.*

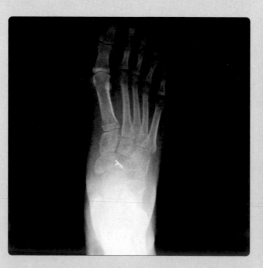
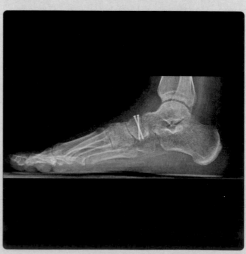

(Left) *Patient had open reduction and internal fixation of the large avulsion fracture. A dorsal approach was used; the fracture was anatomically reduced and fixed with 2 cannulated screws.* **(Right)** *Open reduction and internal fixation of the dorsal avulsion fracture is shown. The anatomic reduction can be seen more readily on this lateral image.*

ANATOMY AND FUNCTION OF MIDFOOT

- The midfoot includes 5 tarsal bones: Navicular, cuboid, and 3 cuneiforms (medial, middle, and lateral). It forms the transverse arch of the foot and is also part of the longitudinal arch.
- The navicular articulates in a mobile relationship with the talus proximally. The articulation distally is with 3 cuneiforms, where stability is more important than flexibility.
- The cuboid articulates in a mobile relationship with the anterior process of the calcaneus proximally. Articulation distally is with the 4th and 5th metatarsal bases. These joints are more mobile than the more medial midfoot joints, as they are analogous to the ring and little finger of the hand, helping provide some measure of "grip" of the ground.
- The cuneiforms articulate with the navicular proximally, 1st-3rd metatarsal bases distally, and cuboid laterally (with lateral or 3rd cuneiform). These articulations are rigid.
- The 2nd metatarsal meets the middle cuneiform in a rigid joint, more proximal than the 1st and 3rd joints, and is referred to as the "keystone" of the midfoot.
- The transverse tarsal, or Chopart, joint is formed by the talonavicular and calcaneocuboid joints. This complex is stiff with hindfoot varus, as in the toe-off phase of gait, and provides a rigid lever for ambulation. Hindfoot valgus "unlocks" the transverse tarsal joint.
- Mobility at the transverse tarsal joint is necessary for normal gait, and fusions are not well tolerated. Temporary spanning fixation of the talonavicular and calcaneocuboid joint in the setting of trauma will not be durable and is often removed once healing of the traumatized foot has occurred.
- Fixation from the 4th or 5th metatarsals into the cuboid also restricts normal foot motion and is not well tolerated. Fixation across these joints is often removed once healing has occurred in the traumatized foot. The remaining midfoot joints (naviculocuneiform and medial 3 metatarsocuneiform) are relatively stable and nonmobile articulations and tolerate permanent fixation well, although hardware that spans those joints will often be removed as well.

NAVICULAR FRACTURES

Introduction

- Navicular injuries include avulsion fractures of the tuberosity and fractures of the body, either extra- or intraarticular.
- Avulsion fractures most commonly occur dorsally, although they can occur anywhere around the navicular. Medial avulsions may be caused by the posterior tibial tendon or the plantar calcaneonavicular (spring) ligament, while most others will be capsular avulsion fractures. An avulsion fracture typically involves a low-energy twisting injury with pain at the medial midfoot and an inability to bear weight afterward.
- Navicular body fractures are less common than avulsion fractures, although they are often greater in severity. They can result from a direct mechanism ("crush") or an indirect mechanism (axial load through foot). Navicular body fractures may present with similar complaints, although a higher energy mechanism may result in a more diffuse midfoot injury in addition to the navicular fracture, and symptoms may correspond to the extent of the injury.
- Physical examination will reveal varying degrees of edema, ecchymosis, and tenderness over the proximal midfoot. Patients will often have significant pain with resisted adduction of the foot. Diffuse edema and ecchymosis about the foot do not negate the possibility of navicular injury; rather, they may be indicative of multiple midfoot injuries.
- Radiographs should include anteroposterior, oblique, and lateral foot radiographs. Navicular avulsion fractures will demonstrate a fleck of avulsed cortex, which is sometimes visualized on only 1 view (increasing the possibility of the injury being missed). This should be differentiated from an accessory navicular, which will be well corticated. Computed tomography (CT) scans can be obtained to further delineate anatomy and pick up subtle findings when plain films fail to show adequate detail.
- Classification of navicular fractures is as follows.
  - Type 1: Transverse coronal plane fracture
  - Type 2: Sagittal plane fracture that often runs dorsolateral to plantarmedial with medial fragment often subluxed and lateral fragment often comminuted
  - Type 3: Fractures with central or lateral comminution and associated with lateral displacement of forefoot &/or occasionally disruption of calcaneocuboid joint or fracture of cuboid

Treatment

- Dorsal avulsion fractures can usually be treated similar to an ankle sprain with progressive weight bearing and functional rehabilitation. Rarely, the avulsed fragment may either include a significant enough portion of the articular surface or remain symptomatic for long enough that operative intervention may be warranted.
- Nondisplaced navicular body fractures are treated with limited weight bearing (usually non-weight bearing) and immobilization in a well-padded short leg splint or cast. Avulsion of the posterior tibial tendon, however, requires surgical correction.
- Type 1 displaced navicular body fractures can be reduced and fixed through a dorsomedial exposure with lag screw fixation from dorsal to plantar.
- Types 2 and 3 fractures require more extensive surgical intervention. The medial fragment, which is often subluxed, must be reduced. An aid to reduction is a medially placed minidistractor. This may also restore the alignment of the medial border of the foot in type 3 fractures.
- Medial to lateral lag screws may be used when there is no lateral fragment comminution. Screws may also maintain reduction by being placed across the naviculocuneiform joints or into the cuboid. Temporary Kirschner wire fixation from the navicular into the talar head may also prove helpful in difficult injuries. Temporary bridge plating across the medial midfoot can be used as an aid to maintaining reduction.

Rehabilitation

- Non-weight bearing is maintained for up to 12 weeks.
- Depending on the individual injury, range of motion exercises may be started at the 2-week mark, although some injuries may require longer periods of immobilization. Temporary Kirschner wires, if necessary, are removed at ~ 6 weeks.
- Removal of implants spanning multiple joints after severe injuries should not occur until healing is complete. Implants spanning naviculocuneiform joints need not be removed, but preservation of motion at the talonavicular joint is desirable.

Outcomes

- There is little in the literature on the results of navicular fractures, as they are relatively uncommon injuries. High-energy navicular fractures lead to a high rate of secondary arthrosis in the hindfoot and have been associated with significant complications in one study. Athletes with navicular fractures in the NFL combine had a greater probability of not being drafted and not competing in at least 2 NFL seasons compared to matched controls.

NAVICULAR STRESS FRACTURES

Introduction

- These are unusual injuries in the general population but are perhaps quite common in high-caliber athletes.
- These are characteristic in athletes participating in sports that require cutting movements (basketball and soccer players) and explosive activity (sprinters and high jumpers). They are traditionally thought to be uncommon in endurance-type activities (distance runners and soldiers), although a recent series noted that 38/62 (61.3%) of athletes with navicular stress fractures were runners.
- It is thought that the mechanism may be related to repetitive force during toe-off phase of gait that is channeled through the rigid lever of the 2nd metatarsal-middle (2nd) cuneiform to the central navicular, which may cause fracture. Other risk factors may include a long 2nd metatarsal or a short 1st metatarsal.
- The classification system proposed by Saxena et al helps to guide both treatment and prognosis.

Evaluation

- The patient often notes an insidious onset of midfoot pain. The pain will characteristically be exacerbated by explosive athletic activity and relieved by rest.
- Physical examination findings will not often include edema or ecchymosis. Tenderness is often localized to the lateral aspect of the navicular. Maintaining a single-limb stance can often be quite difficult. Radiographic evaluation should include standard anteroposterior, oblique, and lateral foot plain radiographs. The fracture line is often invisible, however, on these films. Other conditions should be ruled out. Callus is not always apparent.
- CT is the imaging modality of choice and is least likely to miss a stress fracture. It can often be performed with magnetic resonance (MR) imaging scan to confirm a diagnosis of stress fracture. Fracture lines may be incomplete or nondisplaced, making initial plain radiographs somewhat unreliable.

Treatment

- The mainstay of treatment for navicular stress fractures is rest. Weight bearing is protected for 6 weeks. Cast, splint, or walker boot immobilization is utilized as desired.
- Failed conservative treatment indicates operative intervention, although the morphology of the fracture and Saxena classification may push one to be more aggressive earlier. A dorsal approach is often used. Sclerotic fracture margins are debrided. Autogenous iliac crest bone graft is then placed into the fracture gap, and the navicular is secured with interfragmentary screws.

Rehabilitation

- Postoperative regimen may include immobilization at the surgeon's discretion. Early range of motion exercises are often allowed for the ankle and hindfoot. Weight bearing is restricted for 6 weeks, and athletic activities are restricted for a minimum of 3 months.

CUBOID FRACTURES

Introduction

- Often termed "nutcracker" fractures, these are uncommon injuries. The nutcracker injury results from the violent abduction of the forefoot on the hindfoot, compressing the lateral aspect of the cuboid between the anterior process of the calcaneus and the bases of the 4th and 5th metatarsals.
- Fracture can occur with direct trauma (e.g., crush injury to midfoot). Distraction forces on the medial aspect of the foot may result in associated tear of the posterior tibial tendon or avulsion fracture of the medial tubercle of the navicular (insertion of posterior tibial tendon).

Evaluation

- History may reveal a foot injury with substantial force having been applied to the foot (e.g., motor vehicle crash, fall from a substantial height, crushing injury). Patients may complain of lateral foot pain and inability to bear weight.
- Examination often reveals substantial lateral foot edema, ecchymosis, and tenderness. Deformity in this location may be a consequence of frank cuboid dislocation (rare) or of a complete transverse midfoot disruption (e.g., Lisfranc injury). Medial foot edema can occur, especially with associated navicular or posterior tibial tendon or Lisfranc injury. Any patient with significant foot edema or deformity should be carefully evaluated, especially if a decreased level of consciousness impedes history taking and physical examination.
- Radiographic evaluation should include anteroposterior, lateral, and oblique views. A 30° medial oblique view will allow for full visualization of the cuboid without overlapping structures. CT scanning may be helpful in comminuted fractures or in the absence of adequate plain radiographs.

Treatment

- Nondisplaced isolated cuboid fractures are treated with well-padded short leg splinting or casting and protected weight bearing.

Saxena Classification and Treatment Scheme for Navicular Stress Fractures

Type	Fracture	Treatment
I	Dorsal cortical fracture	Conservative treatment or open reduction and internal fixation in athlete
II	Dorsal fracture propagates into navicular body	Conservative treatment or open reduction and internal fixation in active/athletic patients
III	Fracture penetrates second cortex (either plantar, medial, or lateral)	ORIF

Modifiers are used, which, if present, are generally indications for open reduction and internal fixation.
A = Avascular necrosis (most often seen in type III); C = cystic degeneration (most often seen in type I); S = sclerosis of fracture lines (most often seen in type II injuries).

- Cuboid dislocations should be reduced and splinted. Open reduction through a lateral or dorsolateral incision is usually necessary. Instability after reduction may be treated with Kirschner wires from the base of the 5th metatarsal, spanning the cuboid, and terminating in the anterior process of the calcaneus.
- Displaced fractures (including comminuted crush injuries resulting in lateral column shortening) are treated with open reduction and internal fixation. Failure to treat these fractures appropriately can lead to persistent deformity and pain.
- Exposure of the fracture is accomplished through a lateral longitudinal incision in the interval between the extensor digitorum brevis and peroneal tendons. Articular reduction is accomplished first and provisionally stabilized with Kirschner wires.
- A laminar spreader may then be used to correct lateral column length, if necessary. Alternatively, a lateral small joint distractor, with half-pins placed in the 5th metatarsal diaphysis and the anterior process or tuberosity of the calcaneus, can assist in reestablishing lateral column length. If distraction is necessary, then the resulting defect should be filled with tricortical autogenous iliac crest bone graft or other structural graft as necessary. Structural graft can be held with Kirschner wires, cortical screws, &/or a lateral buttress plate.
- A plate spanning the calcaneocuboid joint &/or the 5th tarsometatarsal joint may be considered if no purchase can be gained in the cuboid itself.

Rehabilitation

- Initially, the operative foot is immobilized in a well-padded short leg plaster splint. Sutures are removed after 2 weeks, and further immobilization with splinting or casting is continued for a total of 6-8 weeks. Weight bearing is protected for a minimum of 6 weeks.
- At the 6- to 8-week mark, the patient may be placed into a walker boot, and range of motion exercises are initiated for the ankle and subtalar joints. Weight bearing is progressed as the clinical situation allows. Any Kirschner wires present can be withdrawn in the clinic at the 6-week mark.
- Implant removal can be accomplished due to irritation of skin or underlying structures or to restore calcaneocuboid &/or 5th tarsometatarsal joint motion (in the case of bridging plates) once healing of the fracture is accomplished.

SELECTED REFERENCES

1. Petrie MJ et al: A new and reliable classification system for fractures of the navicular and associated injuries to the midfoot. Bone Joint J. 100-B(2):176-182, 2018
2. Rony L et al: Clinical and radiological outcomes of a cohort of 9 patients with anatomical fractures of the cuboid treated by locking plate fixation. Orthop Traumatol Surg Res. 104(2):245-249, 2018
3. Saxena A et al: Navicular stress fracture outcomes in athletes: analysis of 62 injuries. J Foot Ankle Surg. 56(5):943-948, 2017
4. Vopat B et al: Epidemiology of navicular injury at the NFL combine and their impact on an athlete's prospective NFL career. Orthop J Sports Med. 5(8):2325967117723285, 2017
5. Coulibaly MO et al: Results and complications of operative and non-operative navicular fracture treatment. Injury. 46(8).1669-77, 2015
6. Borrelli J Jr et al: Fracture of the cuboid. J Am Acad Orthop Surg. 20(7):472-7, 2012
7. Saxena A et al: Results of treatment of 22 navicular stress fractures and a new proposed radiographic classification system. J Foot Ankle Surg. 39(2):96-103, 2000

(Left) *A 40-year-old male patient who was on a motorcycle and was clipped by a car, sustaining a talonavicular fracture dislocation with a fracture of the posteromedial talar body, is shown. Here, we see the talar body fracture ➡ and the navicular fracture with talar head impaction ➡.* **(Right)** *The sagittal component of the navicular fracture (medial component ➡; lateral component ➡) is shown here with impaction fracture of the talar head ➡.*

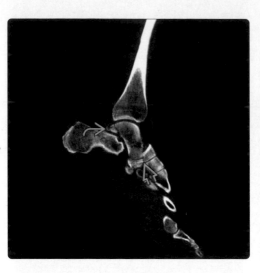
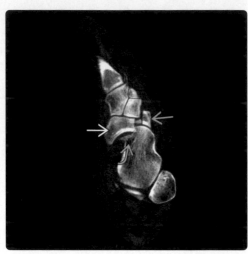

(Left) *Postoperative radiograph shows navicular and talar body open reduction and internal fixation with bridging fixation of the talonavicular joint. Two small hand plates were used for this purpose, as opposed to 1 larger plate. The patient was kept non-weight bearing with the plan to remove the bridging hardware at 12 weeks.* **(Right)** *Lateral image shows some distraction of the talonavicular joint. Two plates were used to make sure that the fixation distracting the joint was sufficiently strong.*

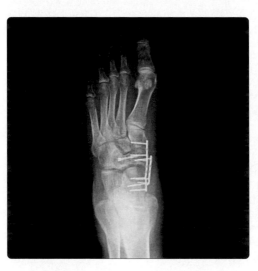
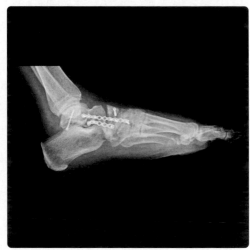

(Left) *Radiograph shows the patient after removal of bridging hardware; stiffness is obviously a concern after an injury and surgery of this nature, although aggressive rehabilitation can return motion to near-normal levels.* **(Right)** *Radiograph shows the patient after removal of bridging hardware; stiffness is obviously a concern after injury and surgery of this nature, although aggressive rehabilitation can return motion to near-normal levels.*

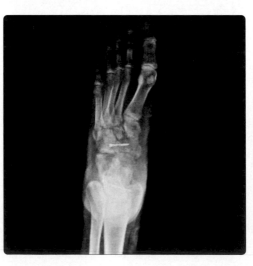
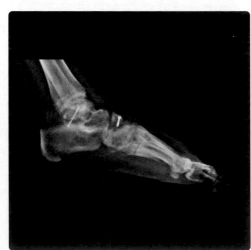

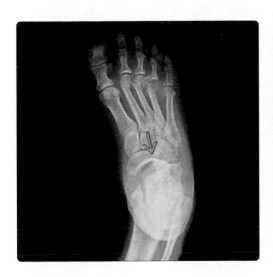

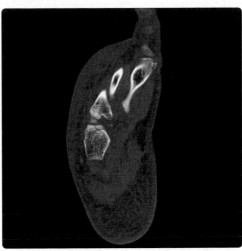

(Left) *A 57-year-old male patient fell and now presents with midfoot pain. A perched talonavicular dislocation ⇨ is shown. This injury was initially missed in the emergency room.* (Right) *CT scan shows the impaction at the cuboid metatarsal articulation. This fracture was relatively small without much displacement.*

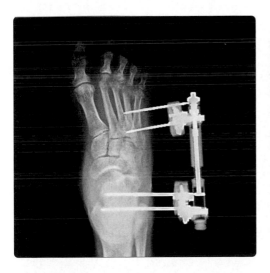

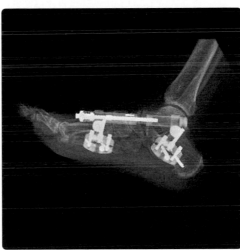

(Left) *Given the significant swelling of the foot (the patient had presented several days after injury), a closed reduction with external fixation was performed. Note that the talonavicular joint is now reduced. The impaction fracture of the talar head was not directly treated.* (Right) *Lateral image shows reduction of the talonavicular joint as well as the external fixator in good position. Two pins were placed in the calcaneus and the 5th metatarsal.*

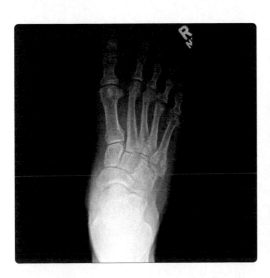

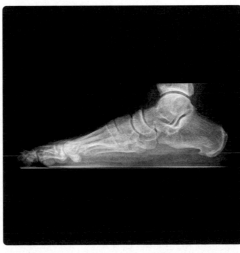

(Left) *One year out from injury, the patient was back working construction with good motion and no complaints of pain in the midfoot. The talonavicular joint remained reduced, and the impaction fracture did not appear to give him trouble.* (Right) *Once again, the talonavicular joint is well reduced, although the cuboid-metatarsal articulation is not well visualized here.*

KEY FACTS

- The midfoot includes 5 tarsal bones: Navicular, cuboid, and 3 cuneiforms (medial, 1st; middle, 2nd; and lateral, 3rd).
- Mobile or "essential" midfoot joints include:
  - Talonavicular
  - Calcaneocuboid
  - Cuboid: 4th and 5th metatarsals
- Nonmobile or "nonessential" midfoot joints include:
  - Naviculocuneiform
  - Metatarsocuneiform
- Navicular fracture outcome is dependent on fracture pattern and restoration of normal anatomy.
  - Restoration of normal anatomical alignment leads to better outcomes in displaced fractures.
  - Increasing comminution tends to result in more frequent poor outcomes.
- Nondisplaced cuneiform fractures, especially without associated midfoot injuries, may be treated conservatively with a well-padded short leg splint.

- Displaced cuneiform fractures require ORIF.
- Injury to the tarsometatarsal joints include a wide spectrum of soft tissue and bony injuries.
  - They may be purely ligamentous or purely fracture or a combination of both (fracture-dislocations).
  - They may be low energy, high energy, or somewhere in between.
- Radiographic evaluation of Lisfranc injuries requires:
  - Weight-bearing anteroposterior, lateral, and 30° oblique views
  - Stress radiographs
- Lisfranc injuries can be surgically treated with ORIF or primary fusion.
- There have been 2 randomized studies comparing primary fusion to ORIF.
  - One suggested improved outcomes with primary fusion.
    - Especially with regard to decreased need for hardware removal surgery
  - The other did not show any major difference in outcome.

(Left) *This patient sustained a type 3 navicular fracture in a motor vehicle crash. Anteroposterior and oblique injury radiographs are shown.* (Right) *Lateral injury radiograph shows dorsal displacement of the fractured navicular with dislocation of both the talonavicular and naviculocuneiform joints. Radiographs tend to underestimate fracture comminution.*

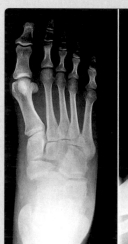
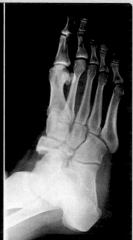
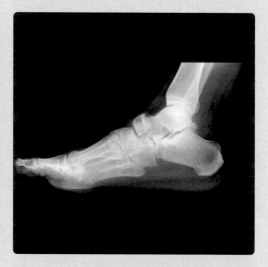

(Left) *Coronal and sagittal CT images, which demonstrate greater detail of the navicular fracture pattern, are shown.* (Right) *Anteroposterior and lateral postoperative radiographs demonstrating internal fixation of anatomically reconstructed navicular, with supporting bridge plate across medial column of forefoot, are shown. The bridge plate was removed ~ 3 months postoperatively.*

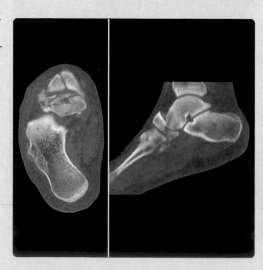
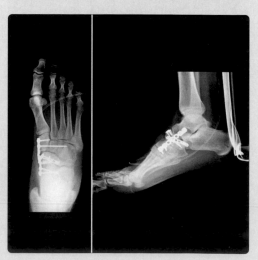

ANATOMY AND FUNCTION OF MIDFOOT

General

- The midfoot includes 5 tarsal bones: Navicular, cuboid, and 3 cuneiforms (medial, 1st; middle, 2nd; and lateral, 3rd).
  - The bases of the metatarsals are also part of the midfoot structure.
- It forms the transverse arch of the foot and part of the longitudinal arch.
- The navicular articulates in a mobile relationship with the talus proximally.
  - Motion at the talonavicular joint is essential for normal foot function.
- The navicular articulate distally with the 3 cuneiforms.
  - Stability at this articulation is more important than flexibility.
- The cuboid articulates with the anterior process of the calcaneus proximally and with the 4th and 5th metatarsal bases distally.
  - Both proximal and distal articulations are mobile.
- The cuneiforms articulate with navicular proximally, 1st-3rd metatarsal bases distally, and cuboid laterally (with lateral or 3rd cuneiform).
  - These articulations are rigid.
- The 2nd metatarsal meets the middle cuneiform in a rigid joint.
  - This articulation is more proximal than the 1st and 3rd joints.
  - This is referred to as the "keystone" of the midfoot.
- The transverse tarsal, or Chopart, joint is formed by the talonavicular and calcaneocuboid joints.
  - This complex is stiff with hindfoot varus during the toe-off phase of gait.
    - It provides a rigid lever for ambulation.
  - Hindfoot valgus "unlocks" the transverse tarsal joint.
- Mobility at the transverse tarsal joint is necessary for normal gait.
  - Fusions are not well tolerated.
  - Temporary spanning fixation of the talonavicular and calcaneocuboid joints in the setting of trauma will not be durable.
    - It is often removed once healing of the traumatized foot has occurred.
- Fixation from 4th or 5th metatarsals into cuboid also restricts normal foot motion and is not well tolerated.
  - If performed, fixation is often removed once healing has occurred in the traumatized foot.
- The remaining midfoot joints (naviculocuneiform and medial 3 metatarsocuneiform) are relatively stable and nonmobile articulations.
  - They tolerate permanent fixation well.

Midfoot Injuries

- Although it is possible to fracture a single bone of the midfoot complex, many injuries are more complex.
- The tight ligamentous connections across the midfoot bones means that displacement of any 1 midfoot bone often must include injury to ligaments or adjacent bones.
  - These injuries will affect the stability and structure of the midfoot.

- The navicular and 3 cuneiforms are packed tightly together and essentially function as a block unit.
- The 2nd and 3rd metatarsals are tightly connected to each other and to the cuneiforms.
- There is a proximal transverse intermetatarsal ligament that connects the bases of the 2nd-5th metatarsals.
  - Medially, it runs to the medial cuneiform, not the 1st metatarsal.
- There is also a distal transverse intermetatarsal ligament that connects the distal end of the 2nd-5th metatarsals.
  - Medially, it inserts on the lateral sesamoids.
  - Again, the 1st metatarsal is not connected.
- The Lisfranc ligament runs from the medial cuneiform to the base of the 2nd metatarsal.
  - It is mostly a plantar structure.
- The 1st metatarsal has ligamentous connections to the medial cuneiform.
  - There is no ligamentous connection to the other midfoot joints.
- The various midfoot injury patterns seen are a reflection of these connections.

CUNEIFORM FRACTURES

Introduction

- Isolated cuneiform fractures are rare.
- They often occur in conjunction with other midfoot injuries.
  - Lisfranc injuries
  - Cuboid fractures
  - Navicular fractures
- They most commonly involve the medial (1st) cuneiform.
- Injuries may occur via a direct mechanism (direct blow) or an indirect mechanism (violent forefoot abduction or adduction)

Evaluation

- Patients may complain of generalized midfoot pain or may isolate their area of maximal pain to the medial midfoot.
  - Patients often are unable to bear weight on the injured foot.
- Physical examination may reveal signs of typical midfoot injury, including the following.
  - Edema
  - Ecchymosis
  - Tenderness
- Skin examination is necessary to rule out impending compromise by bony deformity.
  - This is most likely in the setting of multiple bony or ligamentous injuries.
    - Such as Lisfranc injury
- Be suspicious of compartment syndrome with severe swelling and high-energy mechanisms.

Treatment

- Nondisplaced cuneiform fractures, especially without associated midfoot injuries, may be treated conservatively with a well-padded short leg splint.
  - Protected weight bearing is maintained acutely.
- Displaced cuneiform fractures require open reduction and internal fixation (ORIF).
  - Interfragmentary compression, if possible, may be employed for noncomminuted fractures.

- Incision is often centered dorsally over the interspace between the 1st and 2nd metatarsal bases and the medial (1st) and middle (2nd) cuneiforms.
- Comminuted fractures may be stabilized to adjacent, uninjured cuneiforms with intercuneiform screw fixation.
- Associated midfoot injuries, such as Lisfranc injuries, should also be treated accordingly.
- Temporary bridge plating may be employed for severely comminuted medial cuneiform fractures.
  - It maintains medial column length.
  - It can bridge from the base of the 1st metatarsal to the navicular or talus.

LISFRANC INJURIES

Introduction

- Injury to the tarsometatarsal joints include a wide spectrum of soft tissue and bony injuries.
- The injury may be purely ligamentous, purely bony, or a combination of both (fracture-dislocations).
- Purely ligamentous Lisfranc injuries may lack any radiographic abnormality.
  - However, they may also be characterized by a fleck of bone visible near the base of the 2nd metatarsal.
    - Represents avulsion of Lisfranc ligament
      - Normally courses from medial cuneiform to base of 2nd metatarsal
- Lisfranc injuries can be differentiated into low- and high-energy subtypes.
  - Lower energy pedestrian injuries usually involve a forefoot flexing into plantarflexion as the foot is trapped beneath the leg while walking.
    - May have "springing open" of midfoot with dorsal subluxation of 2nd metatarsal base
    - Injuries are usually limited to 1st, 2nd, and 3rd metatarsal bases
  - Higher energy injuries can occur from motor vehicle accidents.
    - May have much wider separation of any part of midfoot
  - Of course, there are all kinds of possibilities in between.
    - Many sporting injuries in elite athletes fall somewhere in middle
- In cases of lower energy purely ligamentous injuries, the displacement may be subtle.
- Injury may involve entire forefoot dislocating laterally ("homolateral" type) on the midfoot or may involve dissociation of metatarsals from one another ("dissociative" type).
  - A common dissociative injury pattern is a reduced (but injured) 1st tarsometatarsal joint with lateral dislocation of 2nd-5th tarsometatarsal joints.
  - A relatively rare variant has dislocation of the medial cuneiform and 1st metatarsal as a unit, relative to the rest of the midfoot.
- Lack of adequate treatment of these injuries can result in loss of stability of both transverse and longitudinal arches.
  - This leads to deformity, pain, and arthrosis.

Evaluation

- **History**
  - Determination of mechanism is important.
  - Complaints of pain over midfoot
- **Physical examination**
  - Areas of ecchymoses (check plantar foot)
  - Midfoot tenderness
    - Global midfoot tenderness may indicate more severe injury than lateral tenderness alone
  - Skin evaluation for lacerations, fracture blisters, and impending compromise by gross skeletal deformity
    - Important for prioritization of treatment
- Be suspicious of compartment syndrome with high-energy mechanism, even in the setting of open fracture.
  - This may occur when dislocation leads to disruption of the deep perforating branch of the dorsalis pedis artery.
- **Radiographic evaluation**
  - Use weight-bearing anteroposterior, lateral, and 30° oblique views.
  - Comparison views with uninjured contralateral foot may be helpful in subtle injuries.
  - Radiographic clues of purely ligamentous injury are as follows:
    - Loss of alignment of medial border of middle (2nd) cuneiform and medial border of base of 2nd metatarsal
    - Widening between bases of 1st and 2nd metatarsals &/or between base of 2nd metatarsal and medial (1st) cuneiform
    - Dorsal subluxation of 2nd metatarsal base, on lateral view, relative to cuneiform
  - Stress radiographs, perhaps under anesthesia, should be utilized when index of suspicion is high and diagnosis is not apparent on normal screening radiographs.
    - AP view while abduction force is applied to forefoot against stabilized hindfoot and midfoot
  - Positive stress radiograph may show disruption of line that intersects medial borders of navicular, medial (1st) cuneiform, and base of 1st metatarsal.
    - Intercuneiform instability may also be detected.
- Fractures of multiple metatarsal bases, medial cuneiform, &/or cuboid should alert examiner to the possibility of complete tarsometatarsal joint disruption.
  - This is analogous to transradial, transscaphoid, &/or transcapitate perilunate wrist injury.
- Routine use of CT and MR for further evaluation of these injuries is controversial and may not add to evaluation.
  - CT can reveal the injury more clearly but almost never changes the diagnosis or plan.
  - It is common to see additional injuries on MR.
    - Peroneus longus insertion is commonly injured.
      - For which no particular treatment is needed

Treatment

- Weight-bearing and abduction stress radiographs, under anesthesia if necessary, should be considered in all cases of suspicious midfoot injuries.
  - Perform prior to electing nonoperative therapy of these severe foot injuries.
  - The role of nonsurgical therapy for injuries apparent on stress radiographs is unknown at this time.
- Definitive surgical therapy should be delayed until swelling allows.
  - Often 1-2 weeks

- Frank deformities should be urgently reduced to prevent skin compromise.
  - Often, closed manipulative reduction can be employed under sedation in the emergency department.
  - Postreduction nonstress radiographs are appropriate.
  - A well-padded short leg plaster splint with toe plate is appropriate immobilization.
  - Use "RICE" (rest, ice, compression, elevation) to assist with edema control.
- Dorsal dislocation of the lesser metatarsal bases may not be reducible closed.
- Frank dislocations of a single metatarsal or cuneiform, representing more extensive ligamentous injury, may be reducible with closed manipulation.
- Surgical treatment is usually performed with 2 longitudinal incisions.
  - One runs over the medial cuneiform and 1st metatarsal.
    - First and 2nd rays are accessible through this incision.
  - The 2nd runs over the 4th ray.
    - Lateral side of 2nd ray, as well as 3rd and 4th rays, are accessible through this incision.
- The 2nd metatarsal base is reduced to the middle and medial cuneiform and held with wires.
  - The 1st metatarsal is keyed in as well.
- The 3rd metatarsal can then be reduced to the lateral cuneiform.
  - Good reduction of the 2nd ray often carries the 3rd ray close to its normal location.
- Intercuneiform instability should be assessed and stabilized with wires as well.
- Intraoperative imaging, including AP, lateral, and multiple obliques can check for reduction of each of the rays.
- Definitive fixation is traditionally performed with 3.5-mm or 4.0 mm solid screws.
  - One screw passes from the medial cuneiform to the 2nd metatarsal.
    - Usually lagged into place
  - A transarticular screw may be used from the 1st metatarsal to the medial cuneiform.
    - The screw can also be passed from 3rd metatarsal to the lateral cuneiform.
- K-wires are often used to hold the 4th and 5th metatarsals to the cuboid if necessary.
  - These are removed at 4-6 weeks following injury.
- Dorsal bridging plates can be used to minimize injury to the articular surfaces and allow some slight motion.
  - They are commonly used for the 1st ray.
- Comminuted metatarsal base fractures can be bridged with 1/3 or 1/4 tubular plates across the tarsometatarsal articulation, as necessary, to achieve stability.
- Some authors have reported using suture-button implants to stabilize the midfoot.
  - The precise role and results of such fixation has not been reliably proven yet.
  - Historically, less rigid fixation, such as wires alone, was unsuccessful.
- Primary fusion of the 1st, 2nd, &/or 3rd metatarsal base joints can be performed as well.
  - This makes sense in cases of severe articular comminution.
  - It may be preferable with a mostly ligamentous injury.

- Primary fusion does not rely on ligament healing, which is less predictable than bone healing.
- Primary fusion will be less likely to require subsequent hardware removal.
- Primary fusion will be more tolerant of a slight malreduction.
- There have been 2 randomized studies comparing primary fusion to ORIF.
  - One suggested improved outcomes with primary fusion.
    - Especially with regard to decreased need for hardware removal surgery
  - The other did not show any major difference in outcome.
- If early ORIF requires delay due to profuse foot edema, and deformity places skin at risk, emergent closed reduction is required.
  - Failure to maintain this reduction with splinting may require spanning external fixation of the midfoot via medial and lateral frames.
- Complex midfoot injuries with combinations of fractures and dislocations may be treated definitively with a combination of internal fixation and spanning external fixation constructs.
- Well-padded short leg plaster splint with toe plate, with the ankle in neutral position, is an appropriate postoperative dressing.

Rehabilitation

- Initial postoperative care should entail immobilization in a well-padded short leg plaster splint with a toe plate.
  - The patient should be made non-weight bearing on the operative foot.
- Suture removal should occur at ~ 2 weeks.
- A removable cast boot can be used after 2 weeks.
  - Non-weight bearing continues for 2 months or more.
- Weight bearing is progressed as clinically indicated.
  - It begin 6-12 weeks after surgery, in the walker boot.
  - Extensive midfoot reconstructions will often require longer periods of protected weight bearing.
    - Likely 12 weeks
- Hardware removal can be considered once healing is complete.
  - Many advocate waiting 6 months or longer.

Outcomes

- At least 2/3 of athletes will return to preinjury level of competition.
  - There are many anecdotes, with both positive and negative endings, of professional athletes with these injuries.
- Dorsal bridge plating may result in less cartilage injury and may be less rigid (in a good way) than transarticular screws.
  - However, it has not been shown to have better outcomes.
  - Incidence of hardware removal does not appear to be different than transarticular screws.
- Primary fusion has theoretical benefits over traditional ORIF, but this has been difficult to prove.
  - It does have a lower incidence of secondary hardware removal surgery.
- Achievement of anatomic alignment is probably the most important predictor of outcome, regardless of fusion or fixation.

- In one study of long-term follow-up of surgically treated midfoot injuries (2-24 years), 72% had some degree of arthritis on x-ray.
  - However, many were asymptomatic.
  - Nonanatomic reduction of the injury was a risk factor for developing arthritis.

SELECTED REFERENCES

1. Dubois-Ferrière V et al: Clinical outcomes and development of symptomatic osteoarthritis 2 to 24 years after surgical treatment of tarsometatarsal joint complex injuries. J Bone Joint Surg Am. 98(9):713-20, 2016

2. Henning JA et al: Open reduction internal fixation versus primary arthrodesis for lisfranc injuries: a prospective randomized study. Foot Ankle Int. 30(10):913-22, 2009

3. Ly TV et al: Treatment of primarily ligamentous Lisfranc joint injuries: primary arthrodesis compared with open reduction and internal fixation. A prospective, randomized study. J Bone Joint Surg Am. 88(3):514-20, 2006

4. Kuo RS et al: Outcome after open reduction and internal fixation of Lisfranc joint injuries. J Bone Joint Surg Am. 82-A(11):1609-18, 2000

5. Turchin DC et al: Do foot injuries significantly affect the functional outcome of multiply injured patients? J Orthop Trauma. 13(1):1-4, 1999

6. Coss HS et al: Abduction stress and AP weightbearing radiography of purely ligamentous injury in the tarsometatarsal joint. Foot Ankle Int. 19(8):537-41, 1998

7. Arntz CT et al: Fractures and fracture-dislocations of the tarsometatarsal joint. J Bone Joint Surg Am. 70(2):173-81, 1988

8. Myerson MS et al: Fracture dislocations of the tarsometatarsal joints: end results correlated with pathology and treatment. Foot Ankle. 6(5):225-42, 1986

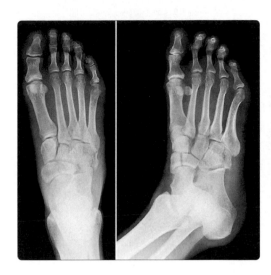

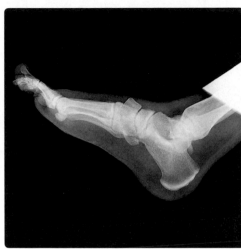

(Left) *Anteroposterior and oblique injury radiographs show navicular and cuboid fractures with middle (2nd) cuneiform dislocation. This patient sustained these injuries in a motor vehicle crash.* (Right) *Lateral injury radiograph is shown demonstrating dorsal dislocation of the middle cuneiform indicating loss of midfoot stability.*

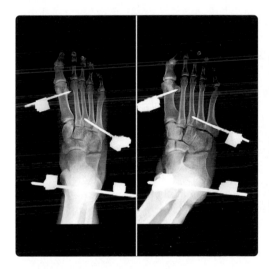

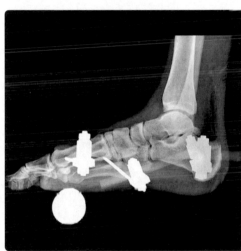

(Left) *Definitive open reduction and internal fixation (ORIF) of this patient's injuries could not be accomplished acutely due to profuse edema. Closed reduction of middle (2nd) cuneiform dislocation and foot alignment was accomplished and held utilizing a through and through calcaneal tuberosity pin, attached via carbon fiber rods to a distal 1st metatarsal pin medially and a proximal 4th and 5th metatarsal pin laterally.* (Right) *Lateral radiograph of the external fixation construct is shown.*

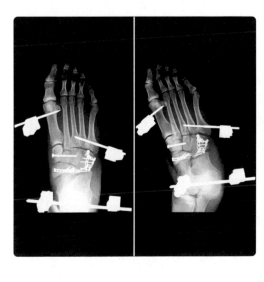

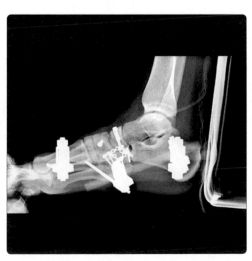

(Left) *Definitive ORIF was accomplished after foot edema was controlled. A single intercuneiform screw holds the middle (2nd) cuneiform reduced. The medial and lateral external fixator was left in place for 6 weeks to supplement fixation support.* (Right) *Plate fixation is noted on the navicular and cuboid, maintaining anatomical reduction.*

(Left) *AP and oblique injury radiographs show a patient that sustained a ligamentous Lisfranc injury in a motorcycle crash. Note wide disruption of 1st-2nd metatarsal interspace without disruption of medial alignment of the 1st metatarsal with medial (1st) cuneiform and disruption of the medial alignment of the 3rd metatarsal with lateral (3rd) cuneiform of the 4th metatarsal with cuboid.* **(Right)** *Lateral injury radiograph is shown. Note the significant dorsal dislocation of lesser metatarsal bases relative to cuneiforms.*

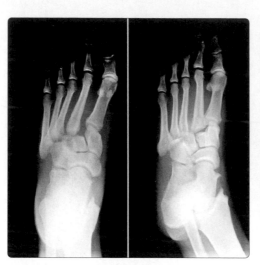 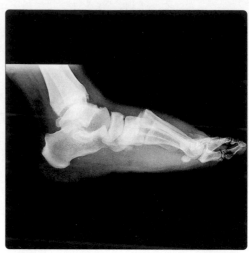

(Left) *Intraoperative fluoroscopic anteroposterior and oblique images demonstrate K-wire provisional fixation of a reduced Lisfranc joint.* **(Right)** *Intraoperative fluoroscopic lateral image demonstrates restoration of the alignment between the metatarsal bases and cuneiforms.*

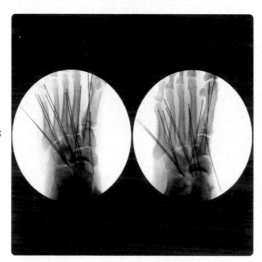 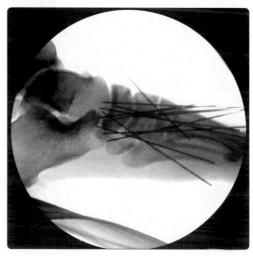

(Left) *Postoperative anteroposterior radiograph demonstrates definitive screw fixation across 1st, 2nd, and 3rd tarsometatarsal joints and K-wire fixation across 4th and 5th tarsometatarsal joints. In most cases, one K-wire across each of the 4th and 5th tarsometatarsal joints is sufficient. Also note the medial to lateral intercuneiform screw, maintaining reduction of disruption between the 1st and 2nd rays.* **(Right)** *Postoperative lateral radiograph is shown. K-wires were removed at 6 weeks.*

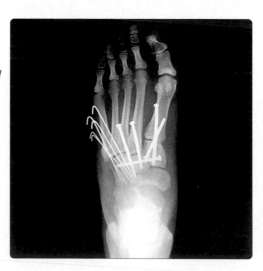 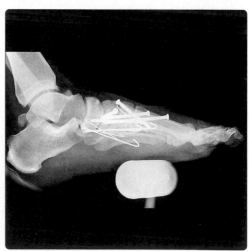

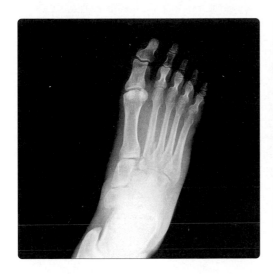

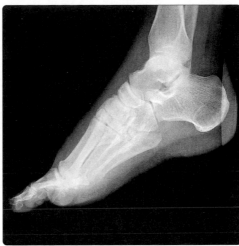

(Left) *Anteroposterior radiograph of a bony Lisfranc injury is shown. This injury was sustained in a motor vehicle crash but is relatively innocuous-appearing on plain injury radiographs.* (Right) *Lateral radiograph is shown, which is again fairly benign-appearing. The typical dorsal displacement of the 2nd metatarsal is not always present.*

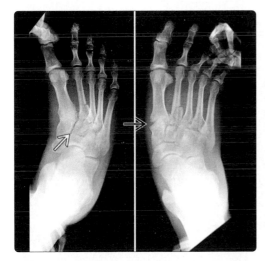

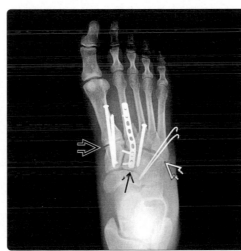

(Left) *Stress radiographs obtained with patient under general anaesthetic is shown. Note disruption of 1st-2nd interspace ➡. Also, note widening of the medial aspect of the 1st tarsometatarsal joint on lateral stress ➡.* (Right) *Postoperative anteroposterior radiograph is shown. The medial ➡ and intermediate ➡ columns of the foot were rigidly fixed, whereas the lateral column of the foot ➡ was temporarily stabilized with K-wires to preserve motion.*

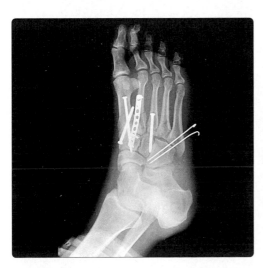

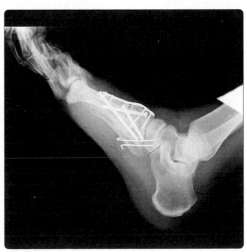

(Left) *Postoperative oblique radiograph demonstrates definitive fixation constructs after anatomical reduction of the midfoot. A bridge plate was utilized across the 2nd metatarsal base fracture due to extensive comminution; this plate was not removed after healing.* (Right) *Postoperative lateral radiograph is shown. K-wires were removed in the outpatient clinic at 6 weeks.*

KEY FACTS

- Toe and metatarsal fractures are the most common fractures of the foot with an incidence of 140 per 100,000 per year.
- The 5th metatarsal is the most frequently fractured metatarsal (23%).
- The metatarsals are affected by stress fractures more commonly than all other sites in the body.
- A majority of metatarsal fractures are low-energy injuries suitable for closed treatment.
  - The intact soft tissues splint the fracture.
- A low-energy metatarsal shaft fracture typically does not disrupt proximal or distal stabilizing soft tissue structures.
  - The metatarsal head remains in the appropriate location for weight bearing.
- A high-energy injury, with disruption of the stabilizing soft tissues proximally or distally, will elevate or depress the metatarsal head.
  - Thus, this may disrupt the normal distribution of weight in the forefoot.

- Altered weight distribution may lead to metatarsalgia and painful plantar keratosis.
- Displacement, shortening, or angulation of the 1st metatarsal in any plane anywhere along the bone can significantly alter the weight-bearing distribution of the foot and is therefore an indication for operative management.
- An isolated, nondisplaced metatarsal base fracture may be stable, but if any uncertainty exists, further evaluation of the midfoot with stress x-rays is necessary.
- High-energy injuries, even when closed, have extensive soft tissue disruption and may require operative treatment.
- Lawn mower injuries are common with an incidence of between 50,000-160,000 each year.
  - They can cause significant morbidity and, rarely, even death.

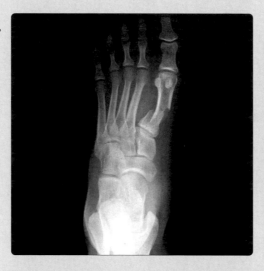
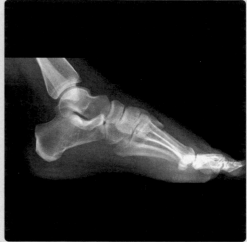

(Left) *This young man's foot was crushed by a large garage door. The 1st metatarsal (MT) shaft is widely displaced.* (Right) *There is not much vertical displacement of the MT head, suggesting that some of the soft tissue connections were intact between the 1st and 2nd MT heads.*

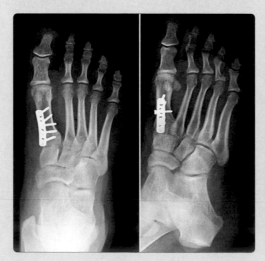
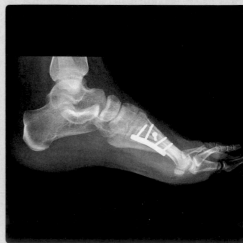

(Left) *Open reduction was performed through a medial incision with a lag screw and neutralization plate.* (Right) *After 6 weeks of non-weight bearing, he went on to a full recovery.*

FOREFOOT STRUCTURE

- The metatarsals are the major weight-bearing structure of the forefoot.
- The 1st metatarsal head and its 2 associated sesamoids bear ~ 1/3 of the body weight.
  - The remainder is distributed among the lesser 4 metatarsals.
  - The 2nd and 3rd frequently bear more than the 4th and 5th.
- The metatarsal bases are rigidly stabilized to the cuneiforms and cuboid in the midfoot.
- The proximal transverse metatarsal ligament runs from the 5th metatarsal base to the 4th, to the 3rd, then the 2nd, and then to the medial cuneiform.
- The distal transverse intermetatarsal ligament runs from the 5th metatarsal head to the 4th, then the 3rd, then 2nd, and then finally to the lateral sesamoid.
- There are no ligaments connecting the 1st metatarsal to the others.
- A low-energy metatarsal shaft fracture does not disrupt these proximal or distal stabilizers, so the metatarsal head remains in the appropriate location for weight bearing.
- A higher energy injury, with disruption of the stabilizing soft tissues proximally or distally, will elevate or depress the metatarsal head.
  - Thus, this may disrupt the normal distribution of weight in the forefoot.
  - Altered weight distribution may lead to metatarsalgia and painful plantar keratosis.
- The 1st metatarsal is intimately associated with the sesamoids, which are held fixed in relation to the lesser metatarsals by attachments to the intermetatarsal ligaments and the 2 heads of the adductor hallucis.
  - Displacement of the 1st metatarsal head in any direction can alter the balance of the entire forefoot.
- The tibialis anterior works to elevate the 1st metatarsal, while the peroneus longus plantar flexes.
  - Either of these muscles may act to deform a 1st metatarsal fracture.
- The flexor digitorum longus, flexor hallucis longus, and intrinsic muscles place plantar flexion stress on the metatarsal heads in distal fractures and can cause plantar flexion deformities.
- The 5th metatarsal, like the 1st, has less soft tissue coverage than the middle metatarsals and has extrinsic muscle attachments, the peroneus brevis and tertius, which attach at its base.
  - It also has a strong attachment to the lateral band of the plantar fascia.
  - It is the most mobile of the metatarsals.

METATARSAL FRACTURES

Mechanism

- Metatarsal fractures result from a wide variety of mechanisms and may range from an isolated single bone fracture to multiple fractures with severe soft tissue compromise.
- Direct trauma with a heavy falling object is common in industrial workers.
- Many low-energy injuries arise from indirect trauma, a twisting force with a fixed forefoot.
- Fractures of the 5th metatarsal base result from avulsion by the lateral band of the plantar aponeurosis.
- Stress fractures occur as a result of repetitive force on the metatarsals and occur frequently in athletes, soldiers, and dancers.

Physical Examination

- Patients with metatarsal fractures present with pain on ambulation or difficulty with weight bearing on the affected foot, swelling, deformity, and ecchymosis.
- Dorsal swelling is typical, because the plantar skin allows little swelling due to the thick fibrous septa within the skin pad.
- Each metatarsal and toe should be carefully and sequentially evaluated.
- Palpation of each digit and each metatarsal shaft usually will elicit point tenderness at the fracture site.
- Subungual hematoma is a hallmark of distal phalangeal fractures and may be associated with open fractures of the distal phalanx.

Imaging

- Radiographs should include anteroposterior, lateral, and oblique views of the foot.
- Metatarsal head alignment can be evaluated further with anteroposterior and lateral weight-bearing views of the whole foot and a tangential view of the metatarsal heads.
  - Unfortunately, these views are difficult to obtain in a patient with a new injury.
- Stress fractures frequently do not appear initially on plain x-ray.
  - Follow-up films 3-4 weeks later will usually demonstrate periosteal reaction or, in the 5th metatarsal, a resorption gap, that confirms the diagnosis.
- Magnetic resonance imaging can identify a stress fracture immediately but is not often needed, because the diagnosis can be made clinically.
- Bone scans also will detect a stress fracture after a few days of symptoms.

Classification

- Metatarsal fractures can be classified according to the location, and thus include head, neck, shaft, and base fractures.
- It is useful to classify 1st and 5th metatarsal fractures separately from the rest, because the treatment options differ widely for these types.
- Second, third, and fourth metatarsal fractures can be grouped together, as the treatment options are similar.
- Proximal 5th metatarsal fractures can be categorized by zone.
- Metatarsal base fractures can occur in isolation.
  - However, it is important to recognize that many, perhaps all, such fractures represent an injury to the midfoot.
- An isolated, nondisplaced metatarsal base fracture may be stable, but if any uncertainty exists, then further evaluation of the midfoot with stress x-rays is necessary.

1st Metatarsal Fractures

- Nondisplaced or minimally displaced fractures of the 1st metatarsal shaft or neck are generally stable and can be treated nonoperatively.
  - Nonoperative options range from a short leg cast with progressive weight bearing over 4-6 weeks to a CAM walker boot to a wooden rocker shoe for very stable fractures.
- Displacement, shortening, or angulation of the 1st metatarsal in any plane anywhere along the bone can significantly alter the weight-bearing distribution of the foot and is therefore an indication for operative management.
- It is important to restore the length and the alignment of the bone anatomically in both the sagittal and transverse planes in order to maintain normal weight bearing through the 1st ray.
- For shaft fractures, the types of fixation are limited due to the thin layer of soft tissue surrounding the bone, necessitating the use of a low-profile device.
  - There is more room for plates on the plantar-medial side of the bone.
- Long oblique fractures may be well treated with multiple lag screws, but most displaced shaft fractures will require a plate.
  - 3.5-, 2.7-, or 2.4-mm implants can be used.
- Common approaches include a longitudinal approach between the 1st and 2nd metatarsals and the medial approach.
  - The superficial peroneal nerve, deep peroneal nerve, and dorsalis pedis artery are at risk with the former approach.
  - The terminal branches of the saphenous vein and nerve are at risk with the latter.
- Comminuted base fractures may occasionally require bridging across the 1st tarsometatarsal joint to maintain proper alignment.
  - Occasionally, fusion of the 1st tarsometatarsal joint may be necessary.
  - So long as the fusion is performed with anatomical alignment of the metatarsal, no long-term consequences should be expected.

2nd, 3rd, and 4th Metatarsal Fractures

- Most low-energy fractures of the middle metatarsals are minimally displaced due to the soft tissue restraints previously described.
- 3-4 mm of displacement in the sagittal plane (elevation or depression of the metatarsal head) can significantly affect the distribution of weight in the forefoot.
  - This results in transfer of load to adjacent metatarsals (if the affected metatarsal is elevated) or overload of the fractured metatarsal (if it is plantar flexed).
- Similarly, shortening of a metatarsal can lead to adjacent metatarsal overload (transfer lesions or intractable plantar keratoses).
- Deformity in the transverse plane (medial or lateral angulation) does not have a large impact on weight-bearing distribution.
  - Thus, a higher degree of deformity, perhaps 4 mm of displacement and 10° of angulation, can be accepted in this plane.

- Nonoperative treatment can be considered for shaft fractures with < 2 mm of shortening, elevation, or depression of the metatarsal head in the sagittal plane.
  - This will be the vast majority of lesser metatarsal fractures.
- Such fractures in the lesser rays can be treated with cast immobilization, a wooden sole shoe, or a CAM walker with progressive weight bearing over 4-6 weeks.
- Fractures that result in significant elevation or depression of the metatarsal head and alteration of the weight-bearing distribution should be treated surgically.
- Closed reduction and percutaneous pin fixation is possible.
  - Pins enter from the metatarsal head.
  - The pins force the metatarsophalangeal (MTP) joints to remain extended while they are in place.
  - This can result in extension contractures at the MTP joints with claw toe deformity.
  - To avoid clawing, the surgeon can place the pins more medially or laterally in the metatarsal head.
    - This is technically more difficult.
    - The pins could enter through the toe and pass across the MTP joint and then across the fracture.
      - This is also difficult.
- Shaft and neck fractures can also be treated with open reduction and internal fixation using mini implants (2.7, 2.4, or 2.0 mm).
- The rare displaced metatarsal head fracture should probably be treated with open reduction and internal fixation.

Multiple Metatarsal Fractures

- It is possible to fracture multiple metatarsals.
- In some cases, the proximal and distal soft tissues will remain intact, so metatarsal head alignment will not be affected.
  - These injuries can be treated closed.
- However, some injuries with multiple shaft fractures may represent a variant of a midfoot (Lisfranc) injury.
- In all cases of metatarsal fracture, especially when there are multiple fractures, midfoot stability should be assessed carefully.

5th Metatarsal Fractures

- There are 4 major types of fractures of the 5th metatarsal.
  - Proximal base (vast majority)
  - Acute proximal metaphysis
  - Distal shaft
  - Stress fractures
- Fractures can be grouped by geographic zone.
  - Zone 2 includes both acute an chronic injuries.

Tuberosity Avulsion Fracture

- Although it was once believed that the avulsion was due to the pull of the peroneus brevis during foot inversion, more recent studies implicate the lateral band of the plantar fascia.
- Almost all tuberosity avulsions can be treated nonoperatively with a walking cast, boot, or hard-soled shoe and weight bearing as tolerated.
  - The majority will heal within 8 weeks, but symptoms may persist for several months.

- Radiographic nonunion is not uncommon, but painful nonunion is rare.
- Some of these injuries will have a larger proximal fragment and may extend into the articulation between the 4th-5th metatarsal bases.
  - Others may be displaced into the articulation with the cuboid.
  - Despite some displacement, all of these acute injuries tend to heal well without surgery.
- The rare, painful nonunion can be treated with excision of the fragment and peroneus brevis repair or bone grafting and intramedullary screw fixation for larger fragments.

"Jones" Fractures

- Jones fractures occur at the metaphyseal-diaphyseal junction, an area of poor vascularity and, therefore, reduced healing potential.
- The textbooks describe the Jones fracture as exiting into the intermetatarsal region between the 4th-5th metatarsal bases.
- It may be more useful to separate these "Jones fractures" into acute fractures of the proximal shaft and chronic stress fractures.
- The literature on these injuries is confusing, mostly because authors have pooled acute and chronic injuries together.
- The acute proximal shaft fracture appears transverse on x-ray with no cortical hypertrophy or periosteal reaction.
  - Although delayed union or nonunion is a concern, this injury can be treated successfully with protected weight bearing in a boot.
  - At least 1 study has shown that immediate weight bearing can result in a good outcome.
- Because of concerns for delayed union or nonunion, some surgeons recommend early surgery for high-level athletes.
  - This allows for more aggressive and confident recovery with possibly less down time.

Stress Fractures

- The chronic metadiaphyseal fracture is very different.
- The patient may present with the same history as for acute fracture: New pain in the foot after an injury.
  - Others may have pain for weeks to months.
- Radiographs show sclerosis, medullary canal narrowing, or periosteal reaction at the fracture site at the time of first presentation.
  - These imaging findings suggest a longstanding bone injury.
- They are most frequently seen in young athletes who have a sudden increase in demand on the foot or who have mild genu varum or heel varus deformities that overload the 5th metatarsal.
- Nonoperative treatment with a short leg walking cast can take from 6-20 weeks and requires a long period of rehabilitation.
  - Refracture and nonunion occur relatively frequently with nonoperative treatment when activity is resumed.
- Most surgeons now advocate operative management for these fractures, especially in athletes.
  - Benefits of operative management are a lower refracture rate and a much quicker return to activity
- Operative treatment consists of intramedullary screw fixation.

- The drilling for screw insertion is thought to increase healing potential, just as with reaming for intramedullary nailing in the tibia.
- A lot of research has studied fixation for these fractures.
  - In the lab, a plate may provide stronger fixation than a screw under cyclic loading.
  - But an intramedullary screw may be stronger in bending.
  - However, more important than simple strength of fixation is augmenting the healing.
    - It is important to stimulate the biology of fracture healing.
  - Some surgeons add bone graft as well.
- In cases of chronic injury, alignment of the foot must be assessed.
  - Patients with a varus hindfoot will overload the 5th ray, leading to stress injury.
  - This can also be seen after varus tibial malunion.
  - If the deformity causing 5th metatarsal overload is not corrected, the fracture may recur.

"Dancer's" Fractures

- Fractures of the 5th metatarsal shaft have been referred to as dancer's fractures, as they occur by "rolling over" the lateral forefoot while up on the toes.
- The fracture is a long spiral fracture, sometimes with comminution.
- The treatment of shaft fractures in the 5th metatarsal differs slightly from that of the medial 4 metatarsals because of the increased mobility of this bone.
  - Thus, a larger degree of displacement and angulation of shaft fractures can be accepted.
- These fractures often appear to have significant displacement.
  - This is especially true on the oblique view.
- Fortunately, most heal quite well.
- Patients can be treated nonoperatively with a walking cast or boot.
- Surgery is indicated for the rare, highly displaced injuries.

Other Metatarsal Stress Fractures

- Stress fractures of the medial 4 metatarsals occur frequently.
- They are commonly referred to as "march fractures" because of their occurrence in new military recruits going for long marches.
- Treatment of these fractures is usually nonoperative and focuses on unloading the affected metatarsal with altered shoewear, orthotics, or a short leg cast for complete fractures.
- It is important to look for underlying causes for the stress injury.
  - Often, none will be found.
- Stress injuries can result from imbalance in the foot (osseous alignment).
- Metabolic causes are also common, such as in the amenorrheic female athlete.

PHALANGEAL FRACTURES

1st Proximal Phalanx Fracture

- Because of the role of the 1st toe in normal gait, deformity in the 1st toe may be less well tolerated than in the other digits.
- The flexor hallucis brevis muscles can act to plantar flex a proximal phalanx fracture.
  - This will lead to a painful prominence on the bottom of the toe, a painful plantar keratosis.
- Nondisplaced or minimally displaced fractures can be treated with buddy taping and a hard-soled shoe and weight bearing as tolerated.
- Displaced fractures should be treated with closed or open reduction and fixation with crossed K-wires, lag screws, or even plating with mini implants.
- Displaced fractures of the MTP joint should be treated with reduction and stabilization.
  - Such fractures often are quite comminuted, and anatomic reduction may be difficult.
- If the MTP joint is functioning normally, then the interphalangeal joint is less important.
  - Posttraumatic arthritis of the interphalangeal joint can be easily treated with fusion, if it develops.

Lesser Phalangeal Fractures

- Diaphyseal fractures in the middle and proximal phalanges are common.
- Usually these are closed injuries and occur as a result of kicking an object, such as a leg of a table or chair, while barefoot.
  - This is a so-called "night walker" fracture.
- The vast majority of these fractures can be treated nonsurgically with buddy taping and weight bearing as tolerated.
- The 5th proximal phalanx is often fractured as a result of an abduction injury.
- For these 5th toe injuries, it is important to correct the lateral angulation with a closed reduction.
  - Persistent angulation will be a problem when the patient goes back into shoes.
- Rarely, closed or open reduction with K-wire fixation is needed for severely displaced fractures.
- Although rare, toes that heal with excessive angulation or abundant callus can irritate adjacent toes (interdigital corn).
  - This rare complication can usually be treated with exostectomy.

Distal Phalanx Fractures and Nail Bed Injury

- Injuries to the distal phalanx typically occur when an object is dropped directly on the digit and are extremely common.
- The majority of distal phalanx fractures can be treated nonoperatively with buddy taping and a hard-soled or wide toe box shoe until pain and tenderness subside.
- Distal phalanx fractures, however, are frequently accompanied by nail bed injuries due to the proximity of the skin and periosteum at the nail root.
- Nail bed lacerations and bleeding from the eponychium should lead to suspicion of an open fracture, which must be treated according to the principles of open fracture management to prevent infection.
- Nail bed injuries can occur without a fracture.

- Subungual hematoma, if painful and tender, can be treated with drainage through a hole bored in the nail plate with a small burr, heated paper clip, or electrocautery device.
- Nail bed lacerations should be carefully cleaned, debrided, and repaired using an absorbable suture material, such as 5-0 or 6-0 catgut.

OPEN FRACTURES AND LAWN MOWER INJURIES

Open Fractures

- Open fractures of the metatarsals and phalanges are not uncommon.
- This is because of the thin soft tissue envelope on the dorsum of the foot and the proximity of the distal phalanx to the skin at the root of the nail.
- As with any open fracture, they should be treated with antibiotic prophylaxis, debridement of nonviable or foreign material, and irrigation.
- Consideration should be given to osseous stabilization with wires to protect the soft tissues from further injury.

Lawn Mower Injuries

- Lawn mower injuries typically occur as a result of mowers that have tipped over and frequently damage both the toe and the metatarsal regions of the forefoot.
- Children riding on the lap of an adult on a riding mower are another source of injury.
- Predisposing factors include a lack of shoewear, insufficient soles, and use of a riding mower on a wet, sloped surface.
- Between 50,000-160,000 injuries occur each year.
- Significant morbidity occurs with eventual amputation frequently becoming necessary.
- The injuries have extensive soft tissue destruction, severe contamination, and degloving of bone and soft tissue.
  - By the Gustilo grading system, these are typically grade 3 injuries.
    - Tetanus prophylaxis and appropriate antibiotics must be administered.
      - 1st-generation cephalosporin plus aminoglycoside
- The foot should be wrapped with a sterile dressing and splinted with abundant soft padding &/or plaster.
- Radiographs in the emergency department are appropriate, but further care should probably be given in the operating room.
- In the operating room, aggressive debridement of foreign material and nonviable tissue is performed, followed by copious irrigation.
- Skeletal stabilization can be achieved with wires, external fixators, or bridging plates (if soft tissue allows).
- Fasciotomies should be performed for those at risk for compartment syndrome.
- The wounds should be left open but protected from desiccation.
  - A return trip to the operating room for further wound care should be planned in 48-72 hours.
- Flap coverage or skin grafting for soft tissue defects is required in ~ 50% of patients.
- Segmental bone loss can be splinted out to length with a bridging plate or wires with structural bone grafting done later, once soft tissues are covered and healed.

Fractures of 5th Metatarsal Classified by Zone

Zone	Location	Description
1	5th metatarsal tuberosity (most proximal)	Tuberosity avulsion fracture
2	Proximal metaphyseal-diaphyseal junction	"Jones" fracture (can be acute or chronic)
3	Diaphysis	Classic "dancer's fracture" of the shaft

Common Etiologies of Metatarsal Stress Fractures

Cause	Examples
Mechanical	1st metatarsal instability Sudden increase in activity Shoe problems Malunion of another metatarsal Overall foot balance (cavus foot)
Metabolic	Osteoporosis Amenorrhea

SELECTED REFERENCES

1. Browner, BD, et al. Skeletal Trauma: Basic Science, Management, and Reconstruction. Philadelphia, PA: Elsevier/Saunders. 2,375-2.492, 2015.

2. Konkel KF et al: Nonoperative treatment of fifth metatarsal fractures in an orthopaedic suburban private multispeciality practice. Foot Ankle Int. 26(9):704-7, 2005

3. Vollman D et al: Lawn mower related injuries to children. J Trauma. 59(3):724-8, 2005

4. Rammelt S et al: Metatarsal fractures. Injury. 35 Suppl 2:SB77-86, 2004

5. Theodorou DJ et al: Fractures of proximal portion of fifth metatarsal bone: anatomic and imaging evidence of a pathogenesis of avulsion of the plantar aponeurosis and the short peroneal muscle tendon. Radiology 226: 857-865, 2003

6. Dameron TB Jr: Fractures and anatomical variations of the proximal portion of the fifth metatarsal. J Bone Joint Surg Am. 57(6):788-92, 1975

(Left) *Graphic depicts common MT fractures. The "march fracture"* →] *is a common fatigue fracture usually of the 2nd or 3rd MT; traumatic fractures are also seen in this region. Fracture of the 5th MT proximal shaft may be due to stress fracture or a traumatic Jones fracture* →]. *The 5th MT tuberosity fracture* →] *is an avulsion injury due to traction by the peroneus brevis tendon and plantar aponeurosis. (DI: MSK Trauma.)* **(Right)** *Lateral radiograph shows an avulsion fracture* →] *of 5th MT base, due to inversion injury of the ankle. (From DI: MSK Trauma.)*

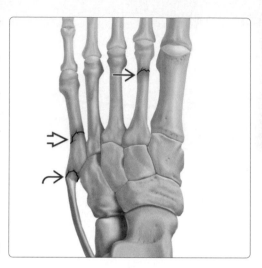
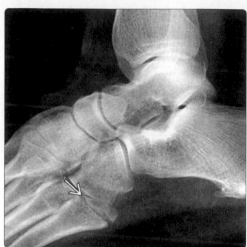

(Left) *Fifth MT tuberosity fractures typically exit close to or in the metatarsocuboid joint* →]. *They are usually mildly displaced and heal well regardless of treatment.* **(Right)** *This older woman had acute onset of pain in the lateral foot after a twisting injury. X-ray shows an acute fracture of the base of the 5th MT. Many of these patients can be treated without surgery.*

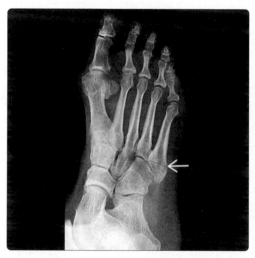
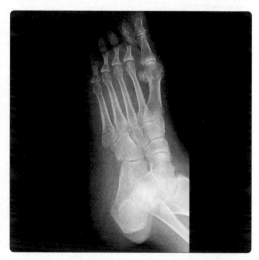

(Left) *The acute fracture must be distinguished from the patient with chronic pain and chronic radiographic changes. This patient presented with indolent pain and an x-ray showing cortical sclerosis. Early surgery may be more appropriate for this patient.* **(Right)** *This woman presented with months of pain in the lateral foot. Her foot was straight and well balanced. The x-ray reveals a chronic fracture of the proximal 5th MT shaft with sclerosis.*

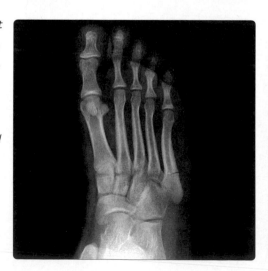
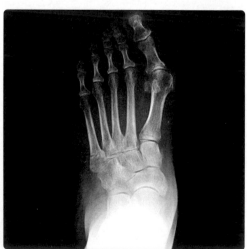

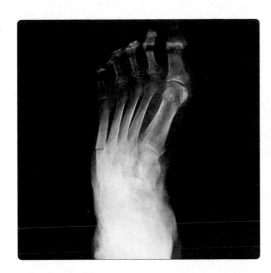

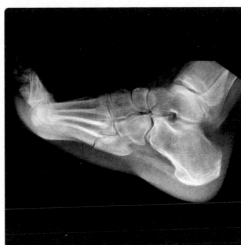

(Left) *Watch for the "Jones" fracture in the varus foot. This patient had a cavovarus foot deformity secondary to a stroke. Chronic lateral foot overload resulted in a 5th MT fracture and subsequent nonunion.* (Right) *The fracture appears incompletely healed after 6 months of symptoms. He underwent surgery, including intramedullary screw placement and hindfoot osteotomy with muscle transfers to balance the deformity.*

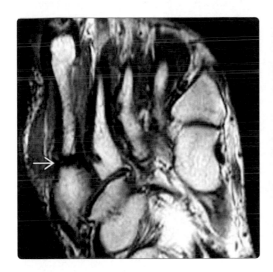

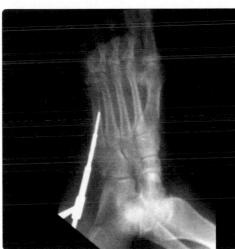

(Left) *Axial T1 MR shows sclerosis at the edges of an ununited proximal shaft fracture of the 5th MT ➡. Proximal 5th MT fractures are at risk for nonunion due to poor vascularity. (From DI: MSK Trauma.)* (Right) *During surgery, the nonunion is "reamed" with a drill over a guide wire.*

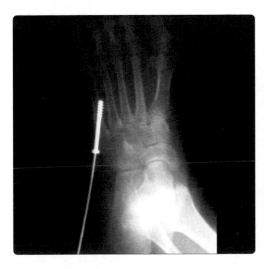

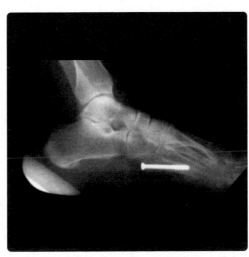

(Left) *A cannulated screw is passed across the fracture. Although most surgeons aim for an intramedullary screw, better distal purchase may be obtained in the medial cortex. Because of the small intramedullary canal, the screw violated the cortex of the shaft, but this presents no problem.* (Right) *On the lateral view, the screw is well placed.*

(Left) *Oblique radiograph shows os vesalianum ➡️, which must be distinguished from a fracture of the tuberosity of the 5th MT. The ossicle is larger than the expected size of the 5th MT tuberosity, triangular, and has rounded, corticated margins. (From DI: MSK Trauma.)* **(Right)** *A spiral fracture of the 5th MT shaft can follow a twisting injury and is sometimes referred to as a "dancer's fracture."*

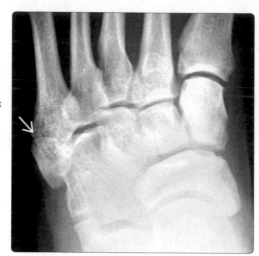
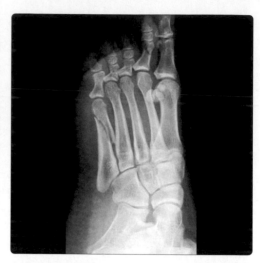

(Left) *This young man twisted his foot while playing basketball. The fractures of the middle MT shafts represent a variant of a midfoot injury, but the fractures are nondisplaced, and the midfoot is stable.* **(Right)** *This young man twisted his foot while playing basketball. The lateral view confirms good foot alignment. He went on to heal the injury well with no restrictions.*

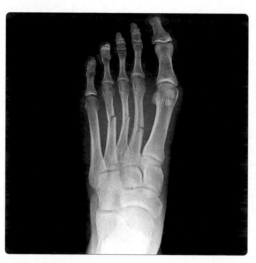
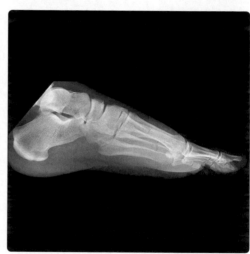

(Left) *AP radiograph shows fractures of the 2nd-4th MTs. There is complete lateral displacement of the 4th MT fracture ⇨ with bayonet apposition of the fragments, while the 2nd MT fracture is nondisplaced. Traumatic MT fractures are commonly multiple. (From DI: MSK Trauma.)* **(Right)** *This young woman presented with forefoot pain and swelling without trauma. X-rays 6 weeks after the pain began reveal a stress fracture of the 2nd MT.*

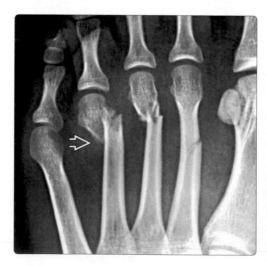
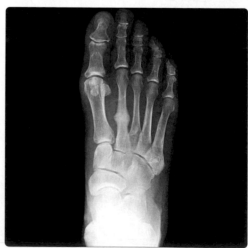

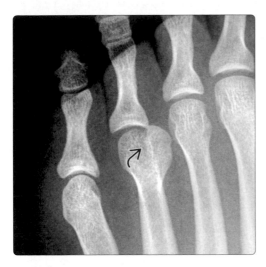

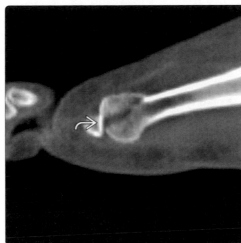

(Left) AP radiograph shows an unusual longitudinal fracture ➡ of the 4th MT head associated with dislocation of the metatarsophalangeal joint. This patient fell off of her bicycle when cycling barefoot. (From DI: MSK Trauma.) (Right) Sagittal CT shows that the fracture bisects the articular surface ➡. Because of the articular injury, the patient was treated with open reduction and internal fixation. (From DI: MSK Trauma.)

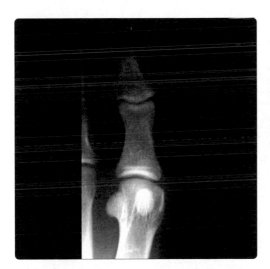

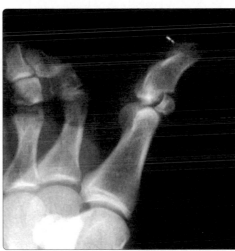

(Left) This young man sustained a trauma to his 1st toe 6 months ago. The anteroposterior view reveals good alignment. (Right) Lateral view reveals a displaced intraarticular fracture of interphalangeal joint. He was bothered by pain at the interphalangeal joint, and stiffness was noted on examination.

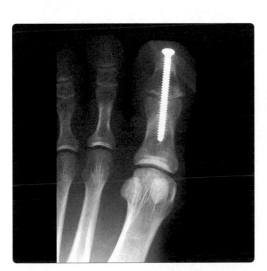

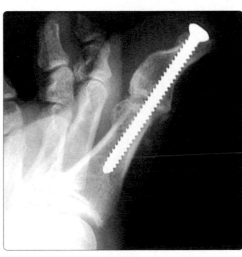

(Left) The patient was treated with fusion of the interphalangeal joint, resulting in a good functional outcome. (Right) The screw head was only slightly prominent at the tip of the toe.

Tumors of Foot and Ankle

- Foot and ankle tumors are relatively rare entities but must be kept in the differential diagnosis of musculoskeletal complaints in that area.
- The overwhelming majority of bone and soft tissue tumors in the foot and ankle are benign, but occasionally, a primary sarcoma will be present. Acral metastases (i.e., below the knee) are uncommon, although they can occur most commonly from breast, lung, thyroid, renal, and prostate primary tumors.
  - Ganglion cysts are likely the most common "tumor" seen in an adult outpatient foot and ankle practice.
- It is imperative that all caregivers be knowledgeable of the common foot and ankle neoplasms, both bone and soft tissue in nature, such that accurate diagnoses, proper treatment, and patient education regarding expected prognosis can occur.

- With that being said, if there is any concern for a malignant tumor, the most appropriate treatment once that reality is recognized is swift transfer of care to a musculoskeletal oncologist.

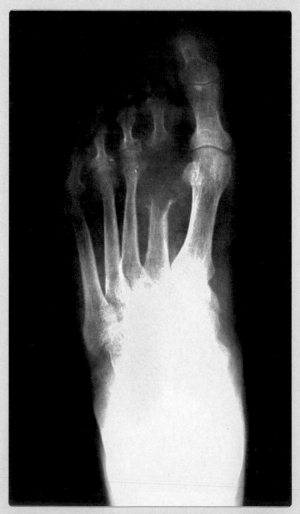

AP radiograph of the foot shows a giant cell tumor of the distal 2nd metatarsal. The destructive nature of the lesion is readily seen here.

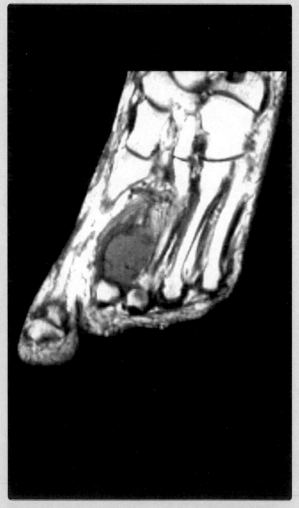

The expansile nature of the giant cell tumor is seen in this T1 MR. Resection of the distal metatarsal is often the most appropriate treatment in this setting.

CLINICAL EVALUATION

History and Physical Examination

- Retrospective analysis of missed or improperly diagnosed malignant lesions often uncovers significant clues in both the clinical history and physical examination.
- A complete physical examination must be undertaken with special attention paid to nodules, adenopathy, masses, skin changes, and local tenderness.
- Although most malignant musculoskeletal tumors metastasize to the lung, some soft tissue sarcomas go to the draining lymph nodes. A careful physical examination of both regional and systemic lymph nodes is required.
- Malignant neoplasms of the soft tissues are ~ 3-4 times more common than malignant tumors of the bone, but both are rare with soft tissue sarcoma comprising < 2% of all malignancies.

BIOPSY AND SURGICAL EXCISION

- If a diagnosis cannot be made with imaging studies, then biopsies can be performed via needle or open approach. If an open biopsy is performed, which may be preferable in the foot so as not to contaminate normal structures, a frozen section analysis should be performed to ensure that diagnostic tissue has been obtained.
- For bone tumors with a soft tissue mass, the soft tissue component is often diagnostic.
- Additional principles for performing a biopsy are as follows.
  - Use longitudinal as opposed to transverse incisions. Keep soft tissue dissection and development of tissue planes at a minimum. Avoid neurovascular planes. Close wound in layers.
  - Use the most direct approach to the lesion through, not between, compartments/muscle.
  - Submit all biopsy samples for bacteriologic analysis should frozen section fail to reveal a neoplasm.
  - Maintain meticulous hemostasis with use of a drain brought out in line with the wound if necessary.
  - Use the smallest biopsy incision that will allow adequate tissue sampling and that can be incorporated into the definitive resection.
  - Do not use Esmarch to exsanguinate if a tourniquet is used.
  - Do not biopsy Codman triangle (new subperiosteal bone that forms when a lesion, such as a tumor, lifts the periosteum away from the bone).

STAGING

Enneking

American Joint Commission on Cancer

- This is used for soft tissue sarcoma.
- The 3 most important prognostic factors are as follows.
  - Grade (most important in staging)
  - Size (> 5 cm) portends worse prognosis
  - Relationship of tumor to fascia (deep to fascia portends worse prognosis)
- In soft tissue sarcomas, almost all metastases occur to the lungs. A chest CT is obtained to stage the tumor. Bone scan is usually not necessary.

- The 5-year survival rate of high-grade soft tissue sarcoma is 50%; of all stages combined, it is 70%.
- The basic work-up of an adult patient with possible metastatic disease is a bone scan; CT scans of the chest, abdomen, and pelvis; and a biopsy of the most accessible lesion. Lesions in the foot are unlikely to be metastatic but if so are usually lung or renal carcinoma.

BONE LESIONS

Benign

- **Synovial chondromatosis**
  - Synovial chondromatosis is a benign condition that involves the synovial lining of joints, bursae, or tendon sheaths and is characterized by the development of multiple osteochondral loose bodies that are the result of metaplasia of the synovium. When it arises in the soft tissues from tendon sheaths, it is called soft tissue chondroma.
  - It is rare in the ankle and can present as tarsal tunnel syndrome. Symptoms include swelling, pain, locking, stiffness, limited joint motion, crepitus, or giving way.
  - On physical examination, an effusion may be present. There may be tenderness of the joint or pain on range of motion. The range of motion may be limited. A palpable tender mass may be present.
  - Until the loose bodies are ossified or calcified, they may be radiographically invisible. Damage to the joint from multiple loose bodies may lead to early degenerative arthritis.
  - The histologic appearance of this process shows well-defined cartilage nests embedded in a layer of synovium.
  - Treatment includes arthroscopic or open debridement of loose bodies ± a synovectomy.
  - Synovial chondromatosis is reported to be a benign, self-limited disease process, although chondrosarcoma of synovium has been described.
- **Giant cell tumor**
  - It is a benign, yet locally aggressive tumor that typically occurs in the 2nd and 3rd decades of life. Giant cell tumor of the foot is rare.
  - It is usually a metaphyseal-epiphyseal, juxtaarticular lesion found most commonly about the knee (50%), shoulder, and distal radius, although it has been reported in virtually all the foot bones.
  - It originates in the metaphysis and extends into the epiphysis following physeal closure.
  - Radiographs reveal a lytic, eccentric, expansile appearance. It typically thins out the cortex, has no internal matrix, and may have a sclerotic rim centrally.
  - It can metastasize, although < 2% metastasize to the lungs.
  - Treatment typically involves biopsy to confirm the diagnosis with intralesional curettage and mechanical burring possibly with adjuvants, such as phenol, cryosurgery, or hydrogen peroxide and subsequent packing of the resultant defect with bone graft or bone cement.
  - When a metatarsal is involved, resection may be more expeditious than reconstruction, depending on the degree of destruction and which metatarsal is involved.
- **Aneurysmal bone cyst**

- An aneurysmal bone cyst (ABC) is a solitary, expansile osteolytic lesion with a thin wall, containing blood-filled cystic cavities. Approximately 30% are secondary to preexisting bone tumors.
- ABCs occur in patients between 10-30 years of age; peak incidence is 16 years of age; 75% are < 20 years of age.
- Radiographs often have a blown out appearance with thin septations. CT and MR characteristically demonstrate multiple fluid-fluid levels within cystic spaces. ABC appears on both T1 and T2 MR images with a low-signal rim encircling the cystic lesion.
- Histology reveals cystic spaces filled with blood. Typically, the fibrous septa have immature woven bone trabeculae.
- ABCs are active lesions that destroy bone and therefore are almost always treated. Treatment consists of curettage and bone graft or, rarely, resection. Local recurrence with curettage and bone grafting can be as high as 25%.
- If a recurrence is detected, a thorough examination of the original radiographs and pathology specimens should be performed to ensure that the primary lesion, if any, is discovered, because this may alter the treatment plan. One unfortunate scenario is to biopsy an ABC, which then recurs and presumably evolves into a telangiectatic osteosarcoma. Once the precise diagnosis is known, local recurrences may be retreated by appropriate methods.

- **Unicameral bone cyst (simple bone cyst)**
  - A unicameral bone cyst (UBC) is a benign radiolucent cavity found within a bone that is filled with straw-colored fluid. It is unifocal and affects patients who are skeletally immature, most frequently in children between 5-15 years of age. The male:female ratio is 2:1.
  - The rarity of the lesion in adults supports a hypothesis of spontaneous resolution. They enlarge during skeletal growth and become inactive after skeletal maturity.
  - Proximal humerus (50%) and proximal femur (40%) account for 90% of UBCs. Less common locations include the pelvis, talus, and calcaneus.
  - Historically, location played a prognostic role. If the cyst is immediately adjacent to the physis, it is active. If it is distant from the physis, it is latent. Recurrence is high for active cysts (50%) and low for latent cysts (10%).
  - Radiographs typically reveal a central lytic metaphyseal lesion with a sclerotic rim and little to no bone expansion. MR/CT are not routinely necessary.
  - Most UBCs are asymptomatic and incidentally discovered. Lesions usually remain asymptomatic unless complicated by fracture. In contrast to ABCs, UBCs are often not treated, such as in the absence of symptoms or mechanical compromise of the involved bone.
  - Treatment should be considered for lesions that have resulted in fracture or marked weakening of bone. Spontaneous healing of a UBC may occur occasionally following fracture. Factors, such as age and lesion location, may strongly influence surgical decisions.

- **Enchondroma**

- Enchondromas are benign cartilaginous tumors of bone that present in patients of all ages. The majority are asymptomatic unless associated with a pathologic fracture. Characteristically, they are found in the intramedullary canal of the central metaphysis. Enchondromas result from failure of normal endochondral ossification below the physis.
- Common sites of involvement include the small tubular bones of the hands or feet (40-65%). With respect to the feet, it most frequently involves the diaphysis of the proximal phalanx followed by the middle phalanx and the metatarsals; it commonly spares the distal phalanx.
- Histologically, it is composed of hyaline cartilage. Radiographs reveal "speckled" or "popcorn" calcifications in this central radiolucent lesion with well-defined margins, endosteal erosion, and no aggressive features.
- The risk of malignant transformation is low: < 2% of asymptomatic solitary enchondromas transform to chondrosarcoma. In contrast, enchondromatosis, i.e., Ollier disease, has a 10-30% risk of malignant transformation. Multiple enchondromas plus soft tissue hemangiomas, known as Maffucci disease, are associated with an increased risk of astrocytoma and gastrointestinal cancer as well as a higher risk of malignant transformation to chondrosarcoma than in Ollier disease. It can be difficult to distinguish an enchondroma from a low-grade chondrosarcoma.
- Asymptomatic solitary enchondromas may be followed nonoperatively with serial radiographs. If an enchondroma becomes symptomatic or begins to enlarge, it may require biopsy to rule out malignancy; curettage and bone grafting is usually adequate for borderline lesions. Pathologic fractures are commonly allowed to heal with closed treatment followed by curettage and bone grafting to prevent refracture.

- **Osteochondroma**
  - Osteochondroma is the most common benign bone tumor. It is a developmental dysplasia of the peripheral growth plate, which forms a cartilage-capped projection of bone found near the metaphysis of long bones, pointing away from the joint. It grows via endochondral ossification of the proliferating cartilage cells and often presents as a firm, nontender, immobile mass arising near the end of a long bone.
  - It frequently occurs in the distal tibia and metatarsals. Specific to the foot and ankle, they may cause angular deformities &/or limit the range of motion of the ankle via syndesmotic impingement.
  - On radiographic analysis, it is classically continuous with the medullary canal of the underlying metaphyseal bone, growing away from the epiphysis. A cartilaginous cap of 2.0-2.5 cm or greater and growth after skeletal maturation may indicate malignant transformation.
  - They may be solitary or multiple, as seen in hereditary multiple exostoses (HMEs), an autosomal dominant condition associated with mutations in *EXT1* &/or *EXT2* genes.
  - Malignant degeneration is the most significant of potential complications. Less than 1% of solitary osteochondromas undergo malignant transformation to a low-grade, secondary chondrosarcoma. In patients with HME, the incidence is higher.

- No intervention is warranted if asymptomatic. Marginal excision of the exostosis, cartilaginous cap, and overlying perichondrium can be done if the lesion is symptomatic. If the osteochondroma continues to grow after skeletal maturity, chondrosarcoma must be ruled out with an MR to measure the thickness of the cartilage cap and to look for an associated soft tissue mass.

- **Osteoid osteoma**
  - Osteoid osteoma is a benign vascular osseous tumor, which occurs primarily in adolescents. The typical presentation is dull pain, often with increased severity at night, classically relieved by prostaglandin E2 inhibitors, such as aspirin or nonsteroidal antiinflammatory drugs (NSAIDs).
  - Most commonly, it is found in the proximal femur (femoral neck = 30% incidence). Other locations include the posterior spine (often causing painful scoliosis) and the talus, navicular, or calcaneus.
  - The pathognomonic radiographic finding is a nidus typically measuring < 1.5 cm in diameter. The nidus is best localized with CT scans with cuts set to 1.0-2.0 mm.
  - They spontaneously resolve with time, and treatment options include medical management with NSAIDs, en bloc excision or curettage, or percutaneous radiofrequency coagulation under CT guidance.

- **Osteoblastoma**
  - Osteoblastoma is a benign osseous tumor typically occurring in the 2nd and 3rd decades.
  - Osteoblastoma presents as a dull, deep pain; however, unlike osteoid osteoma, it is not nocturnal, does not improve with NSAIDs, and is progressive in nature. The size of the nidus is > 1.5 cm (vs. osteoid osteoma, which is < 1.5 cm).
  - The talar neck is the 3rd most common location after the posterior spine and long bones. They can also occur in the metatarsals
  - Treatment typically involves excision and curettage; if it is aggressive in nature, wide excision is favored. Recurrence rate following curettage and bone graft is 10-20%.

- **Chondroblastoma**
  - Chondroblastoma is considered a benign, aggressive tumor, typically occurring in the 2nd decade.
  - In the foot and ankle, the talus and calcaneus are the most frequent locations.
  - Radiographically, it is lytic; histologically, it has chicken-wire calcification and stains with S100 antibody.
  - About 2% metastasize to the lungs. Treatment is curettage and bone graft.

- **Subungual Exostosis**
  - Radiographically, subungual exostosis resembles an osteochondroma. It typically develops on the distal phalanx, most commonly on the medial aspect of the great toe in young children. It is often associated with a history of trauma.
  - Surgical excision is indicated if elevation of the nail leads to deformity &/or pain. The nail bed can usually be preserved.

Malignant

- **Acral metastases**
  - The incidence of skeletal metastasis to primary bone tumor is 25:1. Frequently, the metastatic bone lesion is found before the primary tumor, and it is occasionally mistaken for a primary bone lesion.
  - In general, bones distal to the knee and elbow are very rare sites for metastases. The majority of acral metastases (those distal to the knee or elbow) are from lung and renal carcinoma. Lung is more common than renal.
  - Many of the metastatic bone lesions are multiple, compared with primary bone tumors, which tend to be single lesions. Treatment should always involve consultation with an oncologist.

- **Osteosarcoma**
  - Osteosarcoma is the 2nd most common primary bone malignancy after myeloma. 75% occur in patients between 10-25 years old. It is associated with mutations of the *TP53* and retinoblastoma tumor suppressor genes.
  - Osteosarcoma is usually a metaphyseal tumor. In the foot and ankle, it is most commonly found in the distal tibia with reports of lesions in the metatarsals and tarsals. In a retrospective review of 52 patients with osteosarcoma of the foot by Choong et al (1999), the most common site was the calcaneus.
  - Prior to current treatment regimens, long-term survival was 20%. With present treatment protocols, the mainstay being neoadjuvant chemotherapy and surgical resection, long-term survival is 60-70%.
  - Specific to the foot and ankle, wide surgical resection in the face of close proximity of neurovascular structures can be difficult. Small tumors may be possible to resect with preservation of the foot. Larger tumors may require below-knee amputation.

- **Chondrosarcoma**
  - Chondrosarcoma is a malignant cartilage tumor typically found in patients between 40-70 years of age.
  - In the foot and ankle, this tumor is most often a malignant transformation in patients with Ollier disease or multiple hereditary exostoses.
  - Treatment involves wide excision, as radiotherapy and chemotherapy are ineffective.

- **Ewing sarcoma and peripheral primitive neuroectodermal tumors**
  - Ewing sarcoma is a rare, malignant neoplasm in the small blue round cell family of tumors that is most common in children and adolescents. The peak incidence is between 10-20 years of age. While any bone of the axial or appendicular skeleton can be affected, it has rarely been reported in the bones of hands and feet.
  - The characteristic radiologic findings includes an onion skin &/or moth-eaten appearance of the lesion. Histologically, it consists of sheets of round blue cells separated by bands of stroma. Metastases are common to lungs and other bones.

o Treatment consists of surgery and chemotherapy. Survival is highly dependent on the initial presentation of the disease. About 80% of patients present with localized disease, whereas 20% present with metastatic disease, most often to the lungs, bone, and bone marrow. The overall survival rate in patients with Ewing sarcoma is 60%; however, for patients with localized disease, it approaches 70%. If metastatic, the long-term survival rate is < 25%.

SOFT TISSUE LESIONS

Overview

- Soft tissue masses are common in the foot, and the vast majority are benign. A small number of these will be sarcomas.
- Kirby et al (1989) retrospectively examined the cases of 83 patients who had a soft tissue tumor or tumor-like lesion in the foot or ankle to determine the relative frequency of the lesions and which factors, if any, could be used to identify them preoperatively. 72 (87%) of the lesions were benign with ganglion cysts and plantar fibromatoses being the most common, while 11 (13%) were malignant tumors, 5 (45%) of which were synovial sarcomas. The gender of the patient, a traumatic history, the duration of the symptoms, the size of the lesion, and the presence of pain or of neurologic symptoms were not useful in discriminating a benign lesion from a malignant tumor.
- It is important to have a diagnosis before embarking on treatment of a soft tissue mass. Ganglions, lipomas, plantar fibromas, hemangiomas, and pigmented villonodular synovitis (PVNS) can usually be presumptively diagnosed with MR. Small masses (1-2 cm) can be primarily excised, but larger masses should be biopsied prior to removal.

Benign

- **PVNS/giant cell tumor of tendon sheath**
  - o PVNS is a proliferative disease of the synovium, which has a tendency to bleed and cause hemarthrosis and eventually destruction of a joint.
  - o It is most common in the 3rd-5th decades of life but has also occurred in the ankle in children < 10 years of age. Most series report < 5% occurrence in the foot and ankle.
  - o It may be localized (nodular) or diffuse and can occur either extraarticularly or intraarticularly. It is one cause of periarticular bone erosions.
  - o Symptoms include swelling and stiffness, arthralgia, and a "popping" feeling with movement. The symptoms usually start slowly and may come and go over time. PVNS should be considered in patients with persistent ankle pain and swelling.
  - o On gross examination, it may be nodular or globular and yellow-tan with villous growths associated with synovial membranes. Microscopic findings include hemosiderin deposits, foamy histiocytes, giant cells, and large synovial cells.
  - o MR is useful in delineating the extent of PVNS, as indicated by medium to low signal intensity lesions, often eroding bone and involving synovium of either joints or tendon sheaths.
  - o Treatment generally consists of local resection.
- **Ganglion**

- o Ganglions are mucinous-filled cysts found adjacent to a joint capsule or tendon sheath.
- o They are the most common lesions in the foot and often arise from the tarsal joints. MR can typically confirm the diagnosis.
- o Management typically consists of 3 options: Observation, aspiration, or surgical excision. Aspiration is a temporary treatment, as the recurrence rate is virtually 100%.
- o In a series of 40 patients treated with surgical excision, Rozbruch et al (1998) reported an 86% satisfaction rate and a 10% recurrence rate.
- **Fibromatosis**
  - o Fibromatosis is locally aggressive idiopathic proliferative fasciitis of the plantar aponeurosis that is often (50%) bilateral.
  - o 20% of patients with Dupuytren contracture have plantar fibromatosis. If associated with Dupuytren contractures in the hand &/or Peyronie disease, it is referred to as Lederhosen syndrome and presents as discrete plantar nodules often seen in non-weight-bearing areas (especially medial plantar).
  - o Involvement of adjacent structures is common, reflecting the infiltrative growth pattern often seen in these lesions. MR scans may show characteristic features of prominent low to intermediate signal intensity and bands of low signal intensity representing highly collagenized tissue.
  - o Nonoperative management, consisting of NSAIDs and accommodating orthotics, is the 1st line of treatment. If surgery is elected, excision must include the entire slip of the plantar fascia. Because of the aggressive nature of these fibromatoses, partial or subtotal fasciectomy results in recurrence rates nearing 60%.
- **Nerve sheath and peripheral nerve tumors**
  - o Schwannoma, neurilemmoma, or neurinoma is a benign nerve sheath tumor located within the epineurium, typically of spinal roots and superficial nerves on the flexor surfaces of extremities. It commonly affects patients between 20-60 years of age. 80% are solitary; multiple lesions have been reported and are associated with neurofibromatosis.
  - o Clinical presentation typically involves a painful mass without neurologic impairment; supportive physical examination findings include a positive Tinel sign.
  - o The schwannoma can usually be excised with preservation of nerve fascicles, unlike neurofibromas, which are more infiltrative. Neurofibromas are benign peripheral nerve tumors; 90% are solitary.
  - o Multiple lesions, called neurofibromatosis, consist of 2 types: Neurofibromatosis type 1 (von Recklinghausen disease) involves peripheral nerves; neurofibromatosis type 2 involves acoustic nerves. There is a 10% incidence of development of a malignant peripheral nerve sheath tumor in neurofibromatosis type 1. 50% of neurofibrosarcomas are the result of malignant transformation.
  - o Treatment can be resection if the neurofibroma is sufficiently symptomatic and the functional loss will be minimal, understanding the risk of a painful neuroma and the fact that, due to the intimate association with nerve fascicles, permanent injury to the nerve is likely.
- **Malignant**

- o Soft tissue sarcomas are neoplasms arising from mesenchymal tissues. The most common soft tissue sarcoma in the foot is synovial sarcoma.
- o Treatment of foot sarcomas is complicated by the relative paucity of expendable soft tissues and the need for durable skin able to withstand weight bearing. These limitations may necessitate a more frequent use of amputation than is used for soft tissue sarcoma arising more proximally in the extremity.

- **Synovial sarcoma**
  - o Synovial sarcoma is the most common malignant soft tissue mass in the foot and ankle. It most often occurs in adolescents and young adults and presents as a slowly enlarging, painless mass.
  - o It histologically resembles synovial tissue; it is usually found along fascial planes and in periarticular structures and, rarely, in joints. It is associated with gene translocation (X:18).
  - o All synovial sarcoma are considered high grade. Synovial sarcoma of the foot and ankle frequently is misdiagnosed, which leads to delays in treatment.
  - o Treatment consists of wide resection and usually radiation therapy. Chemotherapy is considered for large, deep, high-grade tumors and for those with metastatic disease. 50% metastasize to the lungs; 30% spread to regional lymph nodes. The 5-year survival rate ranges from 25-55%.

- **Clear cell sarcoma**
  - o Clear cell sarcoma of tendons and aponeuroses is a slow and progressive tumor with a poor prognosis, commonly found in young adults. It is commonly located in the extremities, specifically about and below the knee.
  - o Clear cell sarcoma and conventional malignant melanoma may demonstrate significant morphologic overlap.
  - o A balanced translocation, t(12;22)(q13;q13), has been identified in a high percentage (50-75%) of clear cell sarcomas and is presumed to be tumor specific. Treatment consists of wide local resection and radiotherapy.

- **Melanoma**
  - o Melanoma is the most common primary malignant tumor of the foot, occurring most frequently on the plantar skin. The skin and nails of the foot should be examined as part of the physical examination of the foot with particular attention to the plantar skin.
  - o Malignant melanoma may begin as a benign lesion, the dysplastic nevus. Tumor thickness is the most important prognostic factor.
  - o Treatment involves excision with a 3-cm margin and radiation therapy for those with lymph node metastases. The overall 5-year survival rate is 80%; specific to the foot and ankle, it is 63% (subungual is 16-60%).

SELECTED REFERENCES

1. Choong PF et al: Osteosarcoma of the foot: a review of 52 patients at the Mayo Clinic. Acta Orthop Scand. 70(4):361-4, 1999
2. Rozbruch SR et al: Ganglion cysts of the lower extremity: an analysis of 54 cases and review of the literature. Orthopedics. 21(2):141-8, 1998
3. Kirby EJ et al: Soft-tissue tumors and tumor-like lesions of the foot. An analysis of eighty-three cases. J Bone Joint Surg Am. 71(4):621-6, 1989

Enneking Surgical Staging System

Stage	Grade	Site and Size	Metastasis
IA	Low	Intracompartmental	None
IB	Low	Extracompartmental	None
IIA	High	Intracompartmental	None
IIB	High	Extracompartmental	None
III	Any	Any	Yes

Enneking system is used for bone tumors specifically. Most tumors will metastasize to the lung, although 5-10% do not. Therefore, a chest CT and total body bone scan are necessary for staging.

Types of Surgical Margins

Margin	Definition	Local Recurrence Rate
Intralesional	Dissection plane directly through tumor	100%
Marginal	Dissection plane through reactive zone of tumor	25-50%
Wide	Dissection through cuff of normal tissue	25% but < 10% if radiation therapy is used for soft tissue sarcoma or chemotherapy for bone sarcomas
Radical	Entire compartment containing tumor is resected	Nearly 0%

In practice, intralesional surgery is used for benign bone tumors; marginal surgery is used for benign bone and soft tissue tumors; wide margins are used for bone and soft tissue sarcomas; and radical surgery is of historical interest, except in the foot, since below-knee amputation is still performed for sarcoma.

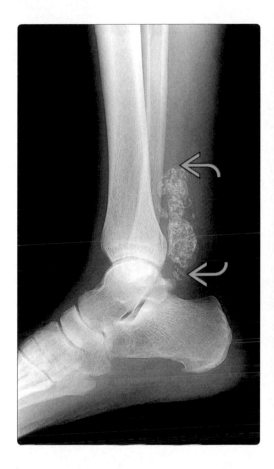

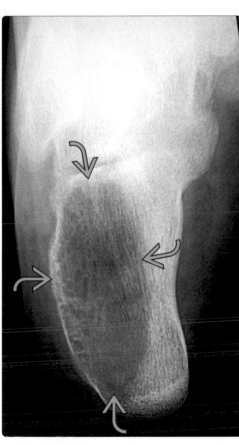

(Left) *Synovial chondromatosis of the ankle is seen here. The lesions are often not visible on x-ray until they become ossified. Here, they have become ossified and are clearly seen extending posteriorly ⇗ out of the ankle joint.* **(Right)** *This cyst is perhaps seen most readily on this axial Harris heel view. The expansile nature of the lesion can be seen here, given the lateral cortical thinning ⇗. The cyst has filled up much of the body of the calcaneus; the risk of a pathologic fracture is even more readily apparent in this setting.*

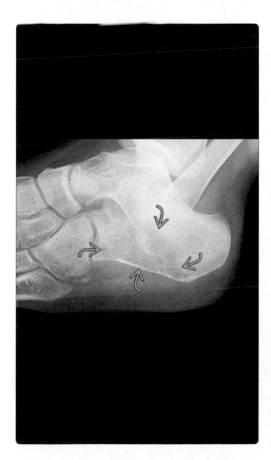

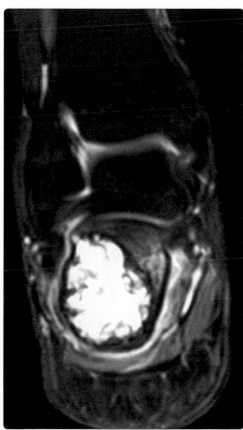

(Left) *An aneurysmal bone cyst is seen in the calcaneus. Note the borders ⇗ of the cyst extending from the midbody to the calcaneocuboid joint laterally and close to the subtalar joint superiorly. Pathologic fracture can readily occur in these cysts.* **(Right)** *The fluid-filled nature of the cyst is readily apparent on this T2 image with fluid density throughout the cyst. The cyst is taking up most of the cross-sectional area of the calcaneus in this image, and the remaining, normal calcaneus demonstrates some edema.*

(Left) *AP view of the foot shows an enchondroma of the distal 2nd metatarsal. They can be common in the phalanges as well as in the hand. Pathologic fracture can occur given the expansile nature of the lesions.* **(Right)** *This patient had significant night pain alleviated by nonsteroidal antiinflammatory drugs. The x-ray shows some abnormality at the central plafond, consistent with an osteoid osteoma. Radiofrequency ablation is the treatment of choice for this bony pathology.*

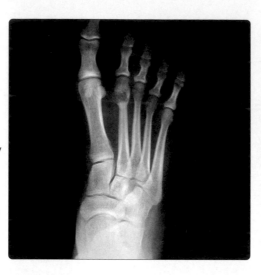
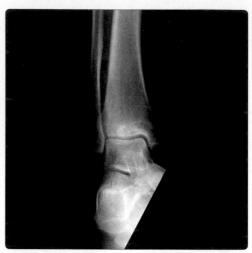

(Left) *The left ankle shows intense focal uptake at the anterior plafond, consistent with the area of abnormality on the x-ray. Radiofrequency ablation was used to address this osteoid osteoma with complete resolution of symptoms.* **(Right)** *Sagittal MR shows a subchondral cyst secondary to pigmented villonodular synovitis (PVNS). Notice the ankle effusion that is also present. PVNS can cause a large effusion in the ankle.*

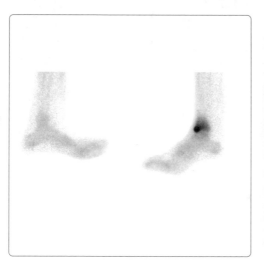
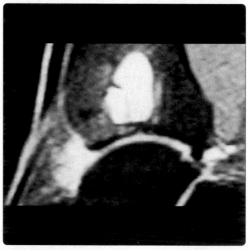

(Left) *This illustration shows a unicameral bone cyst ➔, albeit in the proximal humerus. The cystic cavitation is well demarcated with cortical thinning and mild expansion. The lesions usually contain a clear, serous-like fluid.* **(Right)** *Lateral radiograph shows a lytic lesion in the calcaneal neck. The calcaneus is one of the most common locations of unicameral bone cysts in adults. A paucity of trabeculae in this region, as an anatomic variant, can mimic a bone cyst.*

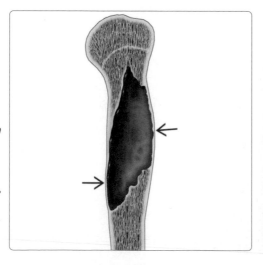
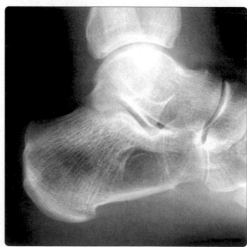

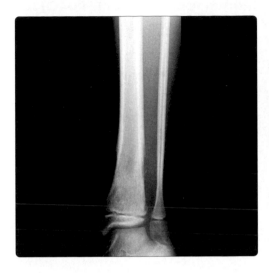
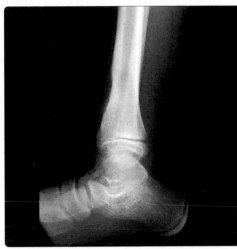

(Left) This skeletally immature patient has metaphyseal and metadiaphyseal abnormality on this AP image. (Right) Ewing sarcoma of the distal tibia is seen here. This patient ultimately underwent limb salvage surgery with resection of the distal tibia and allograft reconstruction.

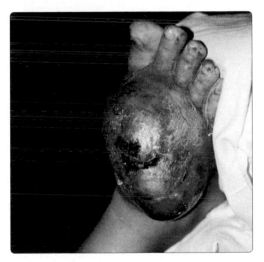
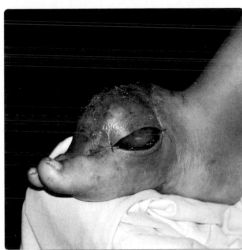

(Left) Dorsal mass of the foot is seen at a significantly advanced stage. This patient had a synovial sarcoma and required amputation. (Right) A lateral view of the foot is seen here, showing just how large and advanced this mass was.

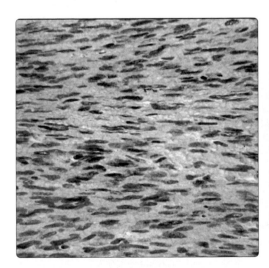
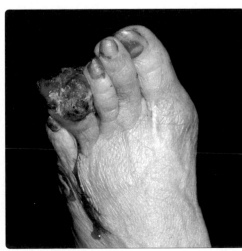

(Left) Slide shows the monophasic spindle cell appearance typical for synovial cell sarcoma. (Right) Melanoma is the most common primary malignant tumor of the foot. This tumor obviously presents at an advanced stage with a significantly exophytic lesion.

KEY FACTS

GENERAL

- Amputation and disarticulation should be viewed as reconstructive procedures and not a failure of treatment.
  - In this manner, one realizes that it is the initial step in getting patients back to their previous functional status.
- Indications for amputation include ischemia, trauma, infection, tumor, and painful dysfunction of the foot and ankle not amenable to further conservative management.
- The goal is to create a modified limb that has a comfortable interface with a prosthesis and offers the most efficient energy-conserving gait as possible.
- A team effort, with a team composed of different medical specialists, is the best way to ensure a good result and restore patients to their optimal level of function.
- It is important to be aware of the psychosocial recovery of the patient with an amputation.
- Functional outcome is generally worse in patients with diabetes or end-stage renal disease.

IMPORTANT POINTS FOR SURGICAL APPROACH TO AMPUTATION

- Team assessment
- Atraumatic soft tissue handling
- Adequate skin flaps
- Myodesis or myoplasty whenever possible
- Nerve transection sharp and at level well above amputation
- Artery and vein dissected free and double ligated
- Closure without tension
- No "dog ear" resection
- Accept delayed primary closure if there is tension

(Left) *USA amputation statistics by cause is shown. [From Adams PF et al. (1999) Current estimates from the National Health Interview Survey, 1996. Vital Health Stat 10: 200.]* (Right) *Myodesis consists of suturing the transected muscle to the bone through drill holes.*

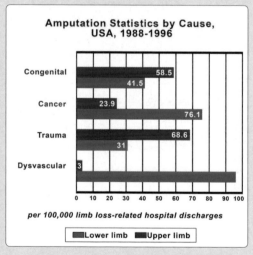

Amputation Statistics by Cause, USA, 1988-1996

Cause	Lower limb	Upper limb
Congenital	58.5	41.5
Cancer	23.9	76.1
Trauma	68.6	31
Dysvascular		3

per 100,000 limb loss-related hospital discharges

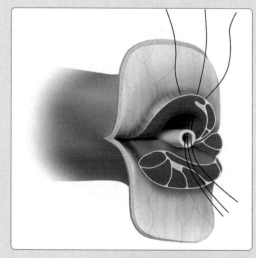

(Left) *The cut ends of antagonistic muscle groups and their fascias are sewn together for myoplasty.* (Right) *Equivalent-length dorsal and plantar full-thickness fish mouth-type skin flaps should be created, thus favoring the tougher plantar skin for the end of the stump.*

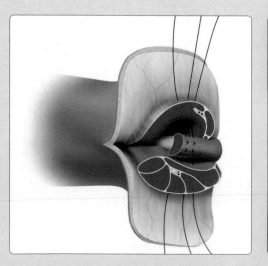

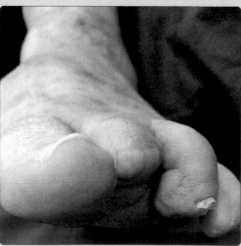

INDICATIONS

Peripheral Vascular Disease

- Peripheral vascular disease (PVD) is the most common reason for amputation.
  - Affects mainly geriatric patients and those with diabetes mellitus.
- Up to 20% of patients with diabetes mellitus will suffer from PVD.
  - Patients are prone to develop foot ulcers leading to lower extremity amputation.
- Peripheral neuropathy increases risk of complications.
  - Loss of protective sensation compromises the likelihood of healing ulcers.
- Prior to considering amputation, vascular studies are useful to determine the following:
  - Possibility of revascularization
  - Level of amputation
- 25% of diabetics who undergo amputation will require an amputation on the contralateral limb within the following 3 years.
- Because of the medical complexity of these patients, optimal management is multidisciplinary with a team composed of a primary care physician, internist, surgeon, physiatrist, physical therapist, prosthetist, and social worker.
  - The input of an infectious diseases specialist may also be required.
- PVD accounts for 90% of amputations with 97% of dysvascular amputations performed on the lower limb.
- African American males are at greatest risk for dysvascular amputation.
  - They are 2-4x more likely to lose a limb than white persons of similar age and gender.
- In amputees with PVD, the 5-year survival rate is between 70-90% with heart disease as the leading cause of death (51%).
  - This is possibly because the coronary heart vessels are subject to the same occlusions as the peripheral arteries.
- Approximately 50% of dysvascular amputees are diabetic.

Civilian Trauma

- Several well-established scoring systems have been developed to help in arriving at a decision to perform an immediate amputation following lower extremity trauma.
- A commonly used scoring system is the Mangled Extremity Severity Score, which consists of 4 categories: Skeletal/soft tissue injury, limb ischemia, shock, and age.
  - A lower number of points indicates a less severe injury.
  - A total score of 7 or below is almost always compatible with limb salvage.
- It is felt by some that soft tissue injury severity has the greatest impact on decision-making regarding limb salvage vs. amputation.
- There are several other proposed limb salvage scoring systems.
- While they may provide guidance for a treating surgeon, none of the scoring systems are considered very reliable in predicting need for amputation.
- In cases of severe limb damage, primary amputation at first surgery may be best for the patient's physical and psychologic well-being.

- In other cases, it may be better to plan an initial attempt at limb salvage and observe.
  - Prolonged attempts at limb salvage lead to severe psychologic and economic burdens on the patient and the family.
- If it is thought that amputation is inevitable, it should be performed as a delayed primary amputation within the first 10-14 days after injury.
- Almost 70% of trauma-related amputations are upper limb amputation.
- The most common causes of lower extremity trauma requiring amputation are lawn mower injuries and motorcycle accidents.
- Traumatic amputees have a better functional prognosis than dysvascular amputees.

Military Trauma

- The changing nature of military conflicts over the past few decades has lead to an increasing number of blast injuries.
  - A mangled extremity is a common combat injury.
- While advances have been made in limb salvage of complex injuries, amputation sometimes offers the best outcome.
- In several studies of wounded soldiers, immediate and delayed lower extremity amputation patients generally have better functional outcomes compared to limb salvage, both physically and psychologically.
  - This is not true for every patient but rather represents a trend for the groups as a whole.
  - Individual decisions are made based on the extent of injury, the experience of the surgeon, and the capabilities of the health care system.
  - Immediate amputation may be necessary for a critically ill patient in a combat zone, whereas the same injury in a stable patient at a tertiary center may be offered limb salvage.

Malignancies

- The most common malignant tumor found in the region of the foot and ankle is synovial sarcoma.
- While metastases to the feet are uncommon, any cancer can metastasize to bone, and any bone can be involved.
- The most common primary tumors that metastasize to the feet are as follows:
  - Carcinoma of lung
  - Adenocarcinoma of colon
  - Genitourinary carcinoma
  - Melanoma
  - Other undifferentiated tumors
- The development of limb salvage procedures, combined with chemotherapy, has reduced the incidence of amputation for primary malignancies of the lower extremity.

Infection

- Life-threatening infection of the lower extremity requires an open amputation.
  - The stump can be closed only when it is certain that the infectious process is under control.
- In some circumstances, repeated debridement and lavage in the operating room is required until the stump is clear of infection and necrotic tissue.

- Chronic osteomyelitis is not an absolute indication for amputation.
  - It can be managed with good preoperative planning and selective surgery, including fistulectomy, sequestrectomy, and similar less invasive procedures.
  - Plastic surgery is often required for coverage of soft tissue defects.
- The ultimate function of the salvaged limb should justify the physical and psychologic costs of the treatment.
- Recurrent infection points to the possibility of PVD.
  - It prevents adequate perfusion of the infected area.
    - Decreased efficacy of antibiotic therapy
- Recurrent infection is common in patients with diminished protective sensation combined with bony deformities leading to abnormal pressure points and recurrent ulcers.
  - Charcot neuroarthropathy involving the foot and ankle is a major cause of recurrent infection.

Dysfunctional Limb

- Painful dysfunction of the limb following several attempts at reconstruction is a rare indication for amputation.
  - A classic example might be a young patient with severe collapse of the talus with avascular necrosis following trauma.
  - If the patient wants to run distances, he or she is more likely to achieve that goal with a transtibial amputation than a pantalar fusion.
- In some cases, consultation with a pain management specialist and a psychiatrist is helpful.
- With the correct indication, a well-healed stump, and a properly fitted prosthesis, many patients with painful dysfunction of the limb will benefit from amputation and regain excellent function with significant pain relief.
- The most common level of amputation for a dysfunctional foot and ankle is a long transtibial amputation, provided that the soft tissues forming the stump are healthy.
- A well-functioning transtibial amputation in a healthy young person will lead to better function than a multiply fused foot and ankle (such as a pantalar fusion).

LEVEL OF AMPUTATION

- Determining the appropriate level of amputation or disarticulation is the most important, and probably the most difficult, part in the treatment of a patient who has no hope for limb preservation.
- If the indication for amputation is a malignant tumor, a life-threatening infection, or an irreparably damaged body part, then the level of amputation must be done proximal to the lesion, in healthy tissues.
- If amputation is performed for PVD, a thorough evaluation of arterial blood flow is essential.
  - Forefoot and toe blood pressure obtained using Doppler devices are of limited value.
    - Artificially high values may be obtained from heavily calcified, hence incompressible, vessels.
- Transcutaneous oxygen measurements (tc$P$o2) can assist in evaluating tissue oxygenation to the dorsal distal metatarsal level.
  - Greater than 30-40 mm Hg indicates wound healing is likely.
  - Less than 20 mm Hg indicates wound healing is unlikely to occur at that level.
- Hyperbaric oxygen chamber therapy with 100% oxygen at 2.5 atm may help wound healing for those patients who are able to increase their tc$P$o2 to 40 mm Hg under the administration of 100% normal baric oxygen via a snugly fitting mask for 20 minutes.
- The presence of palpable pulses does not guarantee healing of the stump.
  - The patient may have heavily calcified arteries or poor peripheral blood distribution due to microangiopathy.
- The presence of hair on the leg or the dorsum of the foot is a positive sign for adequate skin perfusion and secondary wound healing.
- The presence of a thermal gradient from proximal to distal, as well as skin trophic changes, is a clinical sign of poor vascular supply to the soft tissue envelope.
- Lack of protective sensation by itself should not be a factor in considering a more proximal amputation level.
- There is a 2.5x higher complication rate of infection and reamputation in patients who continue to smoke after amputation.
- Platelet function and fibrinogen levels require ~ 1 week of smoking cessation to return to normal levels.
- Perfusion should be optimized by avoidance of vasoconstrictors, such as nicotine and caffeine.
- Serum albumin level below 3.0 g/dL, total lymphocyte count < 1500/mm³, and poor glucose control in patients with diabetes (Hb A1-C > 7% or 8%) significantly decrease wound-healing potential.
- Partial foot amputation is associated with major advantages over higher amputation levels, including:
  - Preservation of weight bearing
  - Improved proprioceptive function
  - Decreased disruption of body image
  - In addition, requires only shoe modifications or limited prosthesis
    - Especially true in older patients or those with diabetes
- A determined effort should be made to save maximum length to enhance function.
  - At the same time, the likelihood of healing should be sufficiently high to avoid the need for repeat surgery.
- In cases of peripheral ischemia secondary to frostbite, vasoconstrictor administration for hypotension, and cryoglobulinemia, it is essential to allow time for completion of tissue demarcation and to keep the necrotic areas dry.
  - In many cases, maximum tissue preservation can be achieved by allowing autoamputation of the necrotic portions.
  - No urgent surgery should be done until the necrotic tissues are well demarcated and the ischemic wounds are dry.
- A contracted knee despite intensive physical therapy is an indication for a knee disarticulation instead of a transtibial amputation.
  - The prosthesis can only partially compensate for the lack of extension of the knee, thus making ambulation challenging.
- A nonambulatory patient requires a level of amputation that will ensure the best chance of healing whenever a lower level might be questionable.

- Split skin grafts should be avoided, especially on surfaces that experience significant shear forces, such as at the end of the stump, where they may ulcerate.
  - In younger children, there will be more remodeling of the soft tissues, and simple skin grafts may be more successful.
- Patients with significant gangrenous changes of the heel pad should have a transtibial amputation.

PHYSIOLOGY OF AMPUTATION: ENERGY EXPENDITURE

- The metabolic demands of walking are increased by the following factors.
  - Decreasing residual limb length
  - Increasing number of amputated joints
  - Increasing number of amputated limbs
  - Dysvascular amputation
- The rates of metabolic energy expenditure ($VO2$, mL/kg per minute) at various amputation levels were compared with those of nonamputees, demonstrating the increased metabolic costs.

SURGICAL TECHNIQUE

- A well-planned amputation or disarticulation conserves all tissue possible according to the diagnosis and good function.
- The skin is the most important tissue for the healing of the amputation wound.
  - It therefore must be handled very carefully with the use of skin hooks.
- The transected muscles should provide an adequate soft tissue mantle for the residual extremity.
- The soft tissue envelope must be mobile, because it will absorb the normal and indirect shear forces during prosthetic usage.
- Myodesis consists of suturing the transected muscle to the bone through drill holes.
- Myoplasty refers to the suturing of the cut ends of the antagonistic muscle groups and their fascias together.
- Bony prominences, such as sharp edges and corners, must be removed and the cut surfaces properly contoured to prevent damage to the soft tissue envelope.
- All transected nerves develop a neuroma, which is painless in the vast majority of patients.
- Neuromas within the weight-bearing area can become painful.
  - Each nerve must be dissected free and sharply transected at a level well above the level of amputation.
- Arteries and veins must be dissected free and doubly ligated before transection.
  - They must be independently ligated in order to prevent the development of an aneurysm or arterial venous fistula.
- Split-thickness grafts may be used occasionally but only over soft tissues and not placed over bone or thick scars.
- Skin grafts are more successful in children than in adults.
- During wound closure, the flaps are trimmed to fit without tension.

SPECIFIC LEVELS OF AMPUTATION AND DISARTICULATION

Toe Amputation or Disarticulation

- Before considering toe amputation, it is essential that the midfoot is sufficiently vascularized to allow for healing of the surgical wound.
  - The tcPo2 is measured at the level of the midfoot.
    - Should never be < 20 mm Hg
    - And ideally > 30 mm Hg
- If more than 1 toe requires amputation in a vascular patient, one should consider performing a transmetatarsal amputation.
- Whenever possible, it is advisable to save the proximal phalanx of the 1st ray.
  - This helps with balance, putting on a shoe, and results in a better gait than after disarticulation at the metatarsophalangeal joint with its accompanying loss of the sesamoids and the flexor hallucis complex.
- Equivalent length dorsal and plantar full-thickness fish mouth-type skin flaps should be created, thus favoring the tougher plantar skin for the end of the stump.
- Extensor and flexor tendons should be transected and allowed to retract.
- "Dog ears" should not be resected, as they will retract and assume a smooth contour.

Ray Resection of Foot

- The most common indication for medial ray amputation is septic arthritis or osteomyelitis secondary to a penetrating ulcer under the 1st metatarsal head.
- First-ray amputation should be as limited as possible for effective orthotic restoration of the medial arch.
  - In 1st metatarsophalangeal joint septic arthritis with a viable great toe, the joint alone can be removed through a medial longitudinal incision.
- The cut 1st metatarsal should be beveled on its plantar and medial aspects to avoid a high-pressure area and permit appropriate fitting of shoes.
- If the length of the 1st metatarsal is too short due to excessive resection, a planovalgus position of the foot may occur secondary to loss of medial column support.
- Both strength and gait can be seriously impaired because of a too short 1st-ray amputation.
- Provided that there is good vascularity on the dorsum of the foot, other single ray amputations are feasible.
- Resection may be carried out through the proximal metaphysis, where the involved ray intersects with the adjacent metatarsals.
- It is not recommended to resect 2 or more central rays.
- If necessary, the 5th metatarsal should be transected obliquely.

Transmetatarsal Amputation

- Transmetatarsal amputation should be considered when:
  - When most or all of 1st metatarsal must be removed
  - If 2 or more medial rays must be amputated
  - If more than 1 central ray must be amputated
- It is the most proximal amputation where patients are able to walk with an almost physiological gait.
  - All the tendons that attach to the midfoot base of the metatarsals are left intact.

- Achilles tendon lengthening or gastrocnemius recession is recommended to further decrease distal plantar pressures.
- The longer the length of the shaft of the metatarsal, the better the function.
- Distal coverage of the metatarsal shafts with a durable plantar flap is of utmost importance.
- To achieve maximum length, the transverse plantar incision is made at the base of the toes.
  - The dorsal incision is made 3-5 mm distal to the metatarsal cuts.
- Metatarsal cuts must be performed in an elliptic manner.
  - Start with the 1st metatarsal and remove as little bone as possible.
  - Lesser metatarsals should be cut roughly perpendicular to the shaft axis.
- Metatarsal shafts should be beveled on the plantar surface to decrease distal plantar pressures.
- Postoperative care includes a well-padded cast with the foot plantigrade or slightly dorsiflexed to prevent equinus.
  - Regular cast changes are needed until the wound is well healed.
  - Change cast to shoe with filler and stiff rocker sole at ~ 6 weeks.
    - When wound is healed

Metatarsal Disarticulation (Lisfranc)

- The indications for amputation at the level of the Lisfranc joint are limited.
  - Trauma and selected cases of foot tumors are the main indications.
- The foot becomes unbalanced because of the loss of forefoot lever and the massive triceps surae overpowering the relatively weaker dorsiflexors.
  - This leads to an equinus contracture.
- Transfer of the distal insertion of the peroneus longus and the tibialis anterior to the medial cuneiform, and leaving a portion of the base of the 5th metatarsal to preserve the insertion of the peroneus brevis tendon, will improve residual foot balance.
- Preservation of the base of the 2nd metatarsal helps maintain the proximal transverse arch.
- Percutaneous Achilles tendon lengthening is recommended to weaken the triceps surae relative to the ankle dorsiflexors.
- Compared with a transmetatarsal amputation, the Lisfranc disarticulation results in a major loss of forefoot length.
  - It correlates with impaired barefoot walking.
- Postoperative care includes a well-padded cast with the foot plantigrade or slightly dorsiflexed to prevent equinus.
  - Regular cast changes are needed until the wound is well healed.
  - Change to shoe with filler and stiff rocker sole at 6 weeks.

Midtarsal Disarticulation (Chopart)

- The disarticulation is performed through the talonavicular and calcaneocuboid joints.
- Even more so than with the Lisfranc disarticulation, the stump has a tendency to develop an equinus posture over time because of severe muscle imbalance between dorsiflexor and plantar flexor muscles.

- The tendency to develop an equinus posture is even greater than with the Lisfranc disarticulation.
  - This occurs due to severe muscle imbalance between dorsiflexor and plantar flexor muscles.
    - Leads to pain &/or ulceration
- The tibialis anterior and long extensor tendons must be inserted into or around the talar neck in order to balance the foot in the sagittal plane.
  - An Achilles tendon lengthening or even complete tenotomy is needed to prevent equinus.
- The main advantage over a more proximal amputation level is that it allows end bearing and does not sacrifice leg length.
- In some cases, it requires only a filler in a regular shoe.
- In the more active patient, however, a formal prosthesis (with a sleeve around the calf) is required because the shoe is unstable.
- Postoperative care should include a well-padded cast in neutral to slight dorsiflexion.
  - At 6 weeks, change to a close-fitting rigid ankle prosthesis/orthosis plus shoe with rigid rocker sole.

Syme Ankle Disarticulation

- Originally described in 1843 by James Syme, it provides an end-bearing stump that allows ambulation without prosthesis over short distances.
  - The heel pad is preserved.
  - It requires a patent posterior tibialis artery.
    - Main source of flow to heel pad
- The limb will be ~ 4-6 cm shorter than the opposite leg.
- Contraindications include the following:
  - Infection or severe traumatic damage to heel pad
  - Inadequate blood flow to heel pad
  - Uncompensated congestive heart failure with pedal and heel edema
  - Psychosis
  - Patient noncompliance
- In the presence of severe foot trauma or infection, a 2-stage amputation is recommended.
  - The wound is initially left open.
  - The viability of the heel flap is established prior to the definitive wound closure.
- Excellent amputation for children, because it preserves the physes at the distal end of the tibia and fibula.
  - About 70% of children with a Syme amputation will participate in sports.
- This level of disarticulation is more energy efficient than a transtibial level.
  - About 70% of adults will be able to return to work.
- The presence of an insensate heel is not a contraindication to a Syme ankle disarticulation.
- Take care to preserve the posterior tibial neurovascular bundle and the integrity of the fat-filled fibrous chambers of the heel pad.
- Iatrogenic disruption of the heel pad during dissection will lead to heel pad atrophy and a dysfunctional weight-bearing stump over time.
  - Heel pad provides shock absorption on heel strike.
  - Bruising of the posterior tibial vessels may lead to thrombosis and loss of the heel pad.

- Before closure, the interior of the heel pad must be carefully palpated for flakes of residual cortical bone.
  - It must be removed to avoid painful bony growth.
- At closure, the heel pad flap must be perfectly centered under the leg and secured to the anterior tibial cortex by suturing the plantar fascia through drill holes.
- Never trim the redundant tissue ("dog ears").
  - It provides vascularity to the distal part of the flap.
- Patients will need a below-knee prosthesis.
  - This can be a molded plastic socket with a removable medial window through which the stump is inserted or a similar type of prosthesis, to which a foot unit is attached.
- Removal of the calcaneus from the heel pad creates a large empty space, and a drain should be inserted to prevent the formation of a large hematoma.
  - It is removed 2 days postoperatively.
- Postoperative care should include a carefully molded cast placing the heel pad in a slightly forward and centered position.
  - Weekly cast changes are performed until the wound is well healed at ~ 4-5 weeks.
  - A temporary prosthesis is then fitted with a walking heel cast, which is changed every 2 weeks (or whenever loose).
  - Final prosthetic application is performed once the limb volume has stabilized.
- There is an alternative to a Syme level for the rare patient with just a bit more soft tissue: Pirogoff procedure.
  - In the Pirogoff procedure, the talus is removed.
  - The anterior process of the calcaneus is transected and removed as well.
  - The distal tibia is cut flat to expose cancellous bone with minimal bone resection.
  - The calcaneal tuberosity is fused to the distal tibia.
    - Preserves more length than Syme procedure but requires ~ 6 weeks of non-weight bearing for fusion

Transtibial Amputation

- As compared with more distal levels of amputation, the following holds true:
  - End weight bearing is no longer possible.
  - Walking will not be feasible without a prosthesis.
- In comparison with a higher level of amputation, the knee joint is preserved.
  - This facilitates ambulation, balance, and walking pace changes.
  - It also decreases the energy expenditure involved in ambulation.
- The ideal length of the bone stump is between 12-17 cm below the joint line of the knee.
  - Shorter stumps up to the insertion of the patellar tendon may still present some benefit to the patient.
- It is the quality of the soft tissue envelope that will determine the length of the stump.
- Careful inspection and clinical evaluation, including tcPo2 measurements, are required.
- Biomechanically, a longer stump provides a better lever arm and hence improved function.
  - However, there is less soft tissue distally to adequately cover the bony stump.

- This can lead to pressure sores, chronic ulceration, and challenging prosthetic fitting.
- Some residual length is necessary to accommodate the pylon and the foot/ankle prosthetic unit.
- Approximately 90% of transtibial amputees successfully use a prosthesis, compared with a rate of < 25% of geriatric dysvascular transfemoral amputation patients.
- The shortest useful transtibial amputation must include the tibial tubercle to preserve knee extension.
- In a very short transtibial amputation, the fibular head and neck should be removed and the common peroneal nerve transected high above the knee.
  - Knee flexion during this maneuver may help achieve a higher transection of the nerve.
- Flap configuration is determined by the soft tissue envelope.
  - Equal anterior-posterior, medial-lateral, or long posterior flaps may all be good options as long as they allow myodesis to the tibia to prevent adherence of skin to bone and to provide good padding.
- Amputation with a long posterior flap, as popularized by Burgess (1971), is most desirable in patients with vascular disease.
  - It leaves the patient with a scar on the anterior aspect of the residual limb.
  - Due to the thick myofasciocutaneous flap, there is very little risk of soft tissue problem at the end of the stump.
- The anterior distal aspect of the tibia must be carefully beveled, removing a significant portion of bone.
- The fibula must be transected 1.5 cm proximal to the level of the tibial transection.
- A knee contracture > 15° that does not respond to intensive physical therapy in a patient with limited ambulatory function is a contraindication to transtibial amputation.
- Postoperative care should include a carefully molded cast extending proximally to the mid- or upper thigh in extension to avoid hamstring contractures.
  - A good supracondylar mold to prevent cast slippage is helpful.
    - Or waist band and suspension strap may be used.
  - After 5-7 days, the cast may be changed to a prosthetic cast if wounds are healed.
  - Serial prosthetic casts should be placed every 7-10 days, or whenever loose, until stump maturity (6-8 weeks).
  - At this time, the transition can be made to a preparatory or definitive prosthesis (requiring fitting).

Knee Disarticulation

- Knee disarticulation allows for end weight bearing through the end of the stump (in a prosthesis).
- Compared with a transfemoral amputation, it maintains a long active lever arm for control of the prosthesis with excellent muscle attachments.
  - The bulbous distal stump enhances suspension (of the prosthesis).
- The prosthesis is end bearing, which avoids the need for the ischial pressure and suspension belts that transfemoral amputation requires.
- In the nonambulatory patient, it provides better balance for wheelchair activities and prevents hip flexion contractures, as compared with transfemoral amputation.

- The skin incisions are not much more proximal than those of a short transtibial amputation.
  - Therefore, before deciding to perform a knee disarticulation, one must be sure that a short transtibial amputation is not indicated.
- Prosthesis tolerance, compliance, and comfort are significantly higher than in those patients with a transfemoral amputation.
- In the past, there have been some concerns with regard to the difference in height of the knee joints between the sound limb and the disarticulated limb.
  - However, with recent prosthetic technologies, this is not an issue sufficient to deny its numerous advantages over a transfemoral amputation.
- The cruciate ligaments are detached from the tibia and retained for suturing to the patellar tendon without pulling the patella over the end of the femur.
- Bone excision is not required, nor is it necessary to remove articular cartilage.
- Medial and lateral sagittal flaps, with an incision extending from distal to posterior, allow the final suture line to stay posterior between the femoral condyles.
  - This eliminates a surgical scar at the end of the stump in the weight-bearing area.
- A method of closure with use of the posterior calf skin and gastrocnemius muscle bellies, as an integral flap has been described with good results.
- Postoperatively, a soft dressing or rigid cast should be applied depending on weight-bearing goals.
  - Casts should be molded in a similar fashion to those in transtibial amputation in order to avoid slippage.
    - Often require suspension belt
  - Once wounds are fully healed, transition to a prosthesis for weight bearing can begin.
    - Serial fittings in 7- to 10-day increments until stump maturity

Transfemoral Amputation

- Transfemoral amputation is associated with a high degree of disability.
- Prosthetic compliance is low in the geriatric population.
  - Most elderly patients do not wear their prosthesis and will remain in a wheelchair.
- Energy expenditure is high and makes ambulation difficult in patients with associated comorbidities, such as cardiopulmonary illnesses.
- Body image is negatively affected to the degree that some patients may become severely depressed.
- In particular, patients undergoing transfemoral amputation will greatly benefit from a multidisciplinary team approach aiming at improving their physical, psychologic, and social outcome.
- Healing is generally very good due to the large amount of soft tissue and rich vascular perfusion in the thigh, even in patients with vascular disease.
- Transfemoral amputation has been the most commonly used amputation level for vascular disease, because of its reliable healing rate.
  - This should no longer be the case in developed countries.

- Patients may benefit from peripheral vascular surgery and objective assessment of skin perfusion through multilevel measurements.
- The technique of transfemoral amputation has evolved over the past decade.
  - Maintenance of the femoral shaft axis close to normal can be achieved by preservation of the adductor magnus and by myodesis of the muscle to the residual femur.
- The 2nd most common complication (after phantom limb pain) is a flexion and abduction contracture of the hip.
  - This will interfere with ambulation and prosthetic fitting.
  - Good surgical technique using myodesis of the adductors and myoplasty of hamstrings to quadriceps, as well as early postoperative physical therapy, will minimize this complication.
- Postoperative care is similar to that of knee disarticulation.

SELECTED REFERENCES

1. Browner BD et al: Amputations in trauma. In Skeletal trauma : basic science, management, and reconstruction. Philadelphia, PA: Elsevier/Saunders. 2613-14, 2015
2. Dillingham TR et al: Limb amputation and limb deficiency: epidemiology and recent trends in the United States. South Med J. 95(8):875-83, 2002
3. MacKenzie EJ et al: Factors influencing the decision to amputate or reconstruct after high-energy lower extremity trauma. J Trauma. 52(4):641-9, 2002
4. Bosse MJ et al: A prospective evaluation of the clinical utility of the lower-extremity injury-severity scores. J Bone Joint Surg Am. 83-A(1):3-14, 2001
5. Bowker JH et al: North American experience with knee disarticulation with use of a posterior myofasciocutaneous flap. Healing rate and functional results in seventy-seven patients. J Bone Joint Surg Am. 82-A(11):1571-4, 2000
6. Myerson M et al: Amputations and disarticulations. In Foot and ankle disorders. Philadelphia: Saunders. 486, 2000
7. Adams PF et al: Current estimates from the National Health Interview Survey, 1996. Vital Health Stat 10. 1-203, 1999
8. Fitzpatrick MC: The psychologic assessment and psychosocial recovery of the patient with an amputation. Clin Orthop Relat Res. 98-107, 1999
9. Gottschalk F: Transfemoral amputation. Biomechanics and surgery. Clin Orthop Relat Res. 15-22, 1999
10. Czerniecki JM: Rehabilitation in limb deficiency. 1. Gait and motion analysis. Arch Phys Med Rehabil. 77(3 Suppl):S3-8, 1996
11. Brakora MJ et al: Hyperbaric oxygen therapy for diabetic wounds. Clin Podiatr Med Surg. 12(1):105-17, 1995
12. McNamara MG et al: Severe open fractures of the lower extremity: a retrospective evaluation of the Mangled Extremity Severity Score (MESS) J Orthop Trauma. 8(2):81-7, 1994
13. Bowker JH et al: The energy expenditure of amputee gait. In Atlas of limb prosthetics : surgical, prosthetic, and rehabilitation principles. St. Louis: Mosby Year Book. 381-7 1992
14. Lind J et al: The influence of smoking on complications after primary amputations of the lower extremity. Clin Orthop Relat Res. 211-7, 1991
15. Pecoraro RE et al: Chronology and determinants of tissue repair in diabetic lower-extremity ulcers. Diabetes. 40(10):1305-13, 1991
16. Russell WL et al: Limb salvage versus traumatic amputation. A decision based on a seven-part predictive index. Ann Surg. 213(5):473-80; discussion 480-1, 1991
17. Helfet DL et al: Limb salvage versus amputation. Preliminary results of the Mangled Extremity Severity Score. Clin Orthop Relat Res. 80-6, 1990
18. Johansen K et al: Objective criteria accurately predict amputation following lower extremity trauma. J Trauma. 30(5):568-72; discussion 572-3, 1990
19. Howe HR Jr et al: Salvage of lower extremities following combined orthopedic and vascular trauma. A predictive salvage index. Am Surg. 53(4):205-8, 1987
20. Gregory RT et al: The mangled extremity syndrome (M.E.S.): a severity grading system for multisystem injury of the extremity. J Trauma. 25(12):1147-50, 1985
21. Burgess EM et al: Amputations of the leg for peripheral vascular insufficiency. J Bone Joint Surg Am. 53(5):874-90, 1971

Amputations

Scoring Systems for Severely Injured Limbs

Reference	Name of Score	Acronym
Gregory et al (1985)	Mangled Severity Extremity Index	MESI
Howe et al (1987)	Predictive Salvage Index	PSI
Helfet et al (1990)	Mangled Extremity Severity Score	MESS
Russell et al (1991)	Limb Salvage Index	LSI
McNamara et al (1994)	Nerve, Ischemia, Soft tissue, Skeletal, Shock, Age Index	NISSSA

Mangled Extremity Severity Score Variables

Variable Group	Description	Points
Skeletal/Soft Tissue Injury		
	Low energy (stab, simple fracture)	1
	Medium energy (open fracture, multiple fractures)	2
	High energy (high-velocity gunshot, crush)	3
	Very high energy (above + gross contamination)	4
Limb Ischemia		
	Pulse ↓ or absent, perfusion normal	1
	Pulseless, paresthesias, ↓ capillary refill	2
	Cool, paralyzed, insensate	3
Shock		
	Systolic blood pressure always > 90 mm Hg	0
	Transient hypotension	1
	Persistent hypotension	2
Age		
	< 30 years	0
	30-50 years	1
	> 50 years	2

Score of 7 or less is nearly always compatible with limb salvage. Ischemia score is doubled for ischemia > 6 h.

Effect of Different Amputation Levels

Level of Amputation	Body Image Disruption	Leg Length Preservation	Preservation of End Weight Bearing	Proprioceptive Function	Ability to Walk Without Prosthesis	Limited Prosthesis	Full Prosthesis	Walking Pace Adaptation
Transmetatarsal	±	Y	Y	Y	Y	Y	N	Y
Lisfranc-Chopart	±	Y	Y	Y	Y	Y/N	Y/N	Y
Ankle (Syme)	+	N	Y	N	Y	N	Y	Y
Transtibial	+	N	N	N	N	N	Y	Y
Knee disarticulation	++	N	Y	N	N	N	Y	N
Transfemoral	+++	N	N	N	N	N	Y	N

Increased Metabolic Costs At Various Amputation Levels

Amputation Level	Increase in Metabolic Cost (%)
Syme	15
Traumatic transtibial	25
Traumatic transfemoral	68
Vascular transtibial	40
Vascular transfemoral	100

(Left) *Transmetatarsal amputation is shown. Distal coverage of the metatarsal shafts with a durable plantar flap is of utmost importance.* **(Right)** *Transmetatarsal amputation is shown. The metatarsal cuts must be performed in an elliptic manner, starting with the 1st metatarsal. Metatarsal length depends on the status of the plantar flap. Ideally, metatarsal length should be as long as possible to give the longest lever arm.*

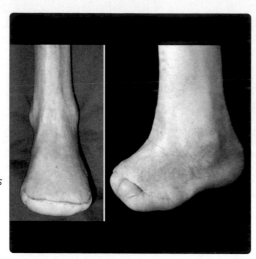
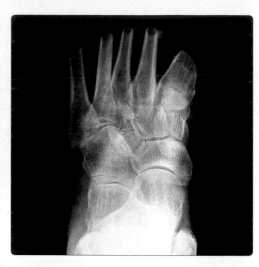

(Left) *AP radiograph shows a Chopart amputation, which is a disarticulation at the calcaneocuboid and talonavicular joints. Note the tunnel ➡ placed for anterior tibial tendon transfer. (From DI: MSK Trauma.)* **(Right)** *Lateral radiograph in the same patient shows the talar tunnel ➡. Despite the tendon transfer, the foot is in equinus, a major challenge with this amputation. The equinus deformity leads to poor biomechanics and predisposes to ulcers and osteomyelitis. (From DI: MSK Trauma.)*

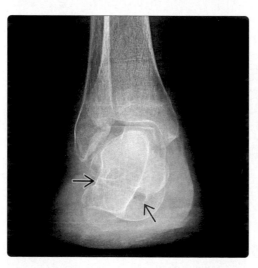
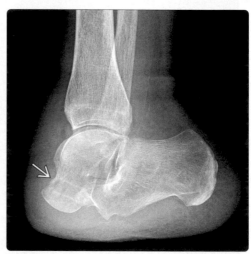

(Left) *The Syme ankle disarticulation (7 days postoperative) provides an end-bearing stump that allows ambulation without a prosthesis over short distances.* **(Right)** *AP radiograph of a Syme amputation is shown. Medial malleolus has been resected. The thick soft tissue flap allows ambulation without a prosthesis. The ends of the stumps are corticated. (From DI: MSK Trauma.)*

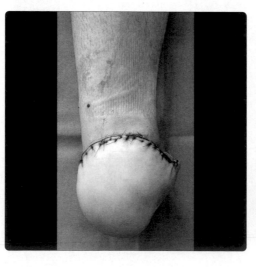
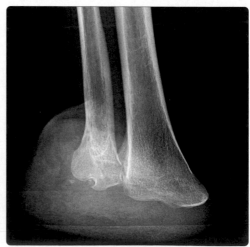

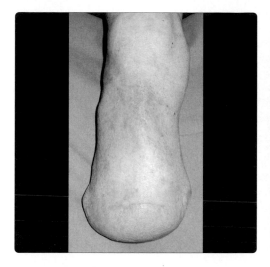

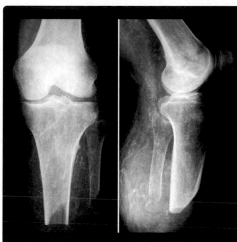

(Left) *Amputation with a long posterior flap is most desirable in patients with vascular disease. It leaves the patient with a scar on the anterior aspect of the residual limb, and due to the thick myofasciocutaneous flap, there is little risk of soft tissue problems at the end of the stump.* (Right) *AP and lateral radiographs show transtibial amputation. The anterior distal aspect of the tibia must be carefully beveled, removing a significant portion of bone. The fibula must be transected 1.5 cm proximal to the level of the tibial transection.*

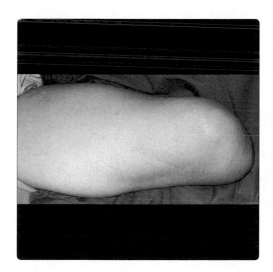

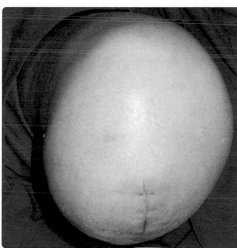

(Left) *Knee disarticulation is shown.* (Right) *Knee disarticulation with posterior suture line is shown. Medial and lateral sagittal flaps, with an incision extending from distal to posterior, allow the final suture line to stay posterior between the femoral condyles. This eliminates a surgical scar at the end of the stump in the weight-bearing area.*

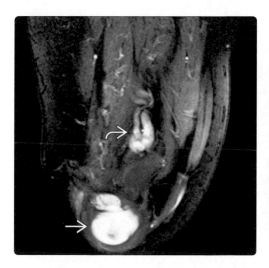

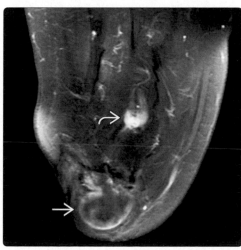

(Left) *Coronal STIR MR of a patient with an above-the-knee amputation shows fusiform enlargement and increased signal intensity of the transected sciatic nerve ➡ characteristic of stump neuroma. A reactive bursa ➡ has formed at the distal margin of the stump. (From DI: MSK Trauma.)* (Right) *Coronal T1WI Gd FS MR in the same patient shows uniform enhancement of stump neuroma ➡. Bursa, in contrast, shows rim enhancement ➡. (From DI: MSK Trauma.)*

KEY FACTS

- Clubfeet can be idiopathic or syndromic.
  - Initial treatment in almost all cases should be Ponseti casting, even if the patient presents outside of infancy, as casting can be quite effective. Surgery is reserved for those cases in whom casting is ineffective.
- Flatfeet are often not pathologic.
  - The Jack toe sign, or Jack test, can be used to show if the patient can form an arch or has a rigid foot.
  - Inserts and physical therapy, especially concentrating on gastrocnemius stretching, can be used to treat those with some pain and potentially prevent future issues.
  - Surgical correction can be considered in severe flatfeet that preclude normal function. The Evans procedure, or lateral column lengthening, has been successfully used, although there are other options as well.
- Tarsal coalitions should be on the differential in the adolescent patient that has multiple ankle sprains.

- Tarsal coalitions can present at a wide array of ages, although traditionally, it presents between 12-16 years of age. However, patients sometimes will not present until into their 20s or 30s.
  - Treatment generally consists of resection or fusion if the coalition involves a large percentage of the joint.
- A congenital vertical talus (CVT) is in some ways the opposite end of the spectrum from a clubfoot.
  - Casting can be attempted for the CVT, although surgery will often prove necessary.
- Physicians should have a heightened awareness of transitional fractures in the appropriate age group.
  - The typical areas for Tillaux fracture and triplane fracture lines should be palpated, and radiographs should be scoured to make sure that these injuries are not missed.

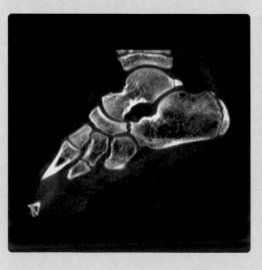
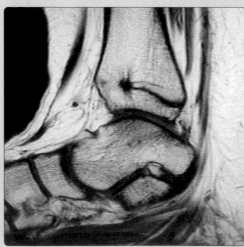

(Left) A child with bilateral clubfeet is shown. This child's condition was diagnosed antenatally by ultrasound, and he was successfully treated with the Ponseti method. (Right) The last cast applied to a patient undergoing serial casting for congenital clubfoot is shown. The foot is dorsiflexed 15°, having just undergone a percutaneous Achilles tenotomy. Note the significant external rotation necessary to avoid recurrence.

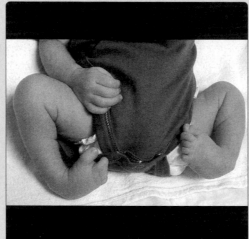
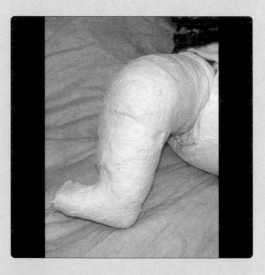

(Left) This 14 year old had multiple ankle sprains over a relatively short period of time. On presentation, the patient had some hindfoot stiffness. This coronal CT shows a fibrocartilaginous calcaneonavicular coalition. (Right) MR scan of a 14-year-old girl who had a Salter-Harris type 2 fracture of the distal tibia 1 year prior is shown. She had a clinical increase in dorsiflexion. The growth arrest can be seen anteriorly. Note the sloping of the physis that resulted from the anterior tether.

CLUBFOOT

Introduction

- Talipes equinovarus (TEV), or clubfoot, is a common disorder seen in roughly 1 in 1,000 live births. 40% are bilateral. TEV may result from intrauterine molding and be completely passively correctable, the so-called positional clubfoot, or it may be rigid.
- Clubfeet may be associated with underlying disorders, such as myelomeningocele, Larsen syndrome, and Streeter dysplasia (constriction band syndrome) as well as other inherited conditions. It may be seen as an isolated condition (idiopathic). Initial treatment consists of ruling out associated conditions, followed by a course of nonoperative treatment with surgery reserved for recalcitrant cases.

Clinical Presentation

- Examination of a baby with TEV requires a thorough evaluation to rule out associated conditions. The spine, hips, and upper extremities should be closely inspected, as should the remainder of the lower extremity. A neurologic examination should be performed to rule out a paralytic clubfoot, as seen in spina bifida.
- Concomitant lower extremity contractures suggest arthrogryposis. Examination of the foot entails evaluation of the forefoot (adduction), midfoot (cavus), hindfoot (varus and equinus), and the amount of internal rotation of the foot. The degree of deformity and its correctability should be determined.

Radiologic Imaging

- Kite angles are most commonly used. These are the talocalcaneal angle measured on the anteroposterior and lateral radiographs. Because of the deformity of the foot, these radiographs should be taken with the beam aligned relative to the hindfoot.
- In a clubfoot, the Kite angle is usually < 20° on the anteroposterior view and < 25° on the lateral view. In essence, the talus and the calcaneus are parallel rather than convergent.
- While radiographs can be used to follow treatment results, there is significant variability in the measurements due to difficulty in positioning the foot, incomplete ossification of the bones of the foot, and difficulty determining the axis of the talus and calcaneus. Clinical examination of the foot must also be used to make treatment decisions.

Nonoperative Treatment

- The initial treatment of TEV is nonoperative. While many descriptions of manipulative treatment exist, the Ponseti method is the most commonly used.

- Casts are applied every 5-7 days until the foot is corrected. First, the forefoot is supinated by dorsiflexing the 1st ray in order to eliminate the cavus deformity. Although the foot appears supinated in a clubfoot deformity, the 1st ray is actually **pronated** with respect to the hindfoot. Rather than pronating the foot, which is the basis of other treatment methods, supinating the foot allows the forefoot to align with the hindfoot. With a thumb applying pressure to the talus (**not** the calcaneus), the foot is externally rotated and then gradually allowed to pronate in order to correct the varus. Finally, the foot is dorsiflexed. Applying a dorsally directed force without sufficient hindfoot flexibility may result in a break in the midfoot, the so-called rocker-bottom deformity.
- Often, a percutaneous Achilles tenotomy is performed in the office to allow the foot to dorsiflex properly. When the foot is in the corrected position, the final cast is left in place for 3 weeks. Straight last shoes connected to a Denis Browne bar are then used full time for 3 months, followed by nighttime use until after walking age.

Surgical Treatment: Primary Procedures

- Given the primacy and overwhelming success of the Ponseti method, the surgical treatment of clubfeet is generally performed less now than it has been historically. Often, those patients that require surgery will be those who had insufficient treatment at a younger age. Not infrequently, in these patients, a trial of casting may be warranted in an effort to minimize the need for surgery.
- The approach will vary depending on age of patient, prior treatment, and degree of deformity.
- Surgery is best performed between 9-12 months of age. This allows proper visualization of anatomic structures, prevents extensive scarring seen with neonatal surgery, and allows the child to be weight bearing soon after surgery, which helps to maintain a plantigrade foot.
- Systematic release of all involved structures is done until deformity is corrected.
- A typical progression begins with a Cincinnati incision. The neurovascular bundle is identified and protected, followed by a release of the posterior ankle and subtalar joints. The foot is then assessed, and the medial portions of the joints released as well, taking care not to cut the deep deltoid ligament.
- The foot is reassessed, and if needed, the talonavicular joint is opened, the spring ligament sectioned, and the navicular reduced. If significant cavus still exists, the plantar fascia can be released. Finally, if a bean shape is still present in the foot, a calcaneocuboid release can be performed.
- Also included may be lengthening of the following tendons: Flexor hallucis longus, flexor digitorum longus, tibialis posterior, and Achilles. **Care should be taken not to overlengthen the Achilles tendon.**
- Pinning of the talonavicular and subtalar joints may be required to maintain position in addition to casting. These are usually removed at 6 weeks, followed by an additional 6 weeks of walking casts. An ankle-foot orthosis may be used following casting in selected patients.

Surgical Treatment: Secondary Procedures and Revision Surgery

- Recurrence of a clubfoot should prompt further investigation to rule out an underlying cause (i.e., tethered spinal cord).
- The choice of procedure depends on the nature of the residual deformity. These secondary procedures are also often needed in the treatment of patients who present for treatment at an older age. The specific components of the recurrent clubfoot should be evaluated to design a surgical plan. Residual forefoot supination, hindfoot varus, internal rotation, equinus, or muscle weakness may all need to be addressed.
- Transfer of the anterior tibial tendon to the midfoot may be helpful in addressing a dynamic supination deformity that is causing overload of the lateral column of the foot. Ponseti and colleagues routinely perform this procedure in patients who have undergone casting and have a residual dynamic supination deformity.
- Weakness of the triceps surae from overlengthening of the Achilles tendon is difficult to overcome. Transfer of various tendons to augment plantar flexion has been described. Unfortunately, normal strength is usually not realized, emphasizing the importance of avoiding overaggressive Achilles lengthening.
- Osteotomy is also a valuable tool. A residual bean shape of the foot can often be corrected via a lateral column shortening. Residual heel varus may be addressed with a Dwyer closing wedge osteotomy.
- For severe residual deformity, gradually correcting the deformity using an external fixator may be helpful in avoiding neurovascular or skin compromise associated with rapid surgical correction.

Complications of Surgical Treatment

- Complications may include inadequate correction of the initial deformity, infection, ischemia with soft tissue loss, and others. The vascularity of the clubfoot is not normal. Often, the anterior tibial artery is hypoplastic or absent.
- A dorsal bunion is seen when the peroneus longus is weakened or cut, leading to unopposed pull of the anterior tibialis combined with "overpull" of the toe flexors. Treatment involves realignment of the 1st ray through tendon release or transfer and osteotomy.
- Subluxation of the navicular can be seen as well, arising from incomplete release or reduction of the navicular, or loss of fixation. Rereduction can be attempted in young children (i.e., < 6 years of age) if treatment for the resulting foot deformity is required.

FLATFEET

Introduction

- Flatfeet are a common cause of concern for parents but usually require no treatment. Of primary importance is distinguishing painless, flexible flatfeet from painful or rigid feet.
- A rigid flatfoot suggests the presence of a tarsal coalition, congenital vertical talus (CVT), or some other pathology. A painful flatfoot may be due to the above as well as an accessory navicular or an inflamed subtalar joint from inflammatory arthritis.

History and Physical Examination

- A good history is paramount. It is important to determine the reason for the visit (i.e., pain, deformity, grandmother's insistence) as well as the onset of the deformity. If painful, the location of the pain is important.
- Angular deformity of the lower extremity should be noted. Young children with physiologic valgus at the knee (3-5 years of age) will often appear flatfooted due to the more proximal deformity. This condition usually resolves as the valgus corrects spontaneously. A neurologic examination should be done to rule out increased muscle tone (i.e., spastic flatfoot) or other neuromuscular condition.
- The examination of the foot should include the following: Presence of an equinus contracture, callus pattern, subtalar motion, arch at rest (non-weight bearing) and with toe raise.
- A flexible flatfoot has a normal arch while sitting as well as with toe raise. During toe raise, the heel should be seen to move into varus as well. This is not the case with a rigid foot seen with a tarsal coalition. The Jack test consists of dorsiflexing the great toe, which should cause the arch to form in a seated patient.
- If an accessory navicular is suspected, an oblique taken with the beam angled 45° medially may be obtained. CT scanning is helpful to rule out the presence of a tarsal coalition.
- Unilateral foot deformities should prompt a thorough neurologic examination, and MR may be indicated to rule out a tethered cord, lipomeningocele, etc.

Treatment

- Treatment options include reassurance, Achilles stretching, arch supports, and surgery. For the majority of patients with flexible flatfeet, no treatment is needed. For those with a tight Achilles tendon, daily stretching may offer some benefit.
- If the feet are painful from collapse of the arch and medial skin irritation, a cushioned arch support may be helpful. A more rigid insert is occasionally helpful for more severe feet, but many children do not tolerate a rigid orthosis.
- Patients with intractable symptoms, despite maximized nonoperative treatment, may benefit from surgery. Arthroeresis, using silicone, silastic, or even metal implants placed through small incisions laterally, has received much attention, as it is an extraarticular, minimally invasive procedure. Although some success has been noted with this procedure, in the author's experience, failure occurs at an unacceptably high rate with pain from the implant &/or migration being consistent concerns.
- As opposed to the adult flatfoot, tendinous and ligamentous pathology is typically not a component of the deformity, and so osteotomy (anterior or posterior calcaneal, 1st metatarsal) is often the procedure of choice. Hindfoot arthrodesis should generally be avoided given the poor long-term results with this procedure in young patients.

TARSAL COALITIONS

Introduction

- Tarsal coalitions occur in at least 1% of the population, but many are not symptomatic. These anomalous connections typically arise between the calcaneus and navicular or between the talus and calcaneus, particularly the middle facet of the subtalar joint.
- Coalitions can also be seen in congenital limb anomalies, such as fibular hemimelia, leading to a "ball and socket" ankle joint. Tarsal coalitions commonly present with painful flatfoot deformities, referred to as the "peroneal spastic flatfoot."
- They are thought to arise as a variation of normal development. Between 50-60% are bilateral. While many may be treated nonoperatively, some may eventually require surgery.

Clinical Presentation

- Symptoms usually begin in early adolescence, possibly as the coalition ossifies and becomes more rigid. The presence of symptoms seems to be correlated with activity; it is possible that relatively inactive patients may not experience symptoms until later in life, i.e., into their 20s or even 30s.
- Pain is usually described as being from the area of the sinus tarsi laterally. It is usually increased with activity, particularly that which stresses the subtalar joint, such as walking over uneven ground.
- Physical examination reveals limited mobility of the hindfoot. Peroneal "spasm" resists inversion. The heel does not move into varus during single-leg toe raise.
- A calcaneonavicular coalition is best seen on the oblique view, while a talocalcaneal coalition may be best seen on a lateral or Harris view.
- Secondary radiographic findings include "beaking" of the talus, narrowing of the posterior talocalcaneal facet, and broadening of the lateral process of the talus.
- CT remains the "gold standard" for tarsal coalitions. Even if a calcaneonavicular coalition is clearly seen on plain radiographs, a CT scan should be obtained to rule out the presence of an additional coalition. MR can aid in the diagnosis of fibrous coalitions.

Treatment

- Patients presenting with coalitions should be initially treated conservatively. Activity modification, antiinflammatory medications, and arch supports or braces designed to reduce hindfoot motion can be helpful. Occasionally, a trial period in a walking boot may be successful. For patients failing these regimens, surgery tailored to the individual coalition can often be helpful.

Calcaneonavicular Coalitions

- Because these do not involve a normal articulation in the foot, wide excision is usually successful. The coalition is excised completely through a lateral incision. The excision should extend from the lateral border of the talonavicular joint to the medial border of the calcaneocuboid joint. In particular, care should be taken not to narrow the excision plantarly; the coalition will often extend down several centimeters toward the sole of the foot. Failure to excise the entire coalition will probably result in an unsatisfactory result.

- After resection, the space between the bones should be filled to prevent recurrence. The extensor digitorum brevis, fat, or bone wax have all been used for this purpose.

Talocalcaneal Coalitions

- Results of surgery are not as predictable as calcaneonavicular coalitions. These coalitions occur through a joint and therefore disturb the normal function of the foot if a large coalition exists.
- Nonoperative treatment should be attempted prior to considering surgery. A preoperative CT scan is mandatory to assess the coalition and estimate the extent of subtalar involvement. Several authors have attempted to quantitate a resectable coalition with some suggesting involvement of < 50% of the posterior facet, while others noted some success with resection if the area of the coalition was < 1/3 of the area of the entire subtalar joint.
- In practice, the measurements described in these studies may be difficult, and parents and patients should be warned preoperatively about the possibility of persistent symptoms requiring further treatment.
- Resection is performed through a medial hindfoot approach. The flexor hallucis longus tendon, which usually is running directly beneath the medial facet coalition must be carefully protected. As above, bone wax or fat can be interposed in the erstwhile coalition. For large coalitions, or in patients who fail to respond to excision, subtalar fusion is indicated.

CONGENITAL VERTICAL TALUS

Introduction

- CVT is a common cause of a rigid rocker-bottom deformity commonly seen in children from birth to 2 years of age.
- The etiology remains unknown, although muscle imbalance or intrauterine positioning has been implicated.
- Rarely appearing independently, CVT is associated with neural tube defects, neuromuscular disorders, and chromosomal abnormalities.

History and Physical Examination

- A patient with a CVT deformity will have a rigid, rocker-bottom foot. The deformity is bilateral ~ 50% of the time. Classically, there is an irreducible dorsal dislocation of the navicular on the talus and a calcaneocuboid joint dislocation.
- The forefoot is abducted and dorsiflexed. A prominent talar head is palpable at the medial convex sole of the foot, and the hindfoot is in equinovalgus.
- Patients may demonstrate a peg leg gait due to limited forefoot push-off. The foot may demonstrate some flexibility; however, it is not passively correctable.

Radiographs

- The diagnosis is confirmed by a lateral x-ray in maximum plantar flexion. In a normal foot, a longitudinal line through the axis of the talus to the 1st metatarsal falls dorsal to the navicular. In a foot with CVT, there is fixed dorsal dislocation of the navicular on the talar neck, and a line through the talus is plantar to the navicular.
- A child < 3 years of age may not have a visible navicular, and so position is identified by position of the metatarsals relative to the talar neck. A screening spine MR should be considered in a child with a unilateral vertical talus.

Treatment

- CVT is usually not amenable to conservative treatment. Long leg casting with the foot in maximum plantar flexion and inversion facilitates surgery by stretching the skin, soft tissues, and extensor tendons over the dorsum of the foot.
- Surgery is the gold standard for treatment of CVT and is usually delayed until ~ 12-18 months old. The goal of surgery is reduction of the navicular on the talar head.
- Release of the bifurcate ligament and calcaneocuboid joint capsule reduces the cuboid on the calcaneus, and Achilles lengthening with posteromedial and posterolateral releases reduces the equinus contracture, talonavicular, and subtalar joints. Finally, in older children, the correction may be stabilized with transfer of the anterior tibialis muscle under the neck of the talus.
- In older children with severe or recalcitrant deformity, excision of the talus or navicular with medial column shortening, or a subtalar or triple arthrodesis, can be utilized to correct the deformity.

ACCESSORY NAVICULAR

Introduction

- An accessory navicular is an ossicle located on the medial side of the foot, proximal to the navicular and in continuity with the tibialis posterior tendon that is often bilateral and is seen in over 20% of people.
- Three types have been demonstrated. In type 1, the ossicle is contained within the tendon, whereas in type 2, the ossicle is connected to the navicular by a cartilaginous bridge. Type 3 is an accessory navicular that has fused with the native navicular.
- Generally, the accessory navicular does not ossify until 9 years of age. Normally, an accessory navicular is not painful, although it can become so through injury.

History and Physical Examination

- The patient with an accessory navicular typically is an active adolescent who may report minor trauma and presents with a flexible flatfoot. The foot should be evaluated for pain or a prominence on the medial side of the foot. Tenderness, swelling, and erythema directly over the prominence of the navicular can be observed.

Radiographs

- A lateral oblique view of the foot is the radiograph of choice to evaluate an accessory navicular, because the standard medial internal oblique view will not show the accessory ossicle in profile. Radiographs may not be helpful if the accessory navicular is not ossified. Although it is actually attached by fibrous tissue or cartilage, the accessory navicular may appear distinct from the navicular on x-rays.

Treatment

- Padding is most appropriate for superficial pain and callus formation. For deep pain, cast immobilization for 6 weeks or an orthosis that relieves pressure over the medial foot and decreases pronation may be helpful. Surgery is indicated for persistent symptoms after conservative measures have failed.

- The Kidner procedure involves removal of the accessory navicular and reinsertion of the posterior tibial tendon, usually with much success. Correction of the flatfoot is not necessary at the same time, although it can be considered in more severe cases.

MISCELLANEOUS FOREFOOT DEFORMITIES

Metatarsus Adductus

- **Introduction**
  - Metatarsus adductus describes a foot with medial displacement of the metatarsals on the cuneiform, leaving the forefoot adducted at the tarsometatarsal joint. The foot has a bean-shaped appearance with a curved, lateral border.
  - Normally, a line bisecting the heel on the plantar surface of the foot will pass through the 2nd toe. In metatarsus adductus, this line moves laterally. Anatomical studies demonstrated medial deviation of the articular surface on the medial cuneiform and adduction of the 2nd-5th metatarsal metaphyses.
  - Typically seen in the 1st year, although capable of presenting at any age, it is the most common congenital foot deformity with an incidence of 1 in 1,000, and the risk of an affected 2nd child is nearly 1 in 20. Bilateral deformity will be present in 50% of patients. Torticollis is common, and developmental dysplasia of the hip is associated 10-15% of the time.

- **History and Physical Examination**
  - The hindfoot is usually normal or in slight valgus, and the 5th metatarsal base is prominent with forefoot deviation. There is usually full range of motion in the ankle and subtalar joints. Internal tibial torsion may contribute to the intoed appearance.
  - Determine whether the forefoot deformity is passively correctable past neutral by holding the heel static and applying a lateral force to the medial border of the 1st metatarsal.

- **Treatment**
  - Over 90% of affected feet will resolve spontaneously without treatment. A foot passively correctable past neutral requires no treatment, although some patients may benefit from passive stretching, stimulation, or straight last shoes. Rarely will any more aggressive treatment be necessary.

Polydactyly and Syndactyly

- **Overview**
  - Polydactyly, a common foot deformity, is a duplication of a toe that occurs bilaterally in 40-50% of patients. Nearly 80% of these patients have postaxial polydactyly (duplication of the 5th toe), which often is not symmetric. Preaxial polydactyly affects the big toe and occurs in 15% of patients, while central duplication comprises the remaining 5% of patients.
  - Often autosomal dominant with incomplete penetrance, polydactyly occurs in 2 out of 1,000 live births. Polydactyly is associated with Down syndrome, trisomy 13, Ellis-Van Creveld syndrome, Apert syndrome, and tibial hemimelia.

○ In older patients, the main complaint is difficult shoewear. The work-up of a child with polydactyly must include weight-bearing anteroposterior and lateral foot radiographs to define the anatomy.

○ Syndactyly, or congenital webbing of toes, is a common deformity usually between the 2nd and 3rd toes, although it can affect any toe. Syndactyly is classified as either simple, when only the skin is involved, or complex, when adjacent toes have not separated. The deformity is further defined as complete, when the webbing extends to the distal end of the toe, or incomplete. The toenails may be united in severe cases.

- **Treatment**
  ○ Syndactyly is a cosmetic issue and usually does not lead to functional problems. Therefore it does not require treatment, except when present with polydactyly or for cosmesis.
  ○ Surgical excision of polydactyly, at 1 year of age, of the most medial or lateral toe will improve cosmesis and shoewear and allows the greatest potential for remodeling. Preaxial excision requires careful soft tissue balancing to prevent hallux varus, a complication of preaxial surgery. Central polydactyly is best treated with amputation of the duplicated central digit and reapproximation of the intermetatarsal ligament, followed by casting to prevent forefoot splaying. Postaxial polydactyly responds very well to simple excision of the duplicated digit.

Curly Toes and Overlapping Toes

- **Overview**
  ○ Curly toes are an autosomal dominant deformity in which there is flexion and medial deviation of the proximal interphalangeal joint of the affected toe. Most commonly seen in bilateral 3rd and 4th toes, lateral rotation at the distal interphalangeal joint leads to underlapping of the adjacent normal toe. Congenital contracture of the flexor digitorum longus and brevis tendons has been shown to cause the malrotation and flexion deformity of the toes. Symptoms of pain and corn formation are a result of abnormal pressure on the tips of the toes.
  ○ Overlapping toes are characterized by dorsal adduction and external rotation of the 5th toe. Contracture of the extensor digitorum longus tendon may occur and in some cases, dislocation of the metatarsophalangeal joint. The deformity is usually asymptomatic. Similar to curly toes, shoewear may be difficult, and pain may be present over the dorsum of the toe with callus formation.

- **Treatment**
  ○ Curly toe deformity in the infant and young child should initially be observed. Percutaneous tenotomy of the long and short toe flexors is recommended at 3-6 years of age. A Girdlestone-Taylor procedure can be utilized for more severe deformity; however, results are similar to those of open flexor tenotomy.
  ○ Overlapping toes can be corrected with a DuVries or Butler correction, which involves release of the extensor digitorum longus tendon, dorsal joint capsule, and medial collateral ligament.

TRANSITIONAL FRACTURES

Introduction

- Due to the progression of closure of the distal tibial physis, certain types of specific distal tibial fractures can occur as the growth plate closes. These injuries generally occur between 12-15 years of age, as the distal tibial growth plate closes.
- The "weak point" in the growing child's ankle is often the physis itself, as opposed to the ligamentous structures about the ankle.
- The 2 types of fractures specific to the adolescent age group are triplane fractures and Tillaux fractures.

Triplane Fractures

- The distal tibial physis closes centrally first with progression medially and finally to the lateral side. As a result of this consistent progression, specific injury patterns tend to occur.
- The triplane fracture consists of a Salter-Harris type 3 fracture of the lateral epiphysis in the coronal plane with a Salter-Harris type 2 fracture of the posterior metaphysis in the sagittal plane.
- The mechanism is often a supination-external rotation-type mechanism, as occurs with many adult ankle fractures.
- Patients with this injury tend to be younger than those with Tillaux fractures, although the 2 occur in a similar age group.
- A CT scan is often necessary to fully appreciate the injury.
- Given the intraarticular nature of the fracture, any step-off necessitates operative intervention for open reduction internal fixation.
- Generally speaking, the physis should not be crossed with screws, and lag screws are typically placed separately in the epiphysis and the metaphysis.

Tillaux Fractures

- These fractures are similar to triplane injuries. However, they only involve the anterolateral distal tibia with the Salter-Harris 3 component of the triplane.
- These injuries are thought to represent an avulsion of the anterior-inferior tibiofibular ligament.
- Treatment proceeds as for a triplane with any step-off necessitating operative reduction and fixation.
- Since these injuries occur as the growth plate is closing, angular deformities and growth arrest are generally not associated with these injuries.

OVERUSE INJURIES OF FOOT AND ANKLE IN CHILDREN

Calcaneal Apophysitis (Sever Disease)

- Heel pain is a common complaint among pediatric athletes. Sever described this phenomenon as an inflammation of the calcaneal apophysis, although others have thought it to be caused by microtrabecular injury in the apophysis due to overuse.
- Patients present with complaints of heel pain, usually bilaterally, which occurs after running sports. Often, the patient may have symptoms on rising in the morning until the feet "loosen up," analogous to plantar fasciitis.

Core Knowledge in Orthopaedics: Foot and Ankle

- The Achilles tendon and gastrocnemius are often found to be tight. There is usually pain to palpation over the medial portion of the distal calcaneus. Patients may avoid pressure on the calcaneus with ambulation and may even toe walk.

- The apophysis may appear fragmented as a normal developmental variant and thus is usually not diagnostic for Sever disease in the absence of a suspicious history and examination. MR may be helpful if stress fracture or tumor is suspected.

- Treatment is divided into several stages. Nonsteroidal antiinflammatory drugs and ice can be helpful for patients with significant pain. An over-the-counter cushioned heel cup may be worn during sports. Often, the most important factor in eliminating symptoms is to improve heel cord flexibility.

- In patients with significant unrelenting pain, cessation of sports activity may be necessary until symptoms abate. The vast majority of patients treated in this manner are able to resume sports without significant discomfort within 4-8 weeks. Prolonged symptoms may require further activity modification and evaluation. In extreme cases, casting is occasionally recommended.

SELECTED REFERENCES

1. Zionts LE et al: Sixty years on: Ponseti method for clubfoot treatment produces high satisfaction despite inherent tendency to relapse. J Bone Joint Surg Am. 100(9):721-728, 2018

2. Kalbouneh H et al: Incidence and anatomical variations of accessory navicular bone in patients with foot pain: a retrospective radiographic analysis. Clin Anat. 30(4):436-444, 2017

3. Jegal H et al: Accessory navicular syndrome in athlete vs. general population. Foot Ankle Int. 37(8):862-7, 2016

4. Seehausen DA et al: Accessory navicular is associated with wider and more prominent navicular bone in pediatric patients by radiographic measurement. J Pediatr Orthop. 36(5):521-5, 2016

5. Shabtai L et al: Radiographic indicators of surgery and functional outcome in Ponseti-treated clubfeet. Foot Ankle Int. 37(5):542-7, 2016

6. James AM et al: Factors associated with pain severity in children with calcaneal apophysitis (Sever disease). J Pediatr. 167(2):455-9, 2015

7. Miller M et al: Congenital vertical talus: etiology and management. J Am Acad Orthop Surg. 23(10):604-11, 2015

8. Park H et al: The relationship between accessory navicular and flat foot: a radiologic study. J Pediatr Orthop. 35(7):739-45, 2015

9. Swensen SJ et al: Tarsal coalitions - calcaneonavicular coalitions. Foot Ankle Clin. 20(4):669-79, 2015

10. Yang JS et al: Treatment of congenital certical talus: comparison of minimally invasive and extensive soft-tissue release procedures at minimum five-year follow-up. J Bone Joint Surg Am. 97(16):1354-65, 2015

11. Choudhry IK et al: Functional outcome analysis of triplane and tillaux fractures after closed reduction and percutaneous fixation. J Pediatr Orthop. 34(2):139-43, 2014

12. Knörr J et al: Percutaneous correction of persistent severe metatarsus adductus in children. J Pediatr Orthop. 34(4):447-52, 2014

13. Pretell-Mazzini J et al: Surgical treatment of symptomatic accessory navicular in children and adolescents. Am J Orthop (Belle Mead NJ). 43(3):110-3, 2014

14. Khoshbin A et al: Long-term functional outcomes of resected tarsal coalitions. Foot Ankle Int. 34(10):1370-5, 2013

15. Talusan PG et al: Fifth toe deformities: overlapping and underlapping toe. Foot Ankle Spec. 6(2):145-9, 2013

16. Wallander H et al: Low prevalence of osteoarthritis in patients with congenital clubfoot at more than 60 years' follow-up. J Bone Joint Surg Br. 94(11):1522-8, 2012

17. Merrill LJ et al: Skeletal muscle abnormalities and genetic factors related to vertical talus. Clin Orthop Relat Res. 469(4):1167-74, 2011

18. Rachel JN et al: Is radiographic evaluation necessary in children with a clinical diagnosis of calcaneal apophysitis (sever disease)? J Pediatr Orthop. 31(5):548-50, 2011

19. Shirzad K et al: Lesser toe deformities. J Am Acad Orthop Surg. 19(8):505-14, 2011

20. Bor N et al: Ponseti treatment for idiopathic clubfoot: minimum 5-year followup. Clin Orthop Relat Res. 467(5):1263-70, 2009

21. Sankar WN et al: Orthopaedic conditions in the newborn. J Am Acad Orthop Surg. 17(2):112-22, 2009

22. Kopp FJ et al: Clinical outcome of surgical treatment of the symptomatic accessory navicular. Foot Ankle Int. 25(1):27-30, 2004

23. Shrimpton AE et al: A HOX gene mutation in a family with isolated congenital vertical talus and Charcot-Marie-Tooth disease. Am J Hum Genet. 75(1):92-6, 2004

24. Ugolini PA et al: The accessory navicular. Foot Ankle Clin. 2004 Mar;9(1):165-80.

25. Barmada A et al: Premature physeal closure following distal tibia physeal fractures: a new radiographic predictor. J Pediatr Orthop. 23(6):733-9, 2003

26. Kanatli U et al: The relationship between accessory navicular and medial longitudinal arch: evaluation with a plantar pressure distribution measurement system. Foot Ankle Int. 24(6):486-9, 2003

27. Zorer G et al: Single stage surgical correction of congenital vertical talus by complete subtalar release and peritalar reduction by using the Cincinnati incision. J Pediatr Orthop B. 11(1):60-7, 2002

28. Davitt JS et al: Plantar pressure and radiographic changes after distal calcaneal lengthening in children and adolescents. J Pediatr Orthop. 21(1):70-5, 2001

29. Horn BD et al: Radiologic evaluation of juvenile tillaux fractures of the distal tibia. J Pediatr Orthop. 21(2):162-4, 2001

30. Sullivan JA: Pediatric flatfoot: evaluation and management. J Am Acad Orthop Surg. 7(1):44-53, 1999

31. Comfort TK et al: Resection for symptomatic talocalcaneal coalition. J Pediatr Orthop. 18(3):283-8, 1998

32. Napiontek M: Congenital vertical talus: a retrospective and critical review of 32 feet operated on by peritalar reduction. J Pediatr Orthop B. 4(2):179-87, 1995

33. Wilde PH et al: Resection for symptomatic talocalcaneal coalition. J Bone Joint Surg Br. 76(5):797-801, 1994

34. Hamer AJ et al: Surgery for curly toe deformity: a double-blind, randomised, prospective trial. J Bone Joint Surg Br. 75(4):662-3, 1993

35. Ray S et al: Surgical treatment of the accessory navicular. Clin Orthop Relat Res. 61-6, 1983

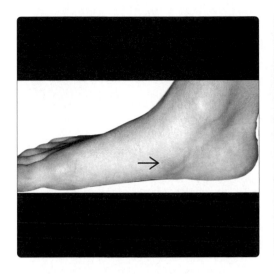

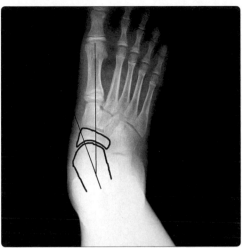

(Left) *Flatfoot associated with an accessory navicular is shown. The arch is flat, and there is erythema, callus formation, and tenderness over the navicular* ➡. (Right) *The talus is significantly uncovered by the navicular due to abduction of the forefoot and becomes a weight-bearing structure, leading to pain. Note the divergence of the talus-1st metatarsal angle.*

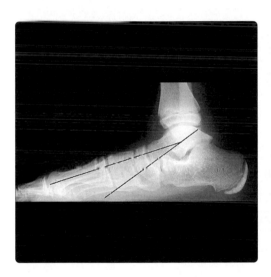

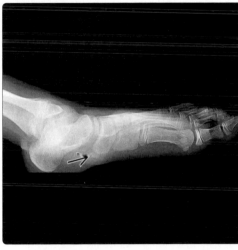

(Left) *Lateral view of the same foot is shown. There is a significant "sag" of the midfoot, measured by an increased talo-1st metatarsal angle, as well as decreased calcaneal pitch. Note the loss of the normal arch.* (Right) *An accessory navicular* ➡ *is more readily apparent on this medial oblique view. Approximately 20-25% of the general population has an accessory navicular, and so its presence is by no means necessarily problematic.*

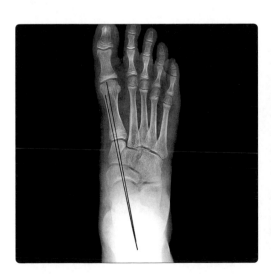

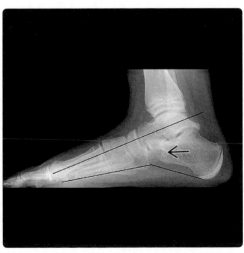

(Left) *Radiograph of the same patient after undergoing percutaneous Achilles lengthening and lateral column lengthening with iliac crest bone graft is shown. The talus-1st metatarsal angle is here restored. The talus is well covered by the navicular and is no longer prominent.* (Right) *The calcaneal pitch and arch are restored. Note the healed lateral column lengthening osteotomy* ➡.

(Left) *This 27-year-old male patient never had symptoms until his 20's, although his hindfoot was always stiff. A calcaneonavicular coalition ⊡ is seen here.* **(Right)** *Talar "beaking" ⊡ and the "C" sign, which represents the fused middle facet ⊡, are shown. Talar beaking occurs as a result of a stiff hindfoot in this talocalcaneal coalition.*

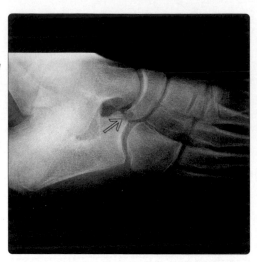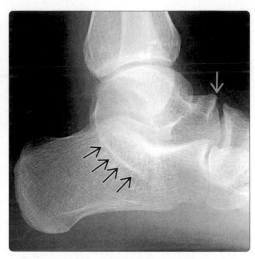

(Left) *This axial view shows the medial facet coalition ⊡. When resecting these coalitions, bone is cleared away from medial to lateral until a more normal joint is encountered.* **(Right)** *A middle facet talocalcaneal coalition ⊡ is seen here with the normal side for comparison. Surgical decision-making is influenced by the degree of coalition, amount of hindfoot motion (or lack thereof), and how much pain the patient has.*

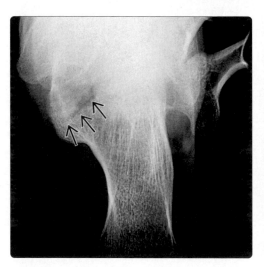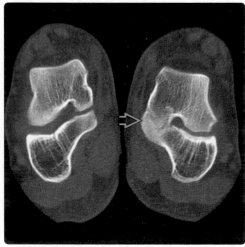

(Left) *An excised calcaneonavicular coalition with the dorsum ⊡ of the resected bone is shown. The superoinferior dimension of the bone is often greater than expected. Some barrier must be placed between the resected ends so that the coalition does not reform.* **(Right)** *A patient after resection of a calcaneonavicular coalition resection is shown. Note the fairly significant defect between the calcaneus and navicular ⊡.*

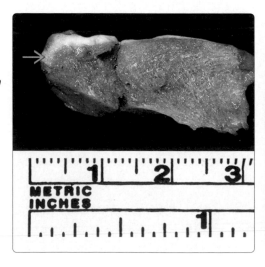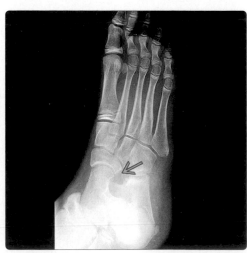

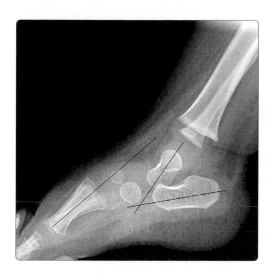

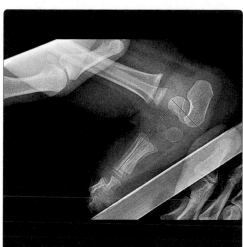

(Left) *Forced plantar flexion view of the foot is shown. The axis of the 1st metatarsal passes dorsal to the talus. The long axis of the calcaneus passes plantar to cuboid.* (Right) *Forced dorsiflexion demonstrates plantar flexion of talus and calcaneus with the forefoot lying dorsally in the subluxed position. As opposed to the calcaneovalgus foot, where the calcaneus is dorsiflexed, here, the calcaneus is plantar flexed.*

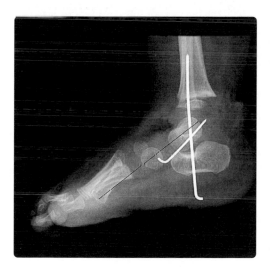

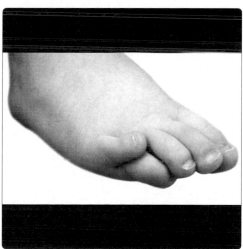

(Left) *Lateral radiograph of the postoperative congenital vertical talus is shown. K-wire fixation of the talus and calcaneus with the axis of the talus no longer passes plantar to the 1st metatarsal.* (Right) *Overlapping 5th toe that caused difficulty with shoewear is shown. The 4th toe is a curly toe and was symptomatic from dorsal pressure from the 3rd toe.*

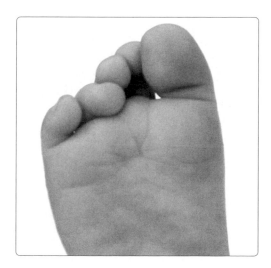

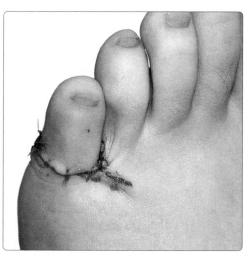

(Left) *Note curly toes at the 4th and 5th toes. This autosomal dominant deformity is notable for flexion and medial deviation of proximal interphalangeal joint of the affected toe.* (Right) *Postoperative foot with straightened 4th and 5th digits is shown. The 4th toe was treated with a simple tenotomy of the toe flexors, and the 5th with a modified Butler procedure, where the extensor tendon is sectioned, metatarsophalangeal joint is released, and toe is reduced using a Y to V advancement of the skin.*

Core Knowledge in Orthopaedics: Foot and Ankle

(Left) *Radiograph of a Salter-Harris type 2 fracture of the distal tibia is shown. This radiograph demonstrates a fracture line of the distal tibia ➥ and distal 3rd fibula fracture ➨.* **(Right)** *Radiograph of a Salter-Harris type 2 fracture of the distal tibia is shown. Lateral radiograph shows tibia ➨ and fibula ➥ fracture lines. As is commonly seen, there is a large Thurston-Holland fragment, and the epiphysis is displaced posteriorly.*

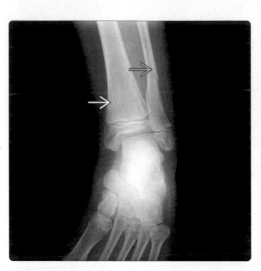
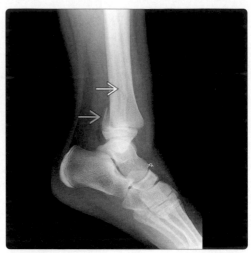

(Left) *AP radiograph of a Tillaux fracture is shown. The anterolateral epiphysis is essentially pulled off by the anteroinferior tibiofibular ligament. The fracture line ➨ is shown here.* **(Right)** *The fractured fragment can be seen more readily on this coronal CT scan. This fracture is a Salter-Harris 3 fracture. Given its intraarticular nature, surgical treatment is often necessary.*

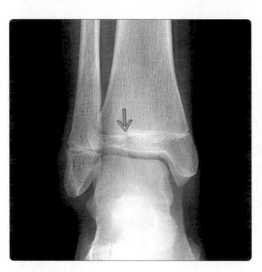
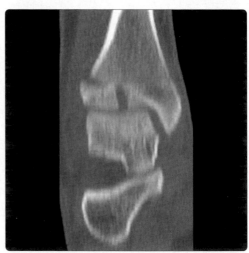

(Left) *Axial MR shows the external rotation mechanism that would lead to this avulsion fracture with the intact anterior-inferior tibiofibular ligament pulling the anterolateral tibial fragment off.* **(Right)** *Postoperative film shows reduction of the fracture using a percutaneously placed cannulated screw. Note that the direction of screw placement is from anterolateral to posteromedial, perpendicular to the fracture line.*

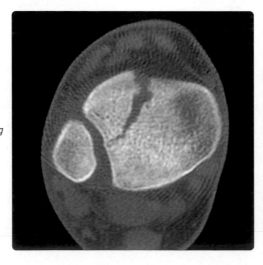
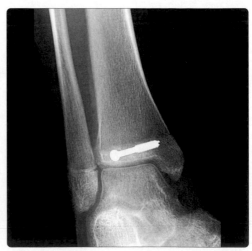

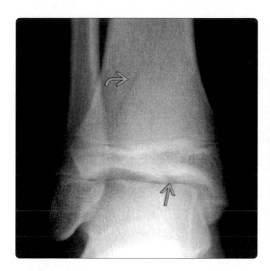

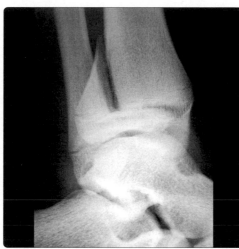

(Left) *Radiograph of the ankle shows a triplane fracture; note the fracture extension ⇨ into the articular surface. This portion resembles a Salter-Harris type 3 component. The posterior fracture of the metaphysis ⇨ is also visible and is more consistent with a Salter-Harris type 2 fracture.* (Right) *This lateral view much more readily shows the Salter-Harris type 2 component posteriorly with the large Thurstan Holland fragment.*

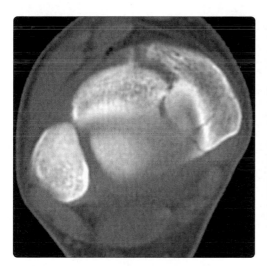

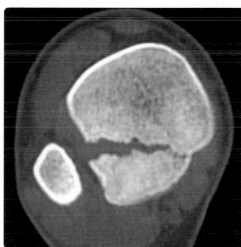

(Left) *The articular component of the fracture is seen on this axial CT with the anterolateral component often seen with a Tillaux fracture as well as a fracture line extending more posterior and medial.* (Right) *This more superior axial cut shows the Thurstan Holland fragment that is very much akin to a posterior malleolus in a skeletally mature individual.*

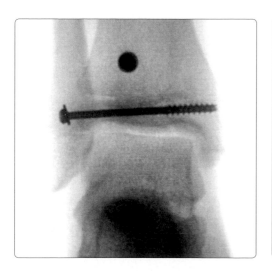

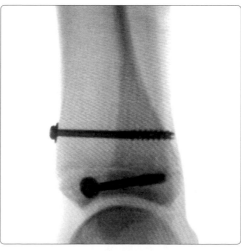

(Left) *Both principle fractures are reduced and fixed with partially threaded, cannulated screws, in this case with washers.* (Right) *Care is taken not to violate the physis in this case. The anatomic reduction of the mortise can be seen here.*

INDEX

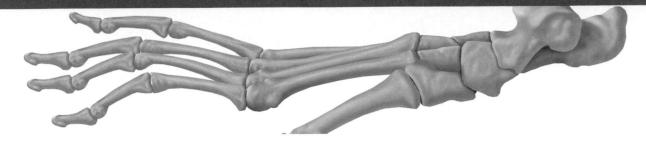

INDEX

INDEX

INDEX

INDEX

INDEX

INDEX

INDEX

INDEX

INDEX

INDEX